Sexualizing Cancer

∴

Sexualizing Cancer

∵

HPV AND THE POLITICS OF CANCER PREVENTION

Laura Mamo

THE UNIVERSITY OF CHICAGO PRESS

CHICAGO AND LONDON

The University of Chicago Press, Chicago 60637
The University of Chicago Press, Ltd., London
© 2023 by The University of Chicago
All rights reserved. No part of this book may be used or reproduced in any
manner whatsoever without written permission, except in the case of brief
quotations in critical articles and reviews. For more information, contact the
University of Chicago Press, 1427 E. 60th St., Chicago, IL 60637.
Published 2023
Printed in the United States of America

32 31 30 29 28 27 26 25 24 23   1 2 3 4 5

ISBN-13: 978-0-226-82927-2 (cloth)
ISBN-13: 978-0-226-82929-6 (paper)
ISBN-13: 978-0-226-82928-9 (e-book)
DOI: https://doi.org/10.7208/chicago/9780226829289.001.0001

Library of Congress Cataloging-in-Publication Data

Names: Mamo, Laura, 1969– author.
Title: Sexualizing cancer : HPV and the politics of cancer
    prevention / Laura Mamo.
Description: Chicago : The University of Chicago Press, 2023. |
    Includes bibliographical references and index.
Identifiers: LCCN 2023008507 | ISBN 9780226829272 (cloth) |
    ISBN 9780226829296 (paperback) | ISBN 9780226829289 (ebook)
Subjects: LCSH: Cervix uteri—Cancer. | Papillomaviruses. |
    Sexually transmitted diseases—Prevention.
Classification: LCC RC280.U8 M244 2023 | DDC 616.99/466—dc23/
    eng/20230414
LC record available at https://lccn.loc.gov/2023008507

♾ This paper meets the requirements of ANSI/NISO Z39.48-1992
(Permanence of Paper).

Contents

The Sexual Politics of Cancer and a New Regime of Cancer Prevention

In the fall of 1999, the *New Yorker* featured an article titled "Contagion," written by Jerome Groopman, a staff writer and Harvard Medical School professor whose scientific research focuses on cancer and acquired immunodeficiency syndrome (AIDS). The piece opened with a diagnosis: "Jennifer," the college-aged daughter of a friend of Groopman's, had received abnormal results from a Pap test; a follow-up colposcopy had shown "severe dysplasia" brought on by a "virulent" strain of "papilloma-infected cells" known as human papillomavirus-16, or HPV-16. "But it hasn't yet progressed to carcinoma," the pathologist who analyzed the cell sample reassured Groopman when he got involved in the young woman's case, touching on a novel and distinct fear that would soon be front and center in the American sexual health dialogue. The "sometimes lethal sexual epidemic that condoms can't stop" referenced in the article's subtitle was upon us, as Groopman, his friend, and Jennifer—as well as all of us readers—were now seeing so clearly. Groopman's article was noteworthy for its candor around sex, and memorable because of the serious long-standing suspicion it invoked: sexual activity and cervical cancer were somehow linked.

The link, a sexually transmitted infection or STI, had been firmly established scientifically, in part due to molecular approaches in viral research. But what the link means socially—for people and their interactions, for their health, and for approaches to prevention—remains less than certain. HPVs are omnipresent, and while some are shown to be oncogenic and can lead to cervical cancer, these HPVs are not *on their own* a certain pathway to cancer. They are necessary but insufficient as a cause, as Groopman signaled through ample use of qualifiers like "sometimes," "may," and "might" with respect to any cancer-causing effects of an HPV infection (Groopman 1999).

The ubiquitous occurrence of HPVs was also signaled in Groopman's dispatch. Relying on expert testimony from Joel Palefsky, a University of

California San Francisco clinical researcher, Groopman painted the statistical landscape: in 1999, ten million young women in their twenties and thirties had "active infection," a million had disease the precise nature of which was unclear, and "perhaps some" of these had "pre-cancer." Today, the vast majority of us likely had or have HPV, although definitive tests and their results are new and are only available and offered in some cases.

What could have provoked Groopman's medical dispatch at this particular moment? How might it signal changes to come in the conceptualization of STIs, cancer, and health risk? Would there be new ways to reduce illness and prevent disease and death? Layering claims of this infection's "common occurrence" over lingering causal uncertainties, he was, in part, normalizing sexual transmission as part of the inherent riskiness of sexual interactions in our lives. He was careful to present the familiar news of this particular risk of sex and disease in medical terms, as something which was always present; yet with a slight refocus of the lens on Jennifer, he also signaled something new for girls everywhere and their future health. Groopman's recounting of the young woman's treatment by the gynecologist who screened her for HPV brought to mind cervical cancer's erstwhile symbolic notoriety as a disease of "bad girls."[1] The doctor at the student health center had shown disbelief at her self-reported sexual history, looking at her skeptically as she told of her sexual encounters and condom use: "He made me feel as if I must be promiscuous," she told her father. Unable to temper the predictable public surprise of a newly real sexual risk, Groopman was also pointing to the unexpected revelation of a well-known "safe sex" tool—the condom—as inadequately protective. There was something lurking that could not be held back. Was everyone—including the "good girls" who "had never had sex or an STI"—now at cancer risk? What might protect against the "sometimes lethal" disease implicated in an unstoppable "sexual epidemic" if not the latex barriers that were the go-to safe sex protection for millions?

The image that appeared close to the headline of the article was of a young, seemingly white woman in sleeping attire who appeared to be somewhat suspended in the air. She is alone, bedposts visible in an otherwise unmarked room; something odd is on the floor: a small (yet prominent) red heart with protruding legs and antennae. But what does it symbolize? Is it a "love bug"? Is it a crab, either the *Pthirus pubis*, of the sexually transmitted variety; or the crab of the zodiac—Cancer? Maybe it is all three. More compelling, seemingly, is the creature's meaning to the young woman in the image, who is obviously getting away from it as fast as she can. Has she just had sex—and caught the bug—or is she leaping out of bed to avoid what lurks below? Her innocence, conveyed by her white nightgown and her feminine confinement in this "room of her own," is juxtaposed with a sense of foreboding, an implied fear of something that is perhaps unavoidable, a proximate or even possibly already embodied risk.

Although Groopman was describing, in his own words, "a sexual epidemic," it was unclear whether the warning was of a bona fide emergency, or, less urgently, of an insufficiently understood but serious health risk.[2] In dispatching the news via his presentation of a single medical "case," he was practicing measured restraint: as a medical doctor, he was already aware of infectious agents and their causative role in diseases, including cancers, and of their capacity to provoke real and unnecessary alarm. He nonetheless focused on his friend's and Jennifer's "surprise" at learning not only that HPV, a sexually transmitted virus, is ubiquitous and thus in practical terms unavoidable (save for people who are completely celibate), but that infection with this pathogen has implications for cancer risk. The article served as a clear warning to sexually active girls like Jennifer, and to their parents (the ostensible readers of the *New Yorker*), as well as, more subtly, to anyone (and everyone) who has sex. Groopman took care to point out to the reader that concern was most particular to sex involving a penis. HPVs are mostly present on skin, such as the shaft of the penis, he wrote. Because of the difficulty in completely covering this area of the body with a condom, he continued, guaranteed protection from transmission is not possible. Safe sex would not be possible; a man who is infected is "a public health risk." Groopman's call was to publicly introduce what lurked below, a viral risk on the loose, and at the same time to express a need for its containment. Though this was a nebulous health risk—"not quite a cancer," and not quite an emergent infectious disease—it was a health risk to be managed nonetheless.[3]

Though the viral pathogen on the loose that the article was calling attention to was neither new nor unknown, and was not presented as something that could render immediate harm or death, what was new was an answer to this problem, and an admittedly significant one: a "pharmaceuticalized" approach that provided what a condom could not—a means to prevent transmission of the pathogen—but also (implicitly in its molecular approach) constituted the basis of a screening tool. Such approaches, however, might be slow to roll out, and if they followed the course of other preventive tools, they would likely be vastly unequal in their financing and thus in the care they provided. The rollout would depend on political will, yet it would likely be dictated by the degree of scarcity, abundance, or something in between for each setting in which it was released. The broader public would soon learn that the contagion Groopman invoked, of an ambiguously understood yet long-surmised link between sex and disease, had gradually come to be understood as a sexually transmitted infection, an STI, with a role in the development of not only early and/or invasive disease, but also in "pre-cancers" as well as more benign genital warts. The newly established risk was also, for many, already present in us.

The US Institute of Medicine had released a report on "The Hidden Epidemic" years earlier (Eng and Butler 1997), calling upon government and private organizations to support prevention activities as a strategy to stave off what they referred to as "STD related cancers." The experts convened to write the report surmised that the secrecy and stigma around STDs (excluding the human immunodeficiency virus, or HIV, but including HPV and others) was contributing to a lack of scientific and medical attention to understanding and, importantly, working to prevent these infections. By the time Groopman wrote the article, a benchmark study of HPV had posited sexual activity as a cause of cancer (Walboomers et al. 1999).[4] Yet, in presenting this risk to the public, Groopman was ushering in a new period in both knowledge about disease causation and the link between infectious disease and cancer, and—most consequentially for the collective path all sexually active people were about to embark on—an incipient approach to preventive medicine. It was a watershed moment when a new narrative of risk, uncertainty, and containment was put into circulation, would soon "go viral," and then would variously shift to include multiple cancers, population groups, and hopes for managing and controlling risk and harm.

"What about . . . husbands?" Groopman then asked a medical "expert," in order to introduce publics to the idea that risk of HPV had never just been for women (like the one in the image who leapt from her bed to avoid the "love-bug")—a question flavored with heteronormative presumption. Palefsky told Groopman that men are a public health risk to other men— saying nothing about whether these men were "husbands," or to whom— and in doing so shifted the source of the threat of infection and riskiness of sexual behavior from women to men, expanding away from its heteronormative presumptions. Palefsky added information about an additional, heretofore hidden threat: a cancer more rare than cervical cancer, but no less a danger to public health. The anal canal, Palefsky told Groopman, is similar to the vaginal canal, and research at UCSF was showing rates of HPV infection in men who have sex with men similar to those seen in women who have sex with men. Palefsky advocated for a prevention approach for men that would function similarly to how the Pap test screens for cellular abnormalities to prevent cervical cancer worked for women.[5] Anal Pap testing on men who have sex with men (and perhaps some high-risk women), he advocated, could be added to the already established preventive approach to cancer. And then he shifted focus yet again, to what he was inferring would be "the best" way to protect against HPV: a vaccine. This approach, he said, looping in women's health concerns, would be "particularly significant in the developing world where women's health services are minimal" (Groopman 1999, 49).

Half a decade after reading Groopman's piece, in 2005, I was drawn to a headline on a magazine at my local gym: "The Coming Storm over a Cancer Vaccine" (Guyon 2005). I grabbed it off the rack. The magazine was *Fortune*, a finance and business publication. The headline's warning of a coming storm was not formed around HPV rates or cancer threats; rather, it warned of a social and political sex panic that could result from the HPV vaccine's imminent introduction. At the heart of the coverage around an "amazingly effective cervical-cancer vaccine" that was on the precipice of being unleashed nationally were questions about whether a vaccine technology designed to prevent an STI could promote girls' sexual activity, "spur promiscuity and undermine abstinence," make them "more inclined to have sex outside marriage," or worse. The *Fortune* editors clearly understood that, from a sociological standpoint, viruses are far more than material entities—they are part of our sociality. As such, these editors considered STIs and their prevention an important part of their biocapital coverage; a new product poised to play a major role in profit-making capital markets was firmly in their wheelhouse. Were the fears raised by the author akin, I wondered, to the fears of getting or passing other STIs, especially in the absence of therapeutic treatments? Were these akin to genital herpes, the "big H" contracted from the HSV-2 virus, or the pox of syphilis? Or, I wondered, would this ignite controversies more like the debates of the 1980s over whether the distribution of condoms might ignite (homosexual) sex among adolescents? Or the worry in the 1990s that sexuality education would promote (heterosexual) promiscuity among "bad" girls?

Groopman's article had concluded on a note of medical hope, the possibility to contain a risk from a viral agent it seemed many of us already had without being aware of it. But by focusing on Jennifer, a young adult woman, in the manner it did—white gowns, scary creatures, and all—the article was rife with subtext about girls' sexuality. Only a few years later, the unease that seemed most visible to me and others in my field was not about cancer or STI risk, but rather about any impending social controversy that might go viral. Calls for containment were focused less on health risk and disease, and more on worries about an "outbreak" of adolescent girls' sexuality, or on the ways such claims could provoke controversy around sex that might not be easily tamed. Seeing these concerns raised in the pages of *Fortune* magazine put a fine point on the potential for any controversy to disrupt profit for Merck and Co.—the maker of the vaccine, referred to as "Merck" throughout—and for their shareholders, which they expected given the money they had already laid out in R&D (research and development) costs. Two companies, Merck and GlaxoSmithKline (GSK), were working to bring HPV vaccines to market under the brand names Gardasil and Cervarix, respectively.

Within the year the first television commercial for the yet-to-be-named vaccine was aired in earnest, imploring viewers to "Know the Link" between a pervasive virus, HPV, and a notoriously deadly cancer, cervical cancer. Advertising medical products to the general public already included products concerning sex. People were accustomed to ads for Viagra that went beyond preventing erectile difficulties to include a plethora of ways this product would ensure better living. Yet appeals to know this link between a virus and cancer were conspicuously without sexual mention. There was no expanded story about STIs or about the uncertain yet known harms to all bodies from the sexual activity they might be engaged in. There was no information about the other cancers that might form when HPVs hide in the crevices of the body. Merck's 2005 "Know the Link" campaign, sanctioned ahead of vaccine approval by the US Food and Drug Administration (FDA), directed particular audiences toward knowledge of specific risk and not inconsiderable concern. The multimedia ads echoed the familiar direct-to-consumer messaging to "Ask your doctor . . . ," which urged consumers—who enthusiastically took note—to take action to improve their own health and to buy the right name-brand pharmaceuticals, from antidepressants (Prozac) to erectile dysfunction drugs (Viagra) to cholesterol-lowering medications (Lipitor) to birth control pills (Seasonale). Yet here, the campaign was calling parents into a concern for their daughters' health risk, and perhaps implicating their own, as they prepared a market for a coming vaccine.

By the late 1990s, vaccines had largely become the purview of Big Pharma and its business model. A half-decade before, vaccines were produced largely with federal funds "for the people," in the words of Jonas Salk describing the development of the polio vaccine. While vaccines are importantly, still supported by early public funding for basic research, they are today part of the political economy of corporate research and development (R&D). Pharmaceutical companies aim to bring blockbuster drugs and devices to market that promise to bring not only "good health" to consumers, but "good returns" to their shareholders.

The pharmaceutical approach to preventing the spread of HPV infection, given the need to inoculate girls prior to sexual activity, would require containing the spread of sexualized controversy. Yet it wasn't just sex, but the ways sex adhered to gender and identity that was in need of containment: would talk of a vaccine to prevent an STI among girls unleash promiscuity among (soon to be) heterosexually active girls? Would such talk about girls' sexuality open the girls, and wider public controversy, to moralism and judgment of their desires and activities? Would discussion of HPV and its disease sequalae be akin to the 1980s, when "To Talk of AIDS" was to talk about two taboos, one of them sex and the other homosexuality (Altman 1986)? In its early years, that epidemic—one of signification, given its early disease pattern (Treichler 1999)—was constructed as a problem predominantly and most visibly for a certain category of people with a particular identity: healthy "homosexual" men. It was the visible lesion of Kaposi's sarcoma, a rare cancer that formed as a result of immunosuppression, that served as an alert that something was amiss for these young men that was entangling their identity with the actions of sex. An early narrative of risky "homosexual" men moved quickly from relative obscurity into a "drama of major discovery" (Wald 2008, 222). Would talk of HPV unleash a stigma for girls as they prevented an omnipresent infection with uncertain risk to their health?

Contagion is also the title of a book by Priscilla Wald (2008)—subtitled *Cultures, Carriers, and Outbreak Narratives*—about disease narratives and the way they are used to make scientific sense of emergent infections. Wald, an English professor at Duke University, analyzed the ways cultural discourse around infectious disease, specifically as outbreak, functions to infer warning and meaning: a means to alert the public to a possible and/or perceived threat, and also a way to understand scientifically what is unfamiliar and uncertain. Similar to the way the now ubiquitous term "viral" evolved to include the spread of ideas and information (real, fake, or otherwise) along with viruses themselves, "contagion" can be both a material manifestation of transmission of microbes (including, of course, viruses, but also bacteria, and myriad other infectious agents like fungi and worms) and a communication and interaction of ideas about the threat and who and what is at risk. As information travels, the narratives of whose bodies, and what lives, are at risk of harm shape accounts of disease emergency; they "promote or mitigate the stigmatizing of individuals, groups, populations, locales (regional and global), behaviors, and lifestyle" (Wald 2008, 3).

An outbreak narrative, Wald argues, carries the characteristics and narrative structures of producing material, symbolic, and social associations as well as consequences. There are profound stakes for people's lives depending on how narratives unfold and the particularities or generalizability that accompany their purported risks and harms. Outbreak narratives are most often applied to pandemic diseases with acute fatal outcomes, from plague, typhoid, and influenza to the novel coronaviruses that cause Middle East Respiratory Syndrome (MERS-CoV) and severe acute respiratory syndrome (SARS-CoV; SARS-CoV-2). They include the unfolding of the emergency of the HIV epidemic in the 1980s, which Wald distinguishes as *the* outbreak narrative—something Groopman, a medical researcher with a background in AIDS, undoubtedly also signaled his awareness of when he alerted the public to a "sexual epidemic that condoms could not prevent." Early configurations of AIDS brought forward associations to "bad boys," as the original nomenclature and narrative applied to the previously unknown illness emerging among young people in twenty US states and seven countries. At first mostly said to be found in "homosexual males" (though there was some acknowledgment that something was amiss among some heterosexual women and bisexual men, too), the acronymic descriptor used was GRID, for "gay-related immunodeficiency" or "gay-related immune disease" (Altman 1982). The "badness" ascribed to this viral risk was shaped less by scientific knowledge of a disease, and more by the structures of anti-gay and anti-sex discrimination and its gendered, as well as racialized, biopolitics.

Outbreak narratives, especially when linked with emergency and de-linked from already established structures of discrimination, can also spur new directions for research as well as biomedical approaches to prevention. Emergency can unlock the sources and levels of financing to do that research, as well as identify where and how to intervene in a coming threat to best contain the scourge of illness and death. The field of epidemiology was invigorated by HIV/AIDS as attention was also bolstered for investigation into communicable disease more generally. The 1990s saw rates of other STIs soar as biomedicine added additional diagnostic tests able to screen for antibodies or other markers that identify the existence of everything from bacteria such as chlamydia, gonorrhea, or syphilis to viruses such as human immunodeficiency virus (HIV) and herpes simplex virus (HSV-2).

Researchers would make decisions about which categories of people to include in their investigations by reproducing assumptions about populations and their social interactions, leading at times to reduced possibilities for other ways of knowing, predicting, and preventing disease. The consequences are multifaceted. HIV galvanized community-action resistance to manage the discriminatory associations with blame (and shame) as gay, lesbian, transgender, and sex worker communities organized into radical protest movements, from ACT UP—the AIDS Coalition to Unleash Power—to medical-student and scientific-medical organizing. Eventually the narrative work of associating who you are with what you do (sexually) was disentangled and de-moralized, as the epidemiology and scientific efforts began to lean into what you do and not who you are. To really "see

AIDS" would be to render visible the discrimination as well as the risk of (inter)actions—from what was called unprotected sex, to sex work and its power dynamics, to the ways intravenous (IV) drug use was a risk. It included seeing how many in these communities suspected that something was already amiss but had been rendered invisible.[6] And it included seeing the ways Black, indigenous, and marginalized people for whom the intersectional workings of racialization, gendering, and/or sexualization obscure their risk by virtue not of their actions, but of the workings of power that sees and acts to protect some people's humanity or existence more than others.[7]

The narrative of a drama of discovery that unfolded around the human papillomavirus, HPV, was unleashed as a pharmaceutical company asked its commercial viewers to "Know the Link" and to act to prevent cancer. The message contrasts with the powerful AIDS-era political slogan "Silence = Death," which called for publics to join a movement (and by doing so, to affirm that the LGBTQ community was already mobilized) to prevent further discrimination.[8] "Know the Link" was a different rallying cry altogether, a marketing pitch produced and placed in circulation in the context of twenty-first-century biomedicalization. This call was forged far from the streets of the West Village and a coalition of diversely gendered and racialized communities of different sexual orientations producing "safe sex" action plans and direct-action and educational responses. These messages were forged under the favorable conditions of loosened FDA guidelines, and deployed by the well-oiled and -financed public relations arms of pharmaceutical companies with intentional tie-ins to community organization and "patient participation." The campaign also included epidemiological evidence, as well as the results of late-stage clinical trials, developed and financed by Merck years earlier as they were securing patent protection for key processes involved in vaccine production. It was the sort of all-hands-on-deck effort AIDS activists might have hoped for when ACT UP members formed the Treatment Action Group (TAG) to call on scientists, research organizations, and the general public to speak up and demand that the development of prevention approaches and treatment plans be fast-tracked to publics in need, in order to put an end to the vast suffering and death in their midst.

Establishing a New Regime of Cancer Prevention

Sexualizing Cancer follows HPV knowledge backward and forward, examining the particular ways sex and cancer intertwine. The book examines the hyphen between a virus (HPV) and disease (its associated cancers) for the ways the linkage effaces and renders visible gendered sexuality and medical and social uncertainties. The book examines how viral causal association with disease establishes certain ways of talking about sex in relation to health, risk, and disease, and how viral infections might lead to distal risk (and the character of that risk) that contributes to the shape of preventive medicine and public health approaches more generally. HPV serves as a bridge from STIs to the diseases of cancer associated with this infectious agent. The new vaccine serves as a jumping-off point to examine questions of how and where it would roll out to those who might need it most, how modifications to its targets and use would be made over time, and ultimately how this admittedly remarkable vaccine would shape prevention politics from vaccination to screening approaches for HPV-associated disease. The analysis focuses on the particular ways gender and sex are managed,[9] whether by desexualizing and degendering or by amplifying the multifaceted ways sexuality and gender punctuate the meaning and thus the practice of a domain of prevention. A guiding contention in *Sexualizing Cancer* is that the ways the linkage of an STI and disease is framed and the science that underlies the evidence for its connection impact the prevention regime that unfolds, and ultimately the people, places, and practices brought into its fold. This includes the conceptualization of risk and disease and the consequences meanings hold for care. The book examines the ways in which HPV knowledge, HPV vaccines promotion, and HPV screening tools become gendered[10] and de-gendered, as well as sexualized and de-sexualized, in ways that suppress and assert these processes and the categories associated with them, thus infusing a disease and prevention domain with various meanings and actions.

The link between "diseases of the womb" and sex had been scientifically suspected for a century, lingering in gendered sex panics around girls and promiscuity. This long association reflects one site of invisible hauntings—or *ghostly matters* (Gordon 2008)—of the ways the prior association between sex and disease found in the cancers now causally associated with HPV lingers. Other viral-disease associations, and more generally other attributions of disease to sexual behavior, also linger and permeate the signification and scientific-medical enterprise that is now shaped around viruses, especially those that are sexually transmitted, and their causal linkages with diseases. My goal is not to reanimate past associations; many of the punitive and racist or sexist underpinnings, as well as some moralistic ones, have been effectively tamed. Rather, I mean to render visible the ways such associations might linger and shape the ways medicine and public health alike now address prevention for STIs, and specifically for the cancers associated with HPV.

The book examines the lingering presence of an epidemiological risk group of men who have sex with men that emerged and became established as a fully entrenched research base following AIDS research in the US in the 1980s and 1990s that has been instrumental in expanding HPV knowledge in general, and specifically knowledge about HPV's role in anal cancer and its risk. The present attention to (now known) HPV-associated oropharyngeal cancer and heterosexually active adult men is examined in terms of how these associations worked backward from molecular knowledge and were able to absorb gendered sexualization. Young, heterosexual men—and their presumed engagement in "liberated" sexual activities including performing oral sex on women—are brought to the fore in a blended narrative of risky actors, and protected from stigma or blame. What remains in the wake of these disease associations—old or new, but each now with molecular certainty—has been materially and socially managed. Sex, gender, and sexuality have variously been suppressed, rendered invisible, or brought into the light. "To study social life, one must study the ghostly aspects of it," argues the sociologist Avery Gordon (2008, 7). To analyze the presence of HPV and its disease associations and how they shape the governance and management of health and illness is to also analyze the hauntings that surround the disease risk.

Groopman's "Contagion" article in the *New Yorker* materialized a threat in the form of a *risk*—in that case, to one young woman—from an unfamiliar and unavoidable source. Yet Groopman's specter of a public health threat called attention to a risk of and for men as well as women. "Disease significations" include representational and disease burdens, as well as stereotypes that linger from discursive configurations attached to words like "infectious" and "contagious." But they also extend beyond those configurations: to the ways they have been linked to "promiscuous" women with diseases of the womb; in small ways to "debauched" men with "bad blood" (referencing men with syphilis as indulging their sexual pleasures with sex worker); and to other non-sexualized outbreak narratives such as Chinese and other immigrants being deemed "carriers" of incurable disease, from smallpox to plague. Science and medicine are sites of discursive and social configurations of gendered disease and of racialized illness that shape everyday lives and everyday medicine. These meanings are forged in intersectional webs of power and discrimination as white heterosexual women are enduringly figured as "pure," and by extension, deserving of care and protection, while often Black, indigenous, and other racialized people continue to be "unseen" or implicitly available for exploitation, experimentation, or neglect.

It is my argument throughout this book that these and other workings of power and its intersectional justifications linger and haunt the framing of HPV, HPV vaccines, and HPV-cancer associations, as well as the ways these are deployed as risks in need of new or better prevention tools and approaches. The scope and shape of the problems of HPV-associated cancers, framed by science, medicine, and many organizational and governmental actors, in turn forge the response, whether that be more research and new or "optimized" tools, or passage of professional or governmental guidelines, or both. These have stakes for whose bodies and lives and what communities are protected and rendered available for monitoring and care.

Conducting the Research

Sexualizing Cancer begins in 2005–2006 as HPV vaccines were being rolled out. A great deal of excellent scholarly work emerged focusing largely on the vaccine rollout effort. I draw especially on an edited volume by historians and social scientists, *Three Shots of Prevention* (Wailoo et al. 2010), and another authored by the anthropologist Samantha Gottlieb, *Not Quite a Cancer Vaccine* (Gottlieb 2018), as well as many others referenced throughout this book. I begin with my own earlier research into pharmaceutical promotion ads that unfolded with public calls to "Know the Link" and then to join a vaccine effort. *Sexualizing Cancer*, however, goes further, following the trail of molecular knowledge and its vaccine product to the latest scientific studies and approaches to disease prevention efforts for "other cancers" and other at-risk groups, and into the tools and approaches to screen for HPV-associated disease.

With a focus on the politics of prevention at the intersection of sex and disease, the book follows HPV talk, HPV research, and HPV clinical practice in pharmaceutical advertising and marketing, at scientific conferences, among patient and public advocacy organizations, and in clinical care.

A new regime of cancer prevention, as theorized, emerges that is distinctly molecular in its scope. The regime is driven by techno-scientific "optimization" of tools already in place. Its scale, like biomedicine itself, is highly uneven in its reach and approach. The much-talked-about and -hoped-for "precision" prevention is deemed necessary for some, less than necessary for others with the same level of cellular risk, and not even conversation-worthy for still others who are altogether outside prevention discourse.

Stratified biomedicalization—the ways biomedicine is driven by tech-noscience, with uneven and inequitable decision points from research and development to clinical practice—is a central analytic lens of the book (Clarke et al. 2010). As the pharmaceutical companies Merck and GSK were busy designing and conducting clinical trial research that would open up a new cadre of potential recipients of an HPV vaccine—including those at risk for cervical cancer, with its newly established causal relationship to HPV—it was patently obvious that an available vaccine could go a long way toward ameliorating suffering and preventing a large number of deaths around the world. At the dawn of the twenty-first century, the second lead-ing cause of morbidity and mortality around the world (after heart disease) was cervical cancer. There were 288,000 cervical cancer deaths in 2000, and 471,000 new diagnoses; 80 percent of all cases were among women in low-resource countries (WHO 2002).[11] Across select regions of Africa, but concentrated in the least resourced countries, cervical cancer was the most common deadly cancer in women.[12] More than half a million Americans die of cancer each year, and of the 273,000 women who die of cancer an-nually, 1.36 percent—approximately 3,700—die of a cancer of the cervix. (72,000 women died of lung cancer, 41,000 of breast cancer.)

In the business model of pharmaceuticals, early adoption and high price points are said to be needed to recoup the early and usually high costs of R&D. To reap their returns, Merck and GSK had plans to introduce and roll out the new vaccines, supported by aggressive advertising and mar-keting campaigns, in high-resource countries first. In Gardasil's first year of availability, in 2006, total vaccine sales were $365 million, immediately propelling Merck's total vaccine market from $272 million to $903 mil-lion (PharmaTimes 2007).[13] Patent protection, which guaranteed Merck's long-term profits by allowing the company to focus sales on potential re-cipients who could purchase the product at a high cost (a minority of 10 percent), would likely limit vaccine expansion, particularly for the other 90 percent of prospective vaccine recipients—the people referred to by the scholar and journalist Steven Thrasher as the "viral underclass" living in low- and middle-income countries—unless governments were able to buy out those patents to ensure mass availability at lower costs. Thrasher's argument, however, is not about place, but about how inequalities ensure that those living in precarity—the poor, the queer, the Black and indig-enous around the world—are also those who bear the largest human cost of a viral scourge (Thrasher 2022).

Meanwhile, the vaccine represented a vital addition to an established arsenal of medical tools designed to screen and prevent invasive cancers of the cervix. Cervical cancer in high-resource countries like the US was considered largely a controllable if not preventable disease, for the majority of those with adequate, affordable, and accessible health care. The Pap test was part of "women's health," in place since the mid-twentieth century around the world. It is said to have effectively decreased cervical cancer deaths by up to 80 percent in the US (American Cancer Society 2005). Despite being considered a basic tool—cheap, and easy to perform and analyze—the Pap test continues to be underutilized and inaccessible in poor countries where women in their prime are most likely to be diagnosed with later-stage cervical cancers, and at times out of reach for people in high-resource countries who have no safety net due to poverty, documentation status, or (health care's) discriminatory and other structural constraints on getting good care. Disparities in cancer rates and deaths, and in cervical cancer, are shaped not by higher rates of HPV or other infections, nor by "deviant" sexual practices or lives, but rather by differences in resources and infra-structures, as well as in the protection of human rights needed to ensure equal and equitable care (World Health Organization 2006; Farmer et al. 2010). As the book reaches its end, a tension is shown between the goals of medical care and the goals of precision public health. Screening tools and vaccination are "commodities of care" for the most well-off and often "worried well," with others in the margins of precarity having less access to the means of preventing early death (Fan 2021). Yet, such an approach is not inherently negative, given the now almost half century of devolution of the public role in health care along with the rights to health care decision making, in reproductive and sexual health especially. The willingness and need to take technologies into one's own hands, for instance with at-home tools and devices or with the guidance of tele-medicine or text-based apps, may be welcome news and relatively accepted (as people's use of at-home screening for COVID antigens has shown). HPV screening as another home tool may be just what many need most, depending on the setting and its social-biomedical contours.

Through a lens of feminist science and technology studies, *Sexualizing Cancer* interrogates the shape of stories, looking for that which lingers, reassembles, and emerges anew as epidemiologists and clinical research-ers seek to understand and address the diseases associated with HPV. The book reveals how the associations between sex, sexual infection, and disease shifted and churned, at times amplifying sex and sexual transmission and at times suppressing them from view. The human papillomavirus's association with disease was not with just any disease, but with one long feared and long regarded as what Siddhartha Mukherjee memorably called the "Emperor of All Maladies": cancer. (Today, up to 20 percent of cancers worldwide are in part attributable to a viral pathogen.) At the same time, HPV is also a sexually transmitted infection, and as such has traveled through multiple variously stigmatized domains: first, as venereal disease or VD; then in the world of sexually transmitted disease or STDs; and now as a neutral and (relatively) stigma-free STI.

By the beginning of the twenty-first century, medical domains focusing on infectious disease and those focusing on cancers would find themselves connecting in particular places, shaping conceptualizations of risk and practices of preventing and governing disease. These ways of understanding and addressing risk are part of a biomedicalization of prevention reflective of the knowledge and practice shifts now consolidated in medicine to approach risk and prevention not only through behavioral approaches to disease prevention (like diet and condom use), but also through molecular and technological approaches of pills, vaccines, and other ways of intervening in health, including sexual health. Once described as two domains on "parallel tracks" (Mukherjee 2010) that intersected only at specific moments in the twentieth century, cancer and infectious disease would not only meet, but gradually fuse together.

As cervical cancer moved from being considered a "silent killer" to a highly visible cancer risk with a "precursor" of high-risk HPV, other HPV-related cancers were either unknown publicly or silenced. At least two "rare" cancers, as designated by their rates of diagnosis, would gradually and differently enter into a narrative of discovery of their own, each with distinct population risk identities and behavioral narrations, and each conjuring claims of "rising epidemics" among well-established and at times new risk groups. Step by step, through research into the scientific and medical literature, observations at professional medical conferences, and interviews with leading experts, I examined the various places, processes, and attributions in which HPV and its cancer linkages were made visible, feared, and contained, specifically through processes of gendering and sexualizing the conceptualizations of risk and governance.

A handful of salient and far-reaching questions emerge: How would this new approach, a vaccine to prevent a viral STI and risk of cancer formation, affect and change clinical biomedicine and its preventive approaches? What is at stake when a biomedical machinery converts patients-in-waiting into enterprising prevention actors, reducing their risks of cancers rhetorically and materially? What happens when sexual risk is invoked, subsumed, or brought to the foreground? Which groups are envisioned and enrolled, and who is left out in this apparatus? What social forces are obfuscated, and what forces are highlighted in the process?

Methodology

This analysis draws heavily on "open-source" and publicly available documents and data, from scientific publications to press releases to web-based content. These are followed up with ethnographic observation of professional meetings and include informal and formal interviews with scientists, researchers, and medical providers. Research was conducted from 2013 to 2020, with the majority conducted in 2018–2021 following an NSF award to focus on precision cancer prevention tools. Scientific meetings were approached first with a request to the organizers for a sociologist to sit among them; once invited, I followed HPV talk into presentations, taking notes on the ways presenters spoke of risk and cause, of sex and gender, and of the possibilities for prevention and care. As I met professional participants and presenters, we would speak informally in the halls outside conference meeting rooms, and some would be contacted for formal interviews to be held at the meeting or later over Zoom.[14] A key part of my fieldwork was observing and meeting the sponsors and industry professionals who purchased space to promote their products. I hung out and accepted their offerings of coffee, candy, pens, and swag bags while perusing the "educational materials" laid out on the showroom tables. When I could, I introduced myself as a sociologist and researcher interested in new and emerging ways to prevent cancers. Back home, I added activists and advocacy groups to my contacts, as well as other experts whose names I heard spoken at the professional meetings.

My fieldwork began at the annual meeting of the National Cervical Cancer Coalition (NCCC).[15] Two days of conversation and presentations were held in a banquet-style room with about ten round tables of mostly women with notebooks out, listening attentively as panelists shared the latest news. While I had introduced myself as a researcher to the roomful of participants at the start of the two-day convening, it was also clear from my rapid note-taking that I was there in a different role than those alongside whom I sat. The back of the room was filled with sponsors and their product displays (Merck, Hologic, Roche, Pure Romance, and others were in attendance), as well as "delegates" from the CDC and smaller advocacy organizations that set out information sheets, some with "Cancer Sucks" buttons.

It was at NCCC that I met an activist (from, I will say, Ohio) who was organizing women around cervical cancer prevention in her hometown— I'll call her Pam. Pam turned to me during the very first presentation on the science of cervical cancer and asked, in a whisper, "Are they saying my aunt died of a sexually transmitted disease?"

I nodded.

She shook her head in affirmation, tightening her lips into a frown.

After the presentation, we talked about her surprise. "Do we need to say that?" she wondered, as she told me about her aunt and their relationship. She hadn't known much about the role of STIs, even as she was introduced to HPV as the (definitive, molecularly established) cause of her aunt's cancer. We wondered together what it meant that HPV was a common infection transmitted through sex, yet had been so shrouded from view. We shared our purpose for being at the meeting and our thinking, as well as stories of the people we knew and had lost from cancers. And then we discussed our individual stakes in the substance of the meeting. The causal association did matter to Pam, she told me as we said goodbye on the second day, "but also, not really." She was energized by the new information and the solidarity formed with other regional representatives she had met during the time at the convening.

Over the next seven years, I would formally interview thirty-one scientists, clinicians, and activists/advocates, and speak informally to many more. I would attend more than fifteen distinct scientific meetings in public health, cancer research, and infectious disease; I also reviewed subsequent meetings via webinars and publicly available materials that did not require registration.[16] These materials were assembled and thematically coded using preliminary assertions about cancer and sex and looking for the disciplinary domain in which they were situated (e.g., oncology, virology, pediatrics). Over time, I got to know some of the major actors and research areas involved. As I listened, I noted with interest as the discourse at the conferences shifted away from cervical cancer to anal cancers, oropharyngeal cancers, and issues of co-infection and their preventive possibilities. I followed these leads and learned that prevention approaches varied, but in each, scientists and advocates navigated uncertainties regarding how to balance infection clearance and medical intervention and to establish what Clarke and Fujimura referred to as the "right tools for the job" of prevention (Clarke and Fujimura 1992a and b). Following the methodology of situational analysis (Clarke 2005), I would come to see how they balanced amplifying sexual transmission and cancer prevention, and how this balancing varied depending on disciplinary domain and specialization. Some would attempt to normalize and suppress talk of sex, while others would work hard to bring this into view.

Sexualizing Cancer has four arguments. The first is that the sexual is always already present, even when subsumed, when talking about researching, treating, and containing STIs and the several cancers associated with them. Sexuality is also always already gendered as well as shaped by dimensions of what we call race and class. This book begins its analysis with the HPV vaccine, and the ways this vaccine and others variously carry matter and meaning (Haraway 1997; Pollock 2008 and 2012). As a vaccine against a sexually transmitted pathogen and virus, this biomedical entity as an STI invites discursive analysis not only of sexual transmission, but of the ways that transmission is gendered and also suppressed a cancer risk, and the ways tools for cancer prevention take hold. As HPV vaccination indications (who would get the vaccine and when) expanded, the workings of sexualization and its suppression changed: HPV grew to be linked with masculine gender and questions were raised about boys and their risk, and whether a direct benefit was needed to secure their adoption of a new vaccine. I examine the places and ways in which sex and sexuality appear, along what intersectional dimensions, and how these renderings provoke either aggressive attempts to banish it from view or efforts to allow its presence to take hold. I use the term *gendered sexualization* to refer to these varied processes and attributions that infuse a domain with overt and intersectional gendered and sexual meaning, and *gendered desexualization* to describe the processes by which domains become disassociated from overt connections to gender and sexuality.

My second argument is that by drawing out these processes along with processes of biomedicalization, not only are scientific ideas and technologies imbued with cultural and symbolic meanings; their narrative shape also holds consequences for the production of specific meanings around risk and the objects in need of prevention. These are part of a politics of knowledge that sheds light on and obscures uncertainty and ambiguity—in this case, in the face of the ways HPV is a necessary but insufficient cause of cancers associated with HPV. How vaccines and cancer screening tools are developed, established as necessary and right, and put into preventive guidelines is shaped through a gendered and sexualized politics of knowledge, and a politics of prevention.

Biomedicalization is a term that reflects the ways social problems are increasingly technologized and scientized and rendered available for new biotechnical approaches. I use it here as I think through the changing landscape of prevention tools, from vaccines to HPV screening tests, and how these are shifting from being used only within biomedical settings to also include at-home or self-administered technologies. It is these processes, whether new, emerging, or cumulative, that are captured by the concepts of risk, governance, and biomedicalization (Clarke et al. 2003; Clarke et al. 2010) that together reveal a pharmaceuticalization of prevention.

A third argument concerns a reengagement with *prevention politics*, to bring forward an assertion that the new regime of prevention is shaped by tensions among precision biomedicine and its individualized approach and the goals of more collective public health approaches. Prevention politics is a term first used to describe the ways prevention favors simultaneously a logic of individualism and a logic of social production and social solutions to health.[17] HPV vaccines reveal a logic of a personal approach in the context of consumer-based medicine, and a logic of a collective approach in the context of a goal of reaching herd immunity. The balance of these logics has shifted over almost fifty years of dis-investment and devolution of the public health and public spheres in favor of privatized and pharmaceuticalized solutions.

Techniques and technologies for HPV screening—of the skin zones where HPV tends to reside (of the anus, the cervix, and the back of the throat) are analyzed for just how HPV knowledge and prevention has transformed clinic-based as well as population-level prevention efforts. I examine how these technologies of vaccination and screening tools travel and are promoted as they move at times into a variety of specialties and settings and at times into the hands of people protecting their health. Along the way, analytic attention is also paid to the ways sexuality and gender are always already present—at times rendered normative and at times viewed as problems and concerns, in health and disease.[18]

Finally, ideas around infectious disease and cancer causation are not two separate propositions; they are shown to be intertwined and mutually co-produced. In terms of preventive medicine, sexual risk reduction, and risk categorization and practices more generally, have permeated the technologies, experiences, and identities of the "healthy" and the management of the "ill." By the close of the book, as I move from vaccines said to prevent cervical cancer, to questions concerning the multizonal nature of HPV's causation, to other cancers (specifically anal cancer and oropharyngeal cancer), I uncover the prevention politics that unfold in science and medicine and among cultural understandings of cancer and STIs. Cervical cancer underwent radical change in its understanding, prevention, and treatment over a 150-year period, largely produced through scientific claims; whether the next shift in cervical cancer might be a restigmatization and sexualization of this disease's understandings and practices was a question posed by the historian of medicine of Ilana Löwy (2011).

Sexualizing Cancer takes on the regime change[19] in the twenty-first century to show how the prevention regime established first by the molecular knowledge of HPV's role in a set of cancers led to a new vaccine that gradually expanded from group to group, subsuming and animating gendered sexual risk along the way. The regime change involved integration of a vaccine into a developing model for screening either for signs of this viral presence or for the virus itself and its specific genotypes. The book argues that inherent tensions among clinical biomedicine and public health, cellular screening and diagnosing the molecular as risk, and clinical expertise and at-home care are each and all producing a new regime of cancer prevention, and are part of the twenty-first-century emphasis on managing the health of patients-in-waiting (Timmermans and Buchbinder 2010). This is not a story of Big Brother or Big Pharma or biomedicalization's control; it is one of new configurations of meaning and practice that includes complex agencies that vary across topographies and settings that structure and shape care and prevention. Some settings are socialized for health to be objects of personal control, responsibility, and ongoing management, while other settings are socialized for scarcity (Benton 2015).[20] These are each and all part of a contemporary prevention regime in which "choice" is structured, yet complex agencies emerge—organizationally and individually—that reflect negotiation. This new regime includes screening tools that are faster and optimized, with processes of molecularization and sequencing, computerization and digitization, and automation that together provide objective risk-based decision making. The transformation includes cellular to molecular risk and prevention made by evidence-based medicine and randomized clinical trials that establish the information and techniques that shape prevention guidelines, and establishment of risk governance. The new regime is animated by a precision imaginary shaping not only prevention biomedicine, but also the ways people perceive and then monitor their health in terms of risk and threat, sexual and otherwise.

CHAPTER ONE

Producing and Protecting Risky Girls

"Tell someone."

"*Tell* someone."

"Tell *someone*."

Teen girls, eyes intent with concern, spoke directly to the camera, addressing millions of television viewers. A handful of their contemporaries respond with their own urgency to the call to communicate what each is ostensibly learning before our eyes: "I didn't know that." "I was stunned!" "I feel like it is my responsibility to tell someone I love." "I just want to tell my sister." "I want to tell my mother." The "it" they are talking about is HPV—the human papillomavirus—which scientists have long suspected and more recently proven with molecular certainty to be a virus that plays an important and causative role in the onset of cancer. "Cancer caused by a virus," the girls said, looking alternately shocked and perplexed, but also confident, newly bolstered by this critical information. In the language of medicine and public health, they had just been made "aware" of a cancer risk they didn't know they had. They stand strong, making direct eye contact to share the news with a subset of the viewing public: other women and girls. As these surprised girls came to know and learn the "facts" of cancer causation, they called on their sisters, mothers, and daughters—literal and figurative—to join them in an open, collective conversation that would soon be pervasive across America: how could a common, seemingly benign adult virus cause the most silent and deadly of diseases—cancer?[1]

"Did you know?" they asked hundreds of thousands of American viewers.

From the outset, both the viral risk and the cancers referenced in these ads were distinctly gendered, associated with girls and women. The narrative joined a virus and a cancer, communicating a risk that was neither new nor imminent. Yet the stakes were clear: a health threat lingered in a cancer scare for girls. With a surprising "I didn't know" came something to learn and manage with careful deliberation. The risk is chilling despite being punctuated by marked uncertainty: though HPV is ubiquitous in sexually active people, the 150-plus genomic types that can be scientifically identified through molecular assays hold widely differing possibilities for one's health: a few are associated with non-cancerous tumors such as genital warts, some are linked to the later onset of cancers and thus considered "high-risk," and many more are either "low-risk" or deemed to be of no risk at all. HPVs remain ambiguous given their uncertain pathways. As the Nobel Prize-winning scientist Michael Bishop added when we spoke at his office at a leading medical center at the University of California San Francisco (UCSF), "We don't have evidence that any human tumor is caused simply by a virus. Other things have to happen." A virus might be necessary, he explained, "but is insufficient to cause later disease." He thought about another virus, the Epstein-Barr virus, stating, "to this day the epidemiological evidence is suspect because the infection is so ubiquitous. It's very hard to get a guilt by association, which is what epidemiology is all about."

Since at least the mid-1950s (but starting earlier in basic science), understanding the role of viruses and their life course and consequences has been part of the projects of molecular biology and tumor virology. HPVs[2] were first identified as causing (genital) warts, leading researchers to differentiate HPV types and identify a subgroup of HPVs closely related to the development of human cancers.[3] While many HPV infections are generally mild and asymptomatic, and most are likely to shed, in a subset of cases HPVs can hide deep in some crevices of the body and persist. This leads to a process of progression in which cells "invade," attach, and divide, and the resulting proliferation of damaged cells can become cancerous.[4]

In the 1980s, scientists, mostly virologists, applied the techniques developed in molecular biology to act on the widely held suspicion that a virus played a role in cervical cancer's progression. They turned attention away from herpes (the herpes simplex or HSV-2 virus) to the papillomaviruses.[5] In 1993 the German virologist Harald zur Hausen was credited with the "discovery" of HPV's link to cancer, for which he received a shared Nobel Prize for Medicine or Physiology in 2008.[6] In part reinvigorated by the HIV/AIDS epidemic, scientists in the field of molecular epidemiology sought to understand the prevalence of HPV in populations and the interactions between these pathogens and external social processes that might explain the rates and routes of disease. Epidemiological research in the 1980s confirmed the transmission of HPV through sexual activity; its prevalence among the vast majority of people; and its association with age, sexual practice, and the later onset of several cancers and other non-cancerous disease.[7] M. Michele Manos, one of the leading researchers to first confirm HPV's role in cervical cancer, described in an interview the scientific and medical innovation: "I put PCR to work," she explained, referencing a new platform (the "polymerase chain-reaction test") used to amplify and thus detect genetic material of the virus. PCR became the gold standard for detecting and typing HPV. "That method," Manos exclaimed, is "what was used to prove the relationship between HPV and cervical cancer, and also to show that HPV is the most common sexually transmitted disease." That HPV is common is highly significant for the narrative plot and the politics of prevention that would unfold around HPV. The scientific association of sex and risk of disease, and the specific links between HPV types and various cancers, obscures the facts that for the vast majority of us, sexual activity results in harmless and continuous transmission and retransmission of the more than 150 genotypes of HPV; that the vast majority of these infections clear on their own; and that for the very rare case where a high-risk strain will persist in our bodies, the life course of virus-to-precancer-to-cancer is largely unknown and, in the case of cervical cancer, has in place an infrastructure of screening for these cellular changes so that they might be identified and effectively treated early to prevent invasive cancer.

The vaccine strategy had "followed the epidemiology very logically," Manos told me. "It is everywhere," she said, and that "allows you to plan your vaccination strategy much better." She explained further: "HPV is everywhere, therefore you need to be protected before you ever get into the backseat of the car with the boy." For Manos, the *you* implicated in the pending threat that needed to be managed was an adolescent girl in need of protection from presumably heterosexual sex. "That's just kind of the storyline there. I think the drug companies were aware that the science was straightforward." She paused, and added, "but perhaps they were not prepared for the controversy." Despite what may have been a clear and easy vaccine strategy to inoculate girls to prevent later disease, drug companies and policymakers confronted controversy around girls and their sexuality. As Manos stated, "all of a sudden parents had to contemplate their adolescents' upcoming sexual activity. And, it turned out, nobody was interested in doing that."

Like all technologies, vaccines are social, and are developed and introduced with multiple considerations that lie far beyond disease burden rates and public health goals. As the historian of medicine Stuart Blume acknowledged early in the HPV vaccine's introduction (Blume 2017), the disease data in the US showed there would be little demand for the vaccine—deaths from cervical cancer were low compared to other cancers; the Pap test was pretty good at finding early disease at a low cost; and most people were relatively unaware of HPV's role in cancer formation.[8] In some ways, there was little need for the HPV vaccine, at least in the US. Merck, the developer of an HPV vaccine, had a balancing act on its hands: on the one hand it was eager to enroll girls and their parents in a commodity market for a vaccine they did not yet know they needed (but that would reduce their risk of disease); on the other hand, the company was careful not to wade into the minefield of "lifestyle" and individual liberty and responsibility that has plagued public debate and opposition around many health prevention approaches. Merck was eager to avert the controversy, for example, that had unfolded around the hepatitis B vaccine when in the 1980s some publics opposed its use by referencing HBV as a disease of irresponsibility, of "junkies," "homosexuals," and other risk-takers.

While vaccines for a little-known risk might be a hard sell, they had also become one of the leading profit products of the late twentieth century. In the 1990s, many companies were in search of vaccines against communicable disease, many in part or exclusively transmitted sexually. STIs were a big concern both in themselves and in the ways they might exacerbate other disease: gonorrhea and chlamydia can cause pelvic inflammatory disease and fertility problems; syphilis is dangerous during childbirth, as bacteria can be passed perinatally; and HIV continues to inflict life-threatening and other disease, including some cancers. With HPV, there are five other known viruses that are also sexually transmitted and associated with the development of cancers. These include two viruses that cause the highest numbers of cancer cases—hepatitis B and hepatitis C (HBV and HCV)—as well as human herpesvirus type 8 (HHV-8), human T-cell lymphotrophic virus type 1 (HTLV-1), and Epstein-Barr virus (EBV). Together, these are believed to account for 12 to 20 percent of cancer cases worldwide.[9] As antibiotics and anti-retrovirals are used to treat these and other infectious agents, some of the agents are developing some antibiotic resistance, creating problems of their own. Vaccines provide solutions to these cascading problems while also producing the profit margins corporations hope for.

The pharmaceutical companies Merck and Co. (Merck) and GlaxoSmithKline (GSK) were busy answering a corporate call for a potentially profitable prevention strategy. A vaccine against cervical cancer, along with an effective business model for securing patent protection and intellectual property rights, would ensure market dominance. Patents provide a guaranteed but limited period of monopoly. While it was researchers in academic institutions and at the National Institutes of Health in the US and Australia who first developed the technology of manufacturing virus-like particles for use in vaccines in the early 1990s, Merck and GSK filed patents on their improvements to these processes.[10] Patents are tools that allow companies to recoup research and development (R&D) investment by locking in (high) prices and reducing competition, thereby also ensuring profit (Padmanabhan et al. 2010).[11] GSK and Merck submitted over 100 HPV vaccine-related patent applications before FDA approvals (Chandrasekharan et al. 2015).[12] By 2018 Gardasil had market dominance, with an average market share of 87 percent in the period 2007–2018; GSK's Cervarix left the US market in 2015.[13]

To reach this blockbuster status required patent protection as well as an effective marketing strategy to ensure adoption and to avert any form of controversy. Merck invested heavily in ensuring marketing success: in 2006, the first year of product advertisements, they allocated US$42.74 million; the next year they allocated US$101.4 million, up 137 percent. The investment paid off; in 2007 the HPV vaccine brought in US$1.5 billion worldwide, up from US$234.8 million in 2006, when it was first approved in the US (Staton 2008).

In the strategy to garner the support of publics, health care providers, and parents alike, Merck and other vaccine supporters produced an early narrative replete with assumptions about gender and sex, risk and disease, and health responsibility. The message was one of a risk of a deadly disease and a responsibility to act to protect oneself from this harm. Girls could avert a risk of cancer by acting now, in adolescence. There was not some imminent thing to be feared by the masses; it was more that there was a distal risk to manage. Merck and its advertisers would not warn publics of girls' sexuality, nor what Manos had euphemistically referred to as the risks of getting "into the backseat of the car with the boy." They did not warn of the risks of diminished sexual agency, power, or consent to protect one's own health. They did not educate about an infectious pathogen that was everywhere and might not be stoppable. Instead, messaging drew on already established discourses of women's reproductive health and preventive responsibility.

Messaging would closely adhere to epidemiological data found in the cancer statistics collected by the National Cancer Institute's (NCI) comprehensive Surveillance, Epidemiology, and End Results (SEER) Program. NCI at the time showed that cervical cancer in the US was relatively infrequent. Deaths from cervical cancer were about 3,700 people each year, compared to the 700,000 deaths from heart disease (Markowitz 2019). Yet, cervical cancer was the second most common cancer among women worldwide, with an estimated 493,000 new cases annually, more than 80 percent of which occur in low-resourced countries in the global south (Ferlay, Bray, and Pisani 2004). The vast majority of deaths from cervical cancer—almost 95 percent—are in low- and middle-income countries (de Sanjosé et al. 2012), highlighting where a new preventive approach could benefit women and people with a cervix the most. At the same time, 1 in

6 people in the US would die of some form of cancer, and the number of "cancer survivors" stood at 10 million in 2005 (Ries et al. 2008), reflecting in part a "remission society" (Frank 2013 [1995]). Cancer was at once a distal fear, a source of suffering, and a cause of much loss and grief.

Advertising would need to tap into the uncertainty and distal risk the virus posed to human health, and into the already established worries among adult parents. Gardasil entered the pharmaceutical market with carefully managed prevention messages about a "woman's cancer" and girls' responsibility (in part due to the FDA approval of the vaccine first for girls). Their message was not aligned with the values, goals, and approaches of many scientists, researchers, and providers. What the public learned as Gardasil hit the consumer market was that girls and their mothers were compelled to know and do something about a virus and its potential harm to their health.

The sales pitch began in 2005 with nonbranded information ads[14] designed and FDA-approved to "educate" viewers—part of a larger multimedia campaign housed on the now inactive website TellSomeone.com. With these ads, a transformation was beginning to take place about the ways certain cancers would be causally understood and prevented. Cancers had long occupied a place of great uncertainty, with little definitive knowledge about their cause. Prevention largely focused on associations with diet, exercise, and tobacco use. Cervical cancer, possibly the most silent and "deadly" among the cancers, was otherwise unique, though, for having long been suspected as having an association with sex. For centuries, a steady dose of shame and blame had been meted out on its sufferers—reprehension that landed on some bodies and lives (with specters of "irresponsibility" inherent in "promiscuous" girls, "wayward" women, and the variety of derogations blaming sex work and workers) with blunter force than others.

These symbolic associations of the attributions of risk were undergoing significant change as the novel idea of a "cancer-causing" virus was introduced to the public. At the same time, the quiet information of the association of that risk with sex, and specifically with a sexually transmitted virus, could upend the ways cancer and prevention were understood altogether. When young people at once declared and questioned the "link"—"Cancer caused by a virus?!"—in the nonbranded ads, they were promoting scientifically evidenced knowledge that a virus (in this case HPV) is causally associated with later onset of several cancers (among them cervical cancer). The public would be drawn into this information gradually and specifically with the introduction, promotion, and availability of a new medical product unlike any other: a vaccine that could prevent, and protect, a viral spread.

With its message to girls, vaccines were shifting from a one-size-fits-all, population-level public health intervention—what the medical ethicist Donna Dickenson (2013) refers to as "we medicine," referring to a collective approach to medical care and health prevention on a mass scale that benefited the "we"—to "me medicine," an approach benefiting individuals or a subgroup. Gardasil would join other medical products in the early 2000s that would be brought directly to consumers, advertised to individuals with appeals to "ask your doctor" if a drug or device or vaccine—often but not always mentioned by brand name—is "right for you." This responsibility to know and choose what is best for you was presumably in the hands of the individual, entering lifestyle choice with decisions laden with the capacity to remake one's (cancer-free) future.

Gardasil's introduction came with a push and pull between individual liberty and public health. Questions of parental choice intersected with government recommendations, and both of these with long-simmering controversies around sex and gendered expectations. As commercials promoted a connection between a little-known virus and a well-known cancer, publics were directed to ask themselves: how does this concern *me*, my body, my family, and our future health? If you are a parent in the US, you will likely recognize yourself in these conversations wherever you might be on the vaccine decision-making spectrum, from wholesale acceptance to balancing interests for your children or in some place of distrust and rejection. No matter where your attitudes lie, you will nonetheless recognize the appeals to look to yourself and your family to consider risk and act to protect. This "personalized" approach is part of an ongoing shift in medicine and public health alike, an era of biomedicalization, wherein medicine no longer only controls sickness by classifying pathology and rendering a treatment and perhaps a cure, but biomedicine—along with its axillary biotech and health tech companies, among others—offers a range of technoscientific fixes aimed at pre-disease, risk of disease, and enhancing one's health.

A slew of medical products were routinely promoted on TV and through other media outlets, from print magazines to product websites, urging consumers to choose the best (i.e., their) product for their individual health. The Food and Drug Administration (FDA), in additional to approving products based on evidence largely submitted to them by the manufacturers, also regulates marketing. They do so by distinguishing between information and product advertising, and they use the terms "nonbranded" and "branded" to distinguish between broader education efforts and a sales pitch for a specific product.[15] Merck blended these approaches in a two-part advertising strategy that began with informational messages and then shifted to more common product promotion messages to promote their first-of-its-kind brand, the Gardasil vaccine.[16] The pharmaceutical company returned frequently to the FDA with new evidence, seeking expanded indications for prevention among different populations, and, at times, for the additional HPV genomic types included in the vaccine itself.

Advertising does multiple forms of work: public health work, medical work, and the cultural work of producing meaning and action. As ads name and describe disease, they communicate an expectation that certain subjects will become aware of a behavioral change they ought to undertake, and will heed the call for preventive action, or at least know that the call exists (Reagan 1997, Wailoo 2011). So, when commercials began appearing for a new vaccine, one that would prevent a deadly cancer, the public was primed to receive, and likely accept, its health care advice as a "cancer prevention" message—for women and girls to first know there is something they can do, and then tell someone what they know. "I feel like it is my responsibility to tell someone I love," say moms and their daughters in the ads.

Despite the widespread airing of commercials for drugs for sexual, reproductive, and genital health—for erectile dysfunction, birth control pills, and incontinence—whether the public was ready to learn of a health risk associated with a sexually transmitted virus had yet to be seen. To avoid any sexual controversy, Merck's advertising would downplay mention of a ubiquitous STI in favor of an overt message of cancer prevention. With direct-to-consumer (DTC) advertising, the mostly young and mostly girl-identified target audience for Gardasil would be introduced to a set of concomitant problems they hadn't previously known they had: a *risk* of developing cervical cancer and a *failure* of current health screening to protect them from this deadly disease. The Pap test had been in use since the 1950s and at this point was well integrated into "women's health" and specialties that address gynecological and reproductive health care. Would publics know that the Pap test had come under scrutiny for its technical lack of sensitivity (the probability of correctly finding those who are positive for disease risk), which has placed limits on its efficacy as a cancer prevention tool? For the girls to whom Gardasil was marketed, the messaging of this new preventive vaccine inferred that it must be a far better preventive approach than the one currently in wide use, and that the Pap test must no longer be the "right enough tool" for the job of protecting their mothers, their future selves, and other people with a cervix from this deadly cancer. The vaccine held both a cancer-free promise and, by extension, potential freedom from an imperfect screening test. This new vaccination would mark the beginning of a new regime of cancer prevention by adding a primary prevention approach, designed to inoculate the host (the person) directly against the virus (HPV) now shown to be necessary in the formation of this cancer.

In their capacity to stimulate an immune response, vaccines had become part of preventive medicine for communicable disease, and research was under way to develop vaccines for many infectious agents. Cancer(s), however, are considered to be noncommunicable diseases, holding little in common with the targets of more than fifteen vaccinations the US CDC's Advisory Committee on Immunization Practices (ACIP) recommends that children receive, mostly at birth and now into their teens. This new vaccine differed from the shots administered to babies and toddlers, for diphtheria or whooping cough, to protect against highly communicable and contagious diseases affecting the lives of children. Given the newly acquired knowledge about the omnipresence of the virus once people became sexually active, the vaccine would be administered early—at adolescence (though not at birth or early childhood). It was shown to be most effective when administered close, but preferably prior, to sexual onset—a period well after the busy early childhood schedule of vaccinations.

Only later would it become clear that this then three-shot regimen (antibody response studies and age would determine the number, and intervals, of shots, gradually moving from 3 to 2 to 1 shot) would not (at first, nor likely ever) be sufficient as a tool for the absolute prevention of either cervical cancer or other diseases associated with HPV. Vaccination would need to be coupled with a screening test, possibly the Pap test or an HPV DNA test in some yet-to-be-determined screening schedule to ensure population protection from disease. As Manos speculated during our interview, "the vaccine will not solve cervical cancer; it will likely make screening more efficient." She clarified that "It will push technology innovation" more than it will affect the global rates of cancer. As screening technologies became more "efficient," to use Manos's term, the interval recommended for this secondary screening tool would undergo change of its own. The combination of vaccination and more efficient Pap tests and HPV tests would promise to reduce cervical cancer, and perhaps eliminate it altogether.[17] As vaccine and other preventive guidelines and approaches shifted with vaccination, sexual dynamics would variously punctuate what I am referring to as a new regime of cancer prevention: a vaccine approved for girls would simultaneously render girls' bodies and their "sexual risk" *part* of this cancer regime, prompting attempts to desexualize girls and thus desexualize this aspect of public health prevention.

As advertising began to flood television and print media to inform publics of this HPV-cancer link, parents of adolescents, specifically girls, were called to join conversations with one another and with health care professionals about cancer risk and cancer prevention. Adults had already been inundated with calls (primarily from TV commercials) to "ask their doctors" about this new medical product. Now, new risk-identities and a preventive practice were placed on the menu of "choices" for consumption. Mothers especially were called upon to be part of a movement of enterprising health care consumers, to join a preventive public health movement to prevent a cancer risk they already had. What was different here was that in doing so, they were also asked to think about and assess their daughters'— and later, their sons'—sexual risk.

Despite attempts to banish sex and sexuality from view, girls and women —as well as many boys and men—wondered how their bodies and lives might be affected by a common virus, a sexually transmitted infection, and whether they might or should enter cancer prevention (Mamo and Epstein 2014). Although viruses have the capacity to penetrate all bodies, it was girls' bodies—already subjects of such discourse and fear, especially of a cancer risk—that parents, professionals, and state actors would seek to determine how best to guard and protect. What unspooled was a range of quiet connections about gender, sex, and sexuality that variously ignited suspicion, controversy, and at times distrust. A vaccine to prevent a women's disease administered to preadolescent (and pre-sexually active) girls for a virus said to be sexually transmittable would unleash sexual anxieties as attempts were made to tame any overt discussion of sex. Elected and other state officials as well as a range of health professions and organizations added skepticism and anxiety as they shared evidence and support for the vaccine's role in preventing cancer. It was immediately clear that Merck would need to overcome a plethora of social and sexual challenges if it was to successfully enter population-level public health on a mass and profitable scale.

(Re)Igniting Sexual Biopolitics: Vaccine Stories Compel and Suppress Sexual Stories

When the French philosopher Michel Foucault (1980) wrote about the operation of power in modern societies, he described power less as the power to kill than as a power to manage. Sexuality in modern societies, he asserted, was characterized less by simple repression of sexuality than by a proliferation of discourses and practices relating to sexuality, health, and the body aimed at managing populations in the service of multiple social goals. Working from this assertion, the places in and conditions under which the appearance of sexuality emerges and then provokes a range of responses are illuminated—from aggressive attempts to banish it from view to the production of a range of possibilities for its circulation. With HPV as a causal agent implicated in various diseases, sexual matters and health concerns become intertwined, as does their management. Controlling lifestyles, behaviors, and beliefs surrounding sex and the body are part of the biomedical gaze. As adolescents' and gendered girls' bodies come into focus in a new regime of cancer prevention, their age, sexual desires, behaviors, and lives, as well as their imagined sexual futures, are brought into discursive production, along with notions of their risk, identities, and actions, and how to manage them.

The historical case of biopower—the transformation of power from exerting influence over death to exerting influence over life—included some of the first instances of "mass" public health (or public hygiene) and surveillance centered on sexuality and reproduction that were increasingly part of the law, sciences, and various other organizational or juridical systems of state and non-state governance. Biopolitical projects (and biopower) refer to the ways knowledge and practices by which life is administered or governed, including its forms of subject-making. Biopolitics had a dual function according to Foucault (1980): to continue providing for the public's health in terms of promoting healthy habitats (e.g., food, water, sewage), and to shift health-promoting activities (and their costs) from the state to individuals.

Vaccines are biopolitical projects that administer life and death and discipline individuals through the exertion of power, managing populations through state and non-state practices—what Foucault calls governmentality. Vaccination programs have long been state projects, largely developed in consultation with, or in entirety by, public-sector institutes. Given that the diseases targeted for vaccination were mostly those that killed or seriously injured children (e.g., smallpox, cholera, tuberculosis, polio, etc.), development of vaccines and the strategies for their adoption held great interest for publics in wealthy localities and poor ones alike. The mid-1950s polio vaccine, said to be designed "for the people," exemplified a strategy of collective, public effort to research, test, fund, manufacture, and then implement vaccination on a mass scale to eagerly awaiting publics that hoped to be part of an end to the well-known and pervasively feared disease that threatened their children. Credibility and support were found early, evidenced by the nearly two million elementary school children enrolled as "polio pioneers" in 1954 even though only half of the children would receive the vaccine, while the other half received a placebo. By 1955 the Salk vaccine had been shown to be safe and effective, and large-scale distribution began (see Reverby 2020) with a dominant thread of welcome news.[18]

The triumph of vaccination was presented as a result of good science and public investment. These were heady times with high hopes for vaccines to improve the life and health of populations. The triumphant narrative was disseminated through public service awareness campaigns, innovative uses of the mass media, and celebrity tie-ins, as well as the work of advocacy organizations and their (fundraising) campaigns, such as the March of Dimes.[19] While vaccine controversy is not new, this good news narrative—with its implicit trust in vaccines—had been dominant for much of the twentieth century. It helped fuel a cancer-cure hope: vaccines offered a means to control and contain human-to-human spread of now identifiable external pathogens, stopping them in their tracks and saving lives. Vaccines were providing a cure for otherwise devastating, intractable diseases (including smallpox, diphtheria, polio, tuberculosis, mumps, rubella, and whooping cough); a cancer-cure possibility was afoot.[20] In 1961 the American Medical Association reported a "fresh approach to the cancer problem"; a 1962 *Life* magazine cover announced to the public "New Evidence That Cancer May Be Infectious," but assured that a "dream of developing a cancer vaccine" could soon come true (Rosenfeld 1962). The US National Cancer Institute had launched a viral research program into cancer, with some incremental but little major success (Scheffler 2019).[21] When a "War on Cancer" was politicized by President Richard Nixon in his 1971 State of the Union address, the cultural and economic investment in prevention was already underway.[22]

Vaccine development would increasingly be privatized (at least following early basic research, which continued to be publicly funded). Immunological, virological, and manufacturing expertise, for example, were part of the "intellectual property" of corporations such as pharmaceutical companies with large investments in R&D, but with commensurately large investments in public relations, promotion, and advertising. Pharmaceutical companies were becoming the new public health, peppering their work of informing publics with product offering tie-ins, and holding themselves accountable more to shareholders than to public stakeholders. As for-profit corporations, they would hope to recoup those investments. They would engage in efforts to "pharmaceuticalize" health prevention, with support from many social entities (including publics) who welcomed the approach as a way to address a variety of problems, challenges, and opportunities. For some, however, the efforts exemplified prioritization of private over public interests, an overreach that eroded trust in medicine as well as vaccines (Abraham 2010; Williams, Martin, and Gabe 2011; Biehl 2006; Bell and Figert 2012).

Over the next few decades, the role of the public sphere would also become a bone of contention, with questions arising over the place and cost of state intervention in what some refer to as private matters, such as parental decision-making or individual choice. As vaccine targets began to shift to include more "mild" and "moderate" diseases (e.g., measles), so too did more and more state mandates to "get the shots" (e.g., public requirements to attend school).[23] Vaccine mandates that applied to children date back to the nineteenth century, when smallpox vaccines were required for school attendance; such requirements were expanded in 1948, when a combined vaccine against tetanus, diphtheria, and pertussis (known as TDaP) became available and was added to the recommended schedule (DeSilver 2021).[24] Control over decision making—whether by parents, doctors, or governments—joined issues of safety and effectiveness as factors in vaccine acceptance, hesitancy, or rejection. At the same time, publics were organizing with demands that science and medicine roll back their paternalism, as well as objections to overt racist, sexist, and homophobic discrimination.

When a vaccine was developed in the 1970s against the hepatitis B virus (HBV)—which is transmitted by blood, during birth, and through sex—as vaccine programs were imagined and developed, controversy ignited over whether such an approach was needed for a disease that affected only some people. The already stigmatized identities and practices—sex workers who work as "prostitutes," "homosexual" or gay men who engage in sex with same-sex and/or multiple partners, and drug users or "junkies" who share needles—each had yet to shed stigmata associated with their lives. 1970s organizations already mobilized around care for sexually transmitted disease provided advocacy, organizing, and the research subjects, in this case gay men, needed for HBV vaccine research, rollout, and the gradual acceptance of this first "cancer prevention vaccine." It would take twenty years for the HBV vaccine to tame its own biopolitics and enter the recommended and accepted childhood vaccines program, which it did in 1984 when it became part of the newborn vaccination protocol.[25]

Merck would need to ensure a smooth path to vaccine acceptance if its new vaccine was to reach the anticipated blockbuster status and commensurate high profitability. It would traverse, and hopefully overcome, several social and cultural challenges in its trajectory from introduction to large-scale adoption. First, certain cancer(s) would need to be reframed from diseases with seemingly random and unknown causes to diseases that were preventable; and cervical cancer, specifically, would first need to be publicly understood as a cancer of major concern for women and people with a cervix in the US and other high-resource countries (despite the overwhelming evidence that this cancer's deadly impact is felt predominantly in low-resource countries and regions, and is exacerbated by policies that limit health care's capacity to prevent and treat it [a topic taken up later in the book]). Second, HPV vaccination would have to sidestep the causal role of anything to do with sex—in this case, sexual transmission and association with an STI. Effacing the role of sex and the causal attribution of a virus that is sexually transmitted would also enable the suppression of other previous associations of disease with sex and the symbolic significance of those associations. Merck wanted to ensure that the cultural politics of HIV—and its associations with stigmatized identities, sexual promiscuity, and safe sex, to name a few—did not adhere in any way to broader vaccination discourse. Given HPV's causal role in not just cancers, but also genital warts, Merck hoped to sidestep any association with an STD. Third, Merck would also need to clearly situate this new preventive tool alongside the well-known and -established women's cancer prevention tool, the Pap test, and its place in the prevailing gendered health care model of "women's (preventive) health." For half a century, women had been told the Pap test was *the* sole essential part of reproductive and sexual health care, and the means to ensure a cancer-free future.

The Pap test—and the apparatus of cervical cancer prevention in general—was born in the history of gynecology and reproductive medicine, and was shaped by its ghostly matters: a history of abuse of Black women and their bodies in the name of science (Murphy 2012, Roberts 1997, Washington 2008). Throughout the twentieth century, it was middle-class white women's bodies that were made the subjects in need of various protections. The Pap test, and its associated pelvic exam for the white women in need of protection, had been opposed early on the grounds not of these atrocities, but for its potential disruption of women's chastity and a fantasy of arousing sexual passion. Opposition to Gardasil, vocal in the context of legislative attempts to require vaccination to attend public school, found some resonance as calls to protect girls' virginity and ensure a "morally responsible" sexuality emerged. These recalled older messages of white women's vulnerability and enrollment in health prevention and "wellness" efforts (Prescott 2010, Reagan 1997, Wailoo 2011). In the twenty-first century, the associated knowledge that abnormal cellular changes (what the Pap test rendered visible) were responsible for cancer precipitated a racist and classist specter of women's "aberrant behaviors" linked to genital cancers (Braun and Phoun 2010, Wailoo 2011), and genital cancers linked to poverty (Wailoo 2011). With the need to continuously monitor cellular changes, a new type of technical entity—the "precancerous" cell—merged two preventive medicine subjects: the figure of women *not yet ill* but *in need* of protection, and an already established figure of *at-risk* women.

In contrast, promotional media for Gardasil asserted that a three-shot vaccine now ensured the possibility of a cancer-free future for girls. To achieve this, adolescent girls would need to be configured as a risk market for this new vaccine. Teen girls occupied a liminal space—too old for the usual vaccines for newborns and early childhood, and too young for the medical surveillance and disease monitoring permitted for adults. There were relatively few adolescent vaccines (a combined booster for measles, mumps, and rubella; and an elective annual influenza vaccine), although the list was growing. The HPV vaccine was also different in that it addressed a sexually transmitted agent, as HPV was neither highly contagious nor deadly for children, and for the most part there was little in the way of sexual health education or provision. In contrast to childhood diseases with vaccination approvals, the HPV vaccine entered disease awareness in relation to an important (though not widespread, at least in the US and other high-resource countries) form of cancer—its actual target was a little-known virus, and a sexually transmitted one: little-known to publics, that is, but well-known medically. Importantly, this virus was transmitted sexually—rather than through airborne transmission of disease material— conjuring questions of how to address or suppress concerns around sex, sexuality, and the body. Finally, because HPV's connection to the onset of cervical cancer later in life is *uncertain*, its presence as a necessary but insufficient cause of the onset of disease was a hurdle in Merck's communication and marketing strategy for Gardasil.

None of these was a small barrier to overcome; together, they could have proved insurmountable. Merck anticipated that they would have a hard time convincing parents that their daughters were at risk of *possibly* developing a disease, and that if they were to be diagnosed with this cancer later in life it would be the result of a sexually transmitted infection *probably* acquired early in their (presently yet to begin) sexual life. They likely were aware of the debates over sexuality health education in schools and the threat to providing teens with the information and the capacity needed to consent to health care—from condoms to contraception. Just how would a pharmaceutical company tackle these obstacles? What would stand in their way, and what would smooth their product's path to acceptance? How would Merck convince the public of the existence of a sexually transmitted infection, HPV, and its causal role in the development of cancer without inflaming gender politics, wading into school-based health controversy, or creating an outright sex panic? Would Merck promote this new product without simultaneously drawing attention to matters of sexual behavior in general, and to girls' sexuality in particular? These questions are about the governing of life through the management of health, and the containment and regulation of sexuality often in the name of health.

When the HPV-cancer link was broadcast and discussed in public discourse in 2005, a cadre of sociologists, anthropologists, historians, and others in feminist studies, including myself, called out the ways the new informational commercials (later followed by product advertisements launched in 2006) were designed and distributed, with specific appeals to gendered norms or attributes and gendered users (Mamo and Epstein 2014; Mamo, Nelson, and Clark 2010; Wailoo et al. 2010; Casper and Carpenter 2008).[26] As with the language and assumptions that accompanied research for the male contraceptive pill studied by the feminist science studies scholar Nelly Oudshoorn (2003), for example, an alignment of "femininity" with HPV and HPV prevention predated this vaccine's introduction to the public. By 2005, reproductive health, including the annual pelvic exam and Pap test, gynecological health care, and (for adolescents and young adults) contraceptive and sexual health counseling, was already firmly entangled with women's health and its alignment with a construct of "femininity." Many adolescent girls were presumably poised to begin their reproductive health care visits to access contraception and prevent unwanted and early pregnancies. While this entanglement offered Merck an opportunity to secure an established medical market, it also presented them with a need to disassociate from the hauntings by ghosts of past gendered abuses and harms of women's bodies, as well as the ways girls, gender, and sex have often been the objects of contestation and debate.

With a virus that is almost always transmitted sexually, and with vaccination aimed at pre- and early-adolescent girls, the vaccine could reignite cultural politics. In the US, these concerns played out against a backdrop of growing cultural preoccupation with the sexuality of young people, reflected in debates about contraceptives, condom use, and efforts to promote abstinence-based sex education programs in the 1990s (Fields 2008, Irvine 2006).[27] The concerns also played out in the shadow of women's cancers, the HIV/AIDS epidemic, and a broad history linking sex and disease that variously produced stigma, panic, and discrimination. Disease narratives dealing with how risk is shaped, on whose bodies and lives, and what identities emerge have implications for how we understand and care for one another. Marshaling already existing alignments of cervical cancer risk with femininity, motherhood, and reproductive health was a double-edged sword of opportunity and political challenge. How then could Merck prevent the intrusion of sexuality, especially as it might cling to the innocence of preadolescent girls? The marketing and mass-vaccination success of Gardasil hinged on the suppression, management, and "taming" of gendered sexual dynamics around sex, sexual health, and sexual risk.

Producing a New Regime of Cancer Prevention: Advertising as Education

In the United States until the late 1990s, advertising for medical products mainly consisted of appeals to medical providers to make the decisions best for their patients. When Congress passed the Federal Food, Drug, and Cosmetic Act of 1938, they had hoped to ensure that nonprescription medical products were deemed safe for consumer use before marketing them to the public. In 1962, Congress gave the FDA added authority to regulate advertisements of prescription medical products, mainly drugs, as well as nonprescription medications. Advertising was targeted almost exclusively to health care providers, mostly physicians, until the 1980s when regulations began loosening, ultimately resulting in a 1997 deregulation that allowed pharmaceutical advertisements to be pitched directly to consumers (DTC).

Merck had been at the forefront of these changes, publishing the first DTC print ad for a prescription medication in *Reader's Digest* in 1981, and then the first televised ad in 1983.[28] This loosening was especially important for the ways it lifted the requirement to list a product's potential benefits and harms: rather than including the vast amount of information about these benefits and harms in the short time of a television commercial advertisement (which would be virtually impossible), this requirement could now be met by the inclusion of a phone number (later a website) where the consumer would be able to get the facts. While still maintaining a "fair balance" between presenting the risks and the benefits, not every risk had to be vocalized, which created an opening to produce compelling, short-format marketing directly to consumers through all media types.[29] When Merck was readying Gardasil to promote to the public, DTC advertising allowed pharmaceutical companies the leeway to refer consumers to "outside sources" for product information. "Ask your doctor" emerged as a familiar slogan.

Merck hired public relations advertising firms and established partnerships with cancer advocacy organizations, as they planned a trifecta of HPV advertising campaigns beginning with two nonbranded disease informational awareness campaigns, "Make the Connection" and "Tell Someone," to be followed by a vaccine product campaign, "One Less." The product ad was on standby, ready to launch within weeks of FDA approval, designed to encourage their newly educated audience to "get vaccinated." This two-part effort by Merck would, if all went well, fully configure a market of potential girl vaccine users: girls who could (and would) take the *right* actions now to prevent a potentially deadly future (Mamo and Pérez 2021). Working as a single campaign, pre-release information tied with product marketing ads, the message first established the knowledge of a virus-cancer link and the will to spread the word—"Tell Someone"—and then, with the product ad, established an action to take charge of not only their own health but the health of the network, to be "One Less" (Mamo, Nelson, and Clark 2010).

"Pharmaceuticalizing" public health took root as Merck mobilized its significant capital to manufacture and promote a health product, but also to become a key source of information, education, and health promotion, suggesting that viewers not just ask their doctor, but turn to www .merck.com to join a "conversation" with patients, experts, and celebrity appeals. The sequence was quick: information ads in 2005 and then product ads in 2006. The CDCs Advisory Committee on Immunization Practices (ACIP) added Gardasil to the federally funded Vaccines for Children (VFC) program in 2006 and created a new VFC immunization schedule. Recommendations for the VFC program are made by a group of scientific and professional experts who review the evidence, determine safety and efficacy,[30] and propose the appropriate timeline and approach for vaccination programs to be administered to publics. ACIP and VFC guidelines are then adopted by states and professional organizations, and passed on to the pediatricians and public health clinicians who administer the vaccines into the arms and bodies of children and, at times, adults.

Marketing mirrored other pharmaceutical promotion efforts that targeted individual risk in the name of public or population health (Aronowitz 2010). The marketing of pharmaceutical drugs had become similar to that of other consumer goods—such as cosmetics or other over-the-counter health products—despite the need for a prescription.[31] Merck ads differed from prior decades' aggressive saturation advertisements for drugs such as Prilosec for depression, Lipitor to lower cholesterol, or Claritin for allergies.[32] Unlike other consumer goods and these heavily marketed medications, HPV vaccines (at that time) consisted of a three-shot protocol, and were not designed to be taken daily throughout one's life—a regimen that ensures a continuous revenue stream. By the time Gardasil came to market, publics may have been growing weary of pharmaceutical companies' ongoing search for profits and expanding drug development programs, with both the escalating cost of prescription medications and what seemed like growing expectations that they accept an ever-expanding list of drugs. At this time (indeed, since 1992) the CDC, which oversaw vaccine guidelines, was also under some scrutiny for potential conflicts of interest as a result of its foundation arm, the CDC Foundation (CDCF), accepting donations of millions of dollars from pharmaceutical and other corporations. A tension was brewing as many publics formed critiques of predatory prescriptions and "disease mongering" by the pharmaceutical industry. Americans, it seemed, were growing tired of not only consuming large quantities of drugs with increased frequency, but also the ways they were being made into bodies-at-risk and patients-in-waiting (Dumit 2012, Timmermans and Buchbinder 2010).

PRE-MARKET PRIMING: ESTABLISHING AND SUPPRESSING SEXUAL RISK

In 2005, a year prior to Gardasil's regulatory approval, Merck hired the advertising firm DDB Worldwide and the public relations firm Edelman (founded in 1952 and known for creating ads for established over-the-counter products such as Vaseline) to design and launch a messaging campaign. The conversation began with Merck's nonbranded *awareness* campaigns "Tell Someone" and "Make the Connection" (later rebranded as "Make the Commitment"),[33] launched on September 30, 2005. The goal of this messaging campaign would be to establish a need by launching a conversation among girls and their mothers about "the HPV cancer link," and at the same time to sidestep any potential cultural opposition (Siers-Poisson 2007).

Through tie-ins with patient groups, nonprofits, and robust web-based content that eventually spread into social media platforms such as YouTube and Facebook, Merck positioned its vaccine in a way very different from many of the standard DTC marketed drugs that came before. Merck was building an infrastructure of support to tame the flow of potential controversy surrounding a vaccine that directly implicated girls' sexuality and presumed future sexual risk. To preempt a moral panic and sidestep the ghostly hauntings of prior gender, sex, and disease associations, Merck constructed the vaccine as a "vaccine against a cancer found in women," thereby gendering HPV, HPV vaccines, and HPV-associated cancer. At the same time, they desexualized the vaccine by discursively separating its message from one of sexual risk (Wailoo et al. 2010, Gottlieb 2018). Girls and their sexuality and sexual health have long been produced as problematic entities in need of protection and regulation; Merck created distance from these narratives while simultaneously using them to ensure successful uptake of Gardasil.

The slick campaigns created by PR firms also involved efforts to partner with nonprofit cancer organizations: the Prevent Cancer Foundation, dedicated to cancer prevention and early detection; and the Step-Up Women's Network, whose mission is to connect and advance women and girls. These strategies worked together to establish a pre-market by leveraging shifts in disease advocacy as well as information technology. The multilingual, multimedia campaigns focused on an awareness and knowledge-sharing message about the link between HPV and cancer, specifically the causative role of HPV in cervical cancer. As these non-product-branded educational campaigns rolled out, Merck's nonprofit organizational partners held nationwide events featuring celebrities making and wearing beaded "Make the Connection" bracelets to promote cervical cancer awareness (Siers-Poisson 2007). As Crosswell and Porter (2018) describe, the 2005 information campaigns generated the knowledge and emotions needed to ensure a willing and able consumer market for a soon-to-be-released vaccine, in ways that evaded a political and especially a sexual firestorm. Merck and partners shifted cancer risk from mothers to their daughters, transferring the fear of cancer held by adult women to their pre-sexually active girls. They also transformed the worry and danger of sexually transmitted infections, like chlamydia and even HIV, into an achievable risk-reduction practice before having to talk about sex: accepting and using a new cancer prevention tool.

The first ads, released in 2005, featured newly enlightened young women speaking directly to the camera. The actors visually make eye contact with viewers as they deliver a personal message that begins with emotional surprise, a sense of "shock" to learn that HPV is common: "I was stunned," and "millions?!" they ask, at once declaring what they have recently learned: millions of women have HPV. By means of their eyes and voices an intimacy is forged with the women and girls who make up the audience: "There is something I want to tell you that could save your life," they state. Viewers are brought into the information: a common virus is placing them at risk of cancer. "Cancer caused by a virus . . . I didn't know that" is the message, spoken with perplexed and worried looks.

Adults join the messaging, also speaking directly into cameras to share new facts about the link between a virus, HPV, and a well-known disease, cancer. Visually morphing into their teenage selves, they ask other former young people, now mothers, with their daughters in the room: "What did you talk about with your girlfriends?" With increased seriousness in tone and form, they implore: "The next time you get together—there is something more urgent to talk about." Girls in the ads are shown with arms entwined or holding hands. Their stance evokes girlhood culture as a period of intense girl-talk and frequent communication, as they share their pre-sexual lives and learn, dream, and grow together.

With the new surprise of potential infection and a cancer risk, these "risky girlhoods" (Mamo, Nelson, and Clark 2010) *could* become a new social collective able to evade these risks altogether. Stylistically, the ads and website draw on a peer-to-peer communication mode with a simu-lated girl sharing knowledge: "Human papillomavirus or HPV is a virus you may not know too much about—but you should," one actor says. "So take a look around" (Merck & Co. 2021b). Girls need to know and gather information for themselves and their peers. Mothers, as parents respon-sible for their children's futures, also need to be aware. Mothers and daugh-ters co-participate in cervical cancer prevention. With their promotion of pledges to "Make the Connection/Make the Commitment," these ads echoed the contemporary virginity pledges of abstinence sexual education: adult women were encouraged to make the "right choice" for health by talking with their doctor about their risk of cervical cancer.

THE CAN-DO GIRLS OF GARDASIL: A VACCINE TO PROTECT AGAINST CANCER

In November 2006, Merck launched phase two of this trifecta campaign. The first product advertisement, the "One Less" campaign, was released as a national print, television, and online advertising campaign for the sale and adoption of the vaccine, Gardasil. Gardasil, a vaccine against a can-cer of major public health risk—however distant that risk might be in the future—effectively converted a viral risk into a normalized, accepted can-cer risk for *all* preadolescent and adolescent girls. The narrative production positioned the vaccine as a technological solution to cancer risk: Gardasil as a new tool in the war against (women's) cancer. In emphasizing cancer control, the vaccine product governed not just the prevention of cancer, but also the possibilities for the meaning and practices around sexuality more generally. This sexual health education was not a type that would al-low young people to learn and flourish as sexually agentic people and com-munities and to reduce sites of potential stigma or shame; nor would it help them to become aware of how sexual behaviors and bodily fluids partici-pate in modes of transmission, or how viruses and viral pathways operate. And it certainly did not act as a message to learn about and take charge of one's sexuality and body. Instead Gardasil diminished references to sex and sexuality, averted direct conversation about STIs, and avoided any specter of sexual risk. Or so it seemed.

"One Less" product ads framed vaccination exclusively as a tool to *pro-tect* girls from a future cancer risk. Inviting girls into a social movement for this goal, the television version of the campaign depicts ethnically diverse girls in action—bike riding, doing double-Dutch jump rope, skateboard-ing, horseback riding, flamenco dancing—speaking directly to the camera. In one commercial, the opening scene is a girl skateboarding and doodling "one less" on her sneaker as she shares some "facts" about cervical cancer. The commercial quickly cuts to two girls playing basketball, then switches to a girl engaging the viewer, and then to a skilled drummer speaking to the viewers: "now there is Gardasil, the only vaccine that may help protect you from the four types of human papillomavirus that may cause 70 percent of cervical cancer." A white-appearing adult woman (presumably a mother) appears to disclose the side effects of Gardasil. As she speaks, we see an image of a white girl, her fictional daughter, juggling a soccer ball. Then we see a Black girl speaking directly to the camera: "Become one less," she says, her words intercut with images of a group of four Black girls dancing. These girls are winners. They not only *can* do it all, they *are* doing it all: designing clothes, winning races, and crafting health education messages. Akin to earlier advertisement for tampons, these young people possess a distinct "girl power," one accessed through biomedical interventions into their risky bodies.

Another ad shows girls confidently holding "one less" signs above their heads with contextual markers for urban (a New York City subway sign) and more rural (a Route 1 road sign) locales as girls join together across regional differences to shout "I want to be one less." The voices chant in harmony. Young girls, appearing as mostly Black, play double-Dutch jump rope as they sing "I want to be one less, one less"; presumably Latinx girls dance the flamenco and declare "una menos"; and white-presenting girls ride skateboards and declare "one less." Across regional and racial ethnic difference, girls are drawn into a larger collective made up of active, en-gaged, and strong girls with healthy risk-free bodies—for now and into the future. Creative entrepreneurial girls—girls from various racial back-grounds, social classes, and regions, with individuated personalities, design clothes, win races, ride horses, dance, and assert their voices. The One Less slogan declares "the girl" as already able to exercise her will and make the "right choice." The commercials imitate the rapid visual cuts characteristic of the "MTV aesthetic," an editing style effective at capturing the attention of young viewers (Messaris 1997, 88). Images of sports and music conjure girlhood empowerment. Shown within "play" contexts (e.g., basketball and jumping rope), social peer groups depict deep girlhood friendship.

The "can do" girls unknowingly stepped into a familiar trope and subject-making: the American ideal of gender and family, with its associated responsibility of mothers to safeguard the future health of their children and country. Cultural expectations and a gendered script linger as normative ideals of responsibility for health cling to girls, invoking earlier generations of the "little mothers' leagues" designed to train young girls in the early twentieth-century promotion of the "science" of infant care and motherhood. In what ways are the Gardasil girls akin to the recipients of scientific health advice, primed to take on the role of future mothers and messengers of American ideals of heteronormative families and parenting roles?[34]

The ads take on the new generation's communication modes and speak to a new century of public health with distinctly different gendered norms. Some girls, especially those Americans raised by the empowered (mostly white) women of movements for sexual liberation and feminist health or the activist (mostly Black and Chicana) movements for racial and social justice, were no longer vulnerable and passive; they were framed instead as ready to take action. The girls of Gardasil, with their confidence and collective social spirit, act in ways that would make any mother proud, and their feminist mother even prouder. The advertisements emphasized the girls' power to make decisions using ALL CAPs reminiscent of more recent health social movements—specifically, the ACT UP aesthetics of 1980s and 1990s HIV/AIDS activism. Merck, it seemed, had co-opted these late-twentieth-century cultural messages of powerful resistance, girl power and strength, and empowered health collectives for a new generation of public health messaging.

Gardasil emerged as a gendered technology produced through already established cultural scripts in sciences and infrastructures of women's health and related concerns around sexuality and education. Merck extended the already gendered responsibility of girls for health and the already established health care markets of pediatrics, in a move to connect with and separate from women's reproductive (and sexual) health care. As a result, the HPV vaccine could easily conjure the ghosts of the past: haunted by the racist and classist sexual stereotypes embedded in the histories of these markets that blamed everything, from rates of disease to infant mortality to the very fabric of the family, on anyone not reflecting a white supremacist image of the doting middle-class heterosexual mother educating her daughters for the health of the future. To divert attention from past symbolic associations between sex and disease, in much of this imagery preteen girls were transformed from passive mothers-to-be who lacked a strong voice (one that could say "no" to sex, heterosexuality, or family) into girls able and willing to say "yes" to vaccination and a technological fix. Dodging the lack of agency that signals girls' weak feminine positions in gendered and sexist contexts (Tolman, Striepe, and Harmon 2003; Holland et al. 1994), these scripts of girlhood no longer include narratives of girls as "objects" of boys' "raging hormones" or men's predation—and thus no longer sexually at risk and in need of that kind of protection or agentic action. They therefore escaped the fear and danger of sexuality in favor of a fear and danger of cancer. Gardasil would be the new health protection for this generation of preteen girls, and it would achieve this status by relying on and simultaneously ignoring or discounting previous sexual risk messaging: sexuality is not an attribute of a "strong girl" persona, then, and neither is sexual risk. There is a contradiction.

While a Merck brochure from 2007 informs that "of the approximately 6 million new cases of genital HPV in the United States every year, it is estimated that 74 percent of them occur in 15–24-year-olds," and ads specify that HPV is contracted within two to three years of what is variously referred to as sexual onset or "debut," honest conversations about sex and sexuality are not part of these campaigns. Instead, the mantra is more like this quote found in a Merck 2006 marketing pamphlet: "Cervical cancer is caused by a virus many people get in their teens and 20s." The ideal users and targets of vaccination are girls prior to sexual agency and as categorically different from older cohorts, and different from the messiness of teens' (specifically girls') sexuality. Instead, the visual imagery draws the viewers into feminine embodiments produced and lived in ways that may be risky but are able to ward off that risk. They are not sexual, but empowered to counter worry with action.

Aligning girls with their mothers was a key component of marketing. Mothers in these ads appear as knowledgeable caregivers, weighing the risks and benefits of vaccination. They are invited to participate in this women's health campaign by feminist activist slogans as mothers and daughters become co-participants in activating their self-behaviors and identities to align with the expectation of the given biomedical intervention—what the sociologist Nikolas Rose (2001) refers to as a "will to health."[35] These moms, likely presumed to be in their late thirties and forties at the time of the early campaigns, came of age with contraceptive and abortion politics, an AIDS crisis, and controversies around sex education. These moms are presumably prepared to bring their daughters to medical offices to receive needed contraceptive care before they "get into the back seat of the car with the boy." Importantly, these moms *are* at risk of cervical cancer, a disease that shows up in middle age, as well as health issues from sexually transmitted infections other than HPV. It is these fears that Merck implicitly targeted with its campaigns. These women can only hope that behavioral approaches such as safe sex practices and annual gynecological exams with Pap test technology will protect them, but their daughters have the opportunity to transform their bodies and potential health risk via a vaccine designed to protect them from cancer. When mothers appear, their implicit role as "experienced experts" garners legitimacy.

To stave off skepticism, the "One Less/Una Menos" commercial refutes potential claims of vaccine harm. A mother stands next to her daughter as she lists the potential side effects of Gardasil. The side effects—pro forma for any injection—are pain, swelling, itching, and redness at the injection site; and fever, dizziness and nausea. They are communicated through the protective role of motherhood, not as a warning but as acceptable risk. The moral imperative of risk reduction and a "will to health" implies that mothers would only expose their daughters to risks of side effects if they believed it was in their daughters' best interests. This not only produces adolescent girls as in need of mother's protection; it simultaneously produces appropriate mothering practices and identities as "good" moms protecting their children.

While ads were distributed strategically across demographics with placement in targeted magazines and across TV networks (*Ebony* with largely Black circulation and *Glamour* with largely white), a "color-blind" use of mother-blame serves as a metaphor for a range of social and political fears, erasing race and class differences regarding the social and cultural capital necessary to cultivate the knowledge and skills to acquire valued health care for one's child (Blum 2007, Lareau 2003). In the ad that appeared in *Ebony*, for example, the power to prevent cervical cancer depends on a responsible mother offering her daughter's arm, and otherwise healthy body (Merck & Co. 2007). The mother is assigned responsibility for her daughter's risk—and valorized for potentially preventing cancer. The daughter or girl in this discourse is disembodied—portrayed as a selfless object, a part of the process of preventing cervical cancer for society.

This overt mother-blame conjured 1990s ideas of "deviant" and risky youth that haunt the reputation of other STIs, often racialized with controlling images (stereotypes—Collins 2004). With Black, Latina, and white girls interspersed throughout the advertisements in a multicultural marketing technique reminiscent of 1990s Benetton ads, demarcations nonetheless separate. Viewers might take on a "color-blind racism" of risk, the prior associations of which construct so-called at-risk teens of past generations. At-risk gendered constructs of the 1990s adhered to deviance— mostly marked on poor or Black or immigrant youth—as somehow being at risk of pregnancy and STIs, presumably due to their sexual promiscuity. This contrasts with the innocent girls—mostly white—at risk of sexual predation by others. Responsible girls emerge relationally through their

juxtaposition with irresponsible others, deviant girls and potentially predatory boys, some queer.[36] The "deviant girls" and boys that relationally
place them at risk for pregnancy, STIs, and HIV lie outside the frame of the
twenty-first-century marketing campaigns, yet they are specters of sexual
risk and harm. In their place, the lead characters are empowered individual
girls brought into a gendered collective with a "will to health." Health, not
cancer, is attainable by offering up your daughter's arm, finding out more
about Gardasil, or rolling up one's sleeve and taking one's turn in protecting
a social body (our nation) from the silent killer.[37]

The entanglement of cancer prevention with sexual risk is always nearby,
despite attempts to banish sex and sexuality from view. With a vaccine solution, Merck advised girls and women in a 2006 marketing pamphlet that
"HPV is easily transmitted, so any exposure puts you at risk. It's estimated
that many people get HPV *within their first two to three years of becoming
sexually active*" (emphasis mine). Girls are warned of the risk of sexual onset and drawn into a politics of fear of sex and the risk such an act poses
not only for contracting HPV, but also potentially for causing cancer. This
implicit fear can be used to activate better sexual judgment, bringing girls
and their parents into conversations not only about reducing cancer, but
also about reducing sexual risk—and at the same time, Gardasil becomes
the right tool for cancer prevention. A narrative of risk and prevention
emerges in which sex and sexuality are present, always entangled, yet sidestepped. It is not girls' sexual agency and capacity to navigate sexual risk,
but girls' empowerment as active consumers, that is activated by Gardasil.
By extension, it is mothers' fear of the danger of cancer and their now vital
role in their daughters' health, the health of children and the nation, that
is activated. Mothers, daughters, and a collective social movement of girls
are mobilized to optimize health and manage cancer risk (Mamo, Nelson,
and Clark 2010).

Governing Preteen Sexuality

Advertisements are sites of a narrative framing of the leading character
identities and bodies deemed to be at risk and made into social actors of
concern. What's at stake when girls—especially sexually free girls—are
made into the lead protagonist? What's at stake when pharmaceutical
companies and motherhood are produced as central information providers as well as decision makers in health? Beginning with the Gardasil
clinical trials, a novel shift toward the governing of girls' sexual risk and
health was developing. US trials ran in the first years of a new century,

from 2001 to 2009. Merck prepared to configure its market for the (soon-to-be) new vaccine product following the 1990s, a decade punctuated by sexual panics and discrimination that took shape around another virus and its declarations of epidemic—HIV/AIDS—and the related debates around abstinence-only sex education and condom distribution. This was a decade of activism fighting discrimination against gay and bisexual men deemed "at risk" for HIV. It was also a time when sex had proliferated in popular and public culture, with extramarital fellatio in the White House followed by presidential impeachment.

Merck introduced their vaccine to a public primed to associate sexual risk with a degree of controversy if not fear, as well as a willingness among some to put sex into discourse and demand sexual liberation as others tried to remove sex from discussion. At the outset, the anticipated vaccine provoked contention over whether it would encourage sex and, specifically, promiscuity on the part of girls (Stein 2005); Merck hoped to preempt any concerns over whether a vaccine against a sexually transmitted infection would ignite sexual controversy over girls' presumed sexual lives. Over the course of the vaccine rollout, sexual dynamics would ebb and flow. Age and gender and sex were entangled in quiet reference to "age of sexual onset," a phrase baked into medical design and the vaccine's claims of when to get the shot. Daughters, in turn, were compelled to inform themselves of their own cancer risk and become health care consumers willing and able to engage in self-reliant practices of risk reduction (Fenton 2019). Merck's partnerships with cancer advocacy organizations would hopefully assist them in framing their coming product as a "cancer prevention" tool, rendering invisible both sex and HPV's causal role in the development of an STI.

While Merck's campaign was effective in molding the discourse to emphasize cancer prevention, any hope of fully desexualizing their vaccine vanished as the vaccine entered school mandate policy. As Merck lobbied state legislators to adopt mandatory vaccination policies in 2006 and 2007, their efforts were met with fierce opposition infused with ideas that any established protections against the so-called dangers of sex for girls would be effaced (Mello, Abiola, and Colgrove 2012). The majority of legislative efforts occurred soon after FDA approval of the HPV vaccine in 2006 (Keim-Malpass et al. 2017). That year, a *Wall Street Journal* Online/Harris Interactive health care poll reported that based on survey respondents, an estimated 70 percent of Americans supported the use of the HPV vaccine, and 44 percent likely believed that abstinence education programs targeting teens were a better way of preventing HPV (Bright 2006). (A case of "HPV vax is great—just not for my kid!") Health advocates focused on cancer prevention found themselves at odds with social conservatives

who favored abstinence-only education and interpreted HPV immunization as the encouragement of adolescent (and even preadolescent) sexual
activity. Parent groups mobilized in opposition to school mandates on the
basis of presumed governmental overreach into their parental rights and
their daughters' bodies and lives, arguing that the vaccines could prompt
youth to have sex at a younger age.

While some opposition to vaccines on religious and moral grounds has
emerged, and despite an increase in anti-vax tendencies in the wake of false
claims about autism, pediatricians and public health policies have mostly
been successful in asking parents to adhere to what is a relatively complex
set of vaccine schedules aimed at infants and young children.[38] Given this
period of development and the sexual issues the vaccination effort is already charged with, opposition manifested easily and rapidly. Unlike other
anti-vaccination positions that rest on (usually spurious) health and safety
claims (or outright conspiracy theories), these positions were based on
the imagined risk of excessive and early sexual activity. The *possibility* of
girls' sexual agency and sexual risk was suddenly propelled into the public
consciousness. Parents were asked not only to imagine their girls as sexually active, but to replace the responsibility of behavioral prevention with
a responsibility for medical intervention. This time, the power of decision-
making was not only entangled with federal guidelines issued by the CDC,
and the state-level policy debates regarding vaccine requirements to enter
school; it was also caught up in projections of an adolescent's—specifically
a teen girl's—sexual future.

Given that HPV vaccination is a vaccine against a sexually transmitted
virus, state mandates hoped for by Merck and others quickly became highly
contentious. Once the CDC recommends a vaccination, it often moves to
state policy discussions. In this case, twenty-two state legislatures saw pro-
posals for school requirements, but rejected these mandates for HPV vaccination in the face of opposition. Eleven states required the provision of
HPV vaccine information but did not require the vaccine to attend school.
And the District of Columbia and Virginia (soon followed by Hawaii and
Rhode Island) passed mandatory vaccine laws for school attendance, with
opt-out clauses for medical and religious reasons (Wailoo et al. 2010).[39] The
controversy came from parents, but also from organizational and state actors largely aligned with socially conservative positions.[40] Merck and many
public health officials were dismayed by the controversy, and by the patch-
work of conflicting and confusing policies left in its wake. Public health
historians like Colgrove, Abiolo, and Mello (2010) argue that these efforts
were contentious because of the situational context of adolescent sexuality
and struggles over abstinence-only education as well as the evolving dis-

comfort with pharmaceutical company involvement in mandate policies. The presumption is that had Gardasil left public policy to public actors and not pharmaceutical companies and doctors, perhaps the dynamics that unfolded would have been quieter or more quickly tamed.

Merck's price point for Gardasil's three-shot approach was about $360 for completion—a prohibitive cost for the uninsured and underinsured in the US. This raised questions of cost and need for insurance coverage, as well as of governmental overreach. Given rising health care costs and the vaccine's price, Merck lobbied for federal Medicaid as well as private insurance coverage for the costs as preventive care. Yet, echoing previous controversy around contraceptive coverage, and the ways some companies and other entities have successfully lobbied for religious and/or personal exemptions, these efforts met with opposition. While Gardasil differed from traditional school-mandated vaccines that inoculated children against highly contagious, even if non-deadly, diseases of childhood such as measles, this opposition was mostly on grounds of parental (versus local or federal), decision-making power. Gardasil provoked strong emotions from parents and state actors; but significantly, opposition also came from conservative and religious organizations expressing concerns on the grounds of discomfort with girls' sexuality (Mara 2010).

As state legislatures and non-state actors alike became part of the vaccine controversy, cultural anxieties arose around adolescent sex and sexuality and to what degree decisions about teens should be in the hands of states, professions, and/or parents. A struggle over girls' autonomy and decision-making, and importantly their capacity to direct their sexual care as well as their sexual lives, was obscured. When then Governor Rick Perry of Texas, a conservative Republican, issued an executive order in 2007 hoping to mandate Gardasil for sixth-grade girls to attend school, his order included a provision to provide free vaccination to uninsured and underinsured girls aged nine to eighteen. Unexpectedly, the policy plan ignited a firestorm from publics as well as from both sides of the two-party political system. The *Los Angeles Times* reported the "Uproar over HPV Vaccine Order" (Hart 2007), while the *Tribune Business News* took a more balanced approach, reporting "Reactions Mixed to Perry's HPV Vaccine Mandate" (Berghom 2007). Yet the news was clear: critics feared the mandate would make every girl in Texas get a shot to prevent a sexually transmitted disease—something that was distinctly unlike the requirements for children to wear helmets to prevent injuries, which parents largely did not oppose, nor believe would increase risk-taking among their children. It was something about the associations with sex and sexuality that drove skepticism. Even though the mandate was proposed by a conservative political party with deep roots in the Christian Evangelical movement, and by a politician who supported abstinence and abstinence-based education, associations with promiscuity and a presumed license to trigger girls' sexual onset began to take hold. The ensuing media frenzy was sweeping, covering issues of sexual activity in teens as well as parental rights, campaign contributions from Big Pharma, and (to a lesser degree) the vaccine's potential adverse impacts on the bodies of girls and women (Mara 2010). Trying to settle debate, the *New York Times* published an editorial endorsing a national school-based vaccine mandate in February 2007 ("A Necessary Vaccine" 2007).

Just as swiftly as sexual politics entered, so too did concerns over undue pharmaceutical company and financial influence. As Perry prepared to issue the executive order mandating the vaccine for all girls in the recommended age group, it was revealed that his former chief of staff, Mike Toomey, was working for Merck. Merck's political action committee had been a major donor to Perry's campaigns for governor and later for president, as well as to the Republican Governors Association, leaving publics to wonder whether Perry was doing Merck's bidding. Texas's large evangelical and abstinence communities reacted with anger to Perry's order, fueling a backlash to vaccine mandates from the right. When the executive order was overturned in May 2007, Perry appeared at a press conference surrounded by women who had been diagnosed with cervical cancer. He admonished that "future deaths of Texas women and teens who succumbed to cervical cancer would be on the heads of the legislators who'd voted against" him. Michele Bachmann, a conservative politician known to be anti-vax and anti-science, accused Perry and his campaign of corruption during her own run against Perry in the Republican presidential primaries. Bachmann claimed that Perry was putting "little girls" at risk by forcing them to get "an injection of what could potentially be a dangerous drug" (West 2011, Gabriel and Grady 2011). Appealing to his conservative contingency, Perry responded with an anti-choice and anti-feminist message. His executive order, he said, was driven by his devotion to life: "Texas, I think, day in and day out, is a place that protects life" (Goodwyn 2011). Again, while the mandate decision was overturned in May 2007 in response to opposition, the political and legal battles around Gardasil continued, marked explicitly by new and old sexual contours. At the same time, other populations of girls were treated differently. These state debates did not stop the CDC Advisory Committee on Immigration Practices from deciding in 2008 to require vaccination for permanent resident applicants, not acknowledging that this requirement was already a de facto policy given the form (form I-693) required to report medical examination and vaccination records in alignment with the US guidelines. For a brief time starting in August 2008, the immigration policy included HPV vaccination in its "special vaccine consideration section (section E)" of the vaccine requirement policy for immigrants. The requirement specified that all new "female applicants ages 11 years through 26 years" must receive an HPV vaccination to receive green cards (US Citizenship and Immigration Services 2021, Jordan 2008). The policy, considered a "mistake" with "unintended consequences" by some legal scholars (Kimbol 2008) and a discriminatory policy by others (Canales 2009, Navin 2015), was reversed in December 2009.

As of 2018, Virginia and Washington, DC remain the only state-level entities to require vaccination for school attendance for girls; Rhode Island requires HPV vaccination for girls and boys (National Conference of State Legislatures 2018). These policy initiatives "capture" some girls through what was viewed as pharmaceutically pressured, if not designed, public mandates in Washington DC and Virginia, and produce a consumption imperative for others. As recently as 2020, a familiar sex panic emerged in the state of New York when legislation (S2985) was introduced (for at least the sixth time) which mandated that schoolchildren be vaccinated with Gardasil.[41] Opposition largely came from parent groups who stormed the New York State Assembly, arguing that a mandate would usurp their parental rights while exposing girls and boys to a questionable vaccine that they do not, and may not, need. The unspoken presumption was that their kids are not sexual, and that when they are their sexuality will somehow be contained, if not in marriage then in relations of respectability somehow free from STIs. The anti-vaccination movement added fuel to parental concerns with a false narrative of unacceptable health risk.[42] These combined with growing concern over corporate overreach shaped opposition to the vaccine. Reporting for the *New York Times* in 2008, Elizabeth Rosenthal described a "Drug Maker's Push" from Merck whereby doctors were recruited and paid as spokespersons, with payment of about $4,500 for promotional talks, allowing some doctors to make hundreds of thousands of dollars. Aggressive political lobbying by the pharmaceutical company and payments to health advocate groups made many weary of the outsized role of what had come to be characterized as "Big Pharma" even among those who were otherwise supportive of the vaccine (Rosenthal 2008).

Arguments against the HPV vaccine were often arguments against girls' sexuality: that vaccination would *promote* sexual activity or make already deviant girls (more) sexually active. These were something to be opposed and/or something to be regulated. Such claims, based on the assumption that the protection conferred would unleash behavioral change, have been an ongoing target of evidence-based damage control via truth-saying to combat myths and false claims. In scientific review articles of more than forty epidemiological studies conducted from 2006 to 2016 on sexual onset and activity post-HPV vaccination, researchers have continuously asserted that no evidence of higher STI rates or riskier sexual behaviors among vaccinated girls exists (Kasting et al. 2016, Madhivanan et al. 2016). In fact, those vaccinated reported lower rates of condom-less vaginal sex and non-use of contraception, and had fewer STIs overall, compared to unvaccinated girls.[43] This suggests an opportunity for HPV vaccination to couple with scientific and medical literacy as well as sexuality education. Researchers pointed to the false rhetorical claims of potential increases in girls' sexual activity as contributing to initial low uptake of the vaccine. It is the persistent stigmatization and discrimination against certain populations, and all things sexual, that are the real risks for people's lives. Proponents of HPV vaccination, accordingly, are quick to blame low vaccine uptake on pharmaceutical and policy failure to tame sexual messaging in favor of cancer prevention claims. Many told me that they too were surprised at just how many parents were not ready to think about sex and their adolescent. Yet it is neither progressives nor conservatives that are to blame, but an unwillingness to find ways to ensure that sexuality is neither erased, nor stigmatized, nor lifted up as some behavior or quality that makes someone at risk.

For many scientists and health care providers, the question of how to address sex and sexuality remains unsettled. Many argue that these topics should be muted in vaccine promotion. This modulation, they surmise, would at best reduce parents' and providers' (e.g., pediatricians') "discomfort" with discussing the sexual practices and desires of adolescents, and at worst desexualize girls altogether while maintaining some form of a disease-free future. Not just Merck, but many health care actors, promote an approach to vaccination that is what Porter and colleagues (Porter et al. 2018) describe as "cervical cancer-salient messaging," designed to emphasize the threat of cervical cancer. Shaping the risk of disease and the threat of cancer, many argue, is the right approach for vaccine uptake.

Parents rather than immature minors (to contrast with the "mature minors" designation used for youth deemed able to make decisions for themselves to ensure their privacy and safety), opponents argued, should be the agents of medical, health, and sexuality knowledge and decision making. Such opposition pivoted around parents' rights and health care of minors, not teachers and school health requirements. Indeed, from disease "awareness" campaigns to product advertisements, Merck positioned Gardasil as an intervention for cervical cancer rather than protection from the consequences of sexuality. In subsequent policy debates and other public controversy over HPV vaccination—which lessened over time and in degree, yet would stretch on for the better part of a decade—girls and their bodies were the object of debate, particularly regarding their need for sexual regulation. As the furor receded, it seemed that risky sex and risky sexual behaviors could be subsumed in favor of governing the innocent, not yet "at risk" bodies of preadolescent girls. Controlling girls and their bodies, it seemed, aligned with many cultural expectations and institutional arrangements already in place.

The 2008 "I Chose" product ads continued to emphasize a will to health, with girls able to choose for themselves a life of cancer risk or a life free from such fears. Left off the menu of good choices available to them were choices to navigate sexual lives safely, understanding how viruses work, which viruses transmit sexually, and any information about which behaviors and protection approaches might work to reduce immediate and distal risk, as well as the uncertainties of potential harm. It was not a comprehensive look at sexuality and its role in the social lives of teens and the health lives of people. This may seem an unrealistic expectation, yet as pharmaceutical companies move into a role as the only or the most vocal health educator, examining what is made visible and what remains invisible is central to understanding the stakes in narrative frames. In this case, through a fresh onslaught of advertisements on television and in print media, on social media platforms, and through highly scripted patient group tie-ins, Gardasil was sidestepping issues of girls' pending if not actual sex lives, transmission risks, and messaging to moms that the Pap test was not "good enough" to prevent cancer.

The approach ensured they would not awaken ghosts from stereotypes of the past that linger in the present, nor of recent culture wars in which girls and contraception or boys and condoms were part of resistance to school-based sexual health education. Instead of conjuring these past associations, girls were made into innocent yet agentic collaborative decision makers with parents at their side. Parental consent was a large presence for the girls at a stage decidedly marked as "pre-onset of sexual activity." These girls were already established as in need of protection and safeguarding against risk, and were made available for monitoring, surveillance, and regulations that might come later. At least for now, their bodies are not yet affected by the risks of HPV and other harms that lurk in the shadows of sexuality and adult life.

The specter of twentieth-century promiscuous and hypersexual women, distinctly racialized and gendered but sharing "aberrant behaviors" and stigmatized identities, occupied causal disease narratives for much of the mid-twentieth century. These would be banished from view (Braun and Phoun 2010, Wailoo 2011), replaced with a cadre of innocent girls protected from the dangers of cancer. In this new generation of girls bonded through girl culture, there are no vulnerable adolescents (or predatory men and boys)—there are only empowered health consumers making the good choices necessary to remove their chances of being another person with cancer. By virtue of their age and a social imaginary of good heterosexuality, these girls would be protected from cancer risk and not from the normative and expected riskiness of their sexuality. The narrative drama of a vaccine against *cancer* and a tool in *cancer prevention*—rather than of a *vaccine against a sexually transmitted infection and a tool in STD prevention*—allowed girls to escape the symbolic associations of past infectious disease as well as the ordinariness of risky sex. That risk had yet to befall them as they reached what epidemiologists and other "experts" would refer to as their "sexual onset," a term suggesting one's risk based on a predicted age of first sexual activity and, I argue, an embedded presumption of the beginning of one's heterosexual adulthood.[44]

Such a health risk discourse aligns with biomedicine's economic imperative and pharmaceutical companies' profit goals as they position their products as solutions to a variety of issues, from lifestyle medications to disease prevention to public health needs, and also as quick fixes for a variety of other problems (Bharti and Sismondo 2022). With claims for patient empowerment and collaborative health care, interventions into risk in the name of "health" are ever expanding. HPV vaccination is part of a cancer risk reduction that transforms worried patients-in-waiting (Timmermans and Buchbinder 2010) into engaged consumers taking steps to protect their health—what the sociologist Janet Shim (2001) calls "enterprising actors," subjects called forward with a moral responsibility to reconfigure their risk and enhance their health. Yet such claims are part of the reproduction of inequalities culturally and in our health care system. Sharing a moral obligation to educate themselves and others and to participate in preventive medicine, girls are bound together in what is at once a new collective subjectivity and a familiar enrollment into gender normativity.

The girls of Gardasil hold a collective moral responsibility as keepers of health. While this framing was consistent in other high-resource countries with HPV vaccine campaigns, some countries did not experience the same "moral dilemmas" around girls and sex as the US. Countries in Europe with less puritanical histories around girls' sexuality were able to construct HPV vaccination as a vaccine against a sexually transmitted infection (Stöckl 2010). In the US, gendered cultural expectations endure: on the way to becoming "normal" adult women, girls must become empowered consumers rationally reducing perceived risks associated with tumultuous adolescence and young adulthood. In this production, preadolescent girls become subjects, bodies, and identities in order to mitigate, if not eliminate, this life-threatening disease and the larger public health crisis associated with it. Issues such as age of consent and barriers to health care services including sexual health care because of concerns about parental judgment and subsequent harms to youth fade away with the cultural work of a vaccine against a woman's cancer.[45] Issues of girls' sexual agency, desires, and practices are left aside in favor of calls for enterprising actors to protect against cancer. This renders invisible questions of equity and justice for vaccine availability, sexual rights, and preventive care: first about whose bodies, in what regions of the world, and with what proximity and access to biomedical infrastructures with preventive and cancer care are most at risk of developing and dying from cervical cancer; second, about how this vaccine, with such potential to lessen suffering from a deadly disease, is being made available to the people and in the places that may need it most; and third, about how this virus and its vaccine are linked with other issues of concern for sexual lives and practices as well as sexual rights and freedoms.

The U.S. was primed for corporate and patient-movement tie-ins insisting that women not yet ill—who were already "monitoring their health in the form of risk through their cellularity" (Murphy 2012, 113), for instance by annual Pap testing—pave the way for the enterprising girls of what Elena Conis (2015) calls a modern "Vaccine Nation." Much of the world was primed to rely on narratives of technoscientific innovation and self-driven "participation" that accompanied a logic seemingly accepting of early adoption. The logic was that to garner profit, new technologies must first sell to affluent buyers and systems, before rolling out to the world's less well-resourced people and places. Together, these produced a narrative of a modern HPV vaccine adopted by enterprising consumers to ensure health, while others without access and financial resources could only hope to reduce their risk of death through whatever antiquated medicine might be available (Murphy 2012). Yet, especially in the US, what had once been public health campaigns using public service announcements had devolved into biopolitical projects shaped by multinational corporations or through public-private partnerships.[46] Merck was the lead actor in privatizing and pharmaceuticalizing public health in ways that reflect ongoing discomforts and well-worn expectations of what makes a good gendered and sexual life for girls.

CHAPTER TWO

"What's In It for the Boys?"

An episode of the HBO show *Girls*, aired on April 29, 2012, valiantly tried to tackle the silencing around sex and sexuality in the public-facing information about HPV. The show was written and produced by Lena Dunham,[1] who also played Hannah, the lead character. In this episode, Hannah learns—she says from the results of an STD test panel—that she has contracted HPV. The news clearly unsettles Hannah and propels her angrily into a "who gave this to me" quest for answers about its source, despite her friend Jessa's assurance that she, too, has "several strains" of the virus. "All adventurous women do," Jessa adds cavalierly.

The story renders sex, as well as boys, visible subjects in the risk narrative—and specifically as a source of HPV's sexual transmission. Despite Jessa's reference to HPV as something all adventurous girls have, Hannah is undeterred in her search for a cause. She confronts her current (hetero)sexual partner, Adam. She then suddenly changes course, seemingly realizing she likely "got it" years earlier, and shifts her accusations to her ex-boyfriend, Elijah, whom she hasn't seen nor had sex with in years. When confronted, Elijah presumes the confrontation is around his sexuality as an out gay man, leading to a mix-up of issues. Elijah confronts Hannah's lack of knowledge, telling her that Adam lied about being tested for HPV—there is no test to detect the disease in men, he tells her.

The episode raises the specter of sexual risk for these characters and, by extension, in the thousands of viewers watching the show: Was HPV something to fear and worry about? Were Hannah and her friends too old to have been vaccinated against HPV, and in the limbo between protected girls and at-risk women? And what about the boys—gay and straight alike? Dunham sets out to provide some information. She informs her viewers of the latency of HPV. She uses the language of "adventurous" girls to signal both a feminist, empowered sexuality and a normalized risk. Yet the speculation about the source of this STD brings suspicion, and potentially "blame," to Elijah, a man about to move in with his boyfriend. Who was the target audience of the episode, we are left to wonder? Was it meant for post-college-aged girls like Hannah and her friends, or for women slightly older who may have missed the protection Gardasil offered? Or perhaps it was meant for the boys, to prompt them to wonder about their role in transmission as well as their potential risk for HPV.

Despite some factual inaccuracies, what is brought forward in the episode is the ways STIs—the infections caused by bodily fluid exchange as well as close friction in bodily contact—continue to be somehow mysterious, feared, and potentially stigmatizing. The episode conjures a generation of girls' panic: fears about what it is, who you got it from, and what it means for your health.[2] Although sex establishes itself as a risk, not from pregnancy but from STIs, and HPV is declared to be one of them, the episode is careful not to associate either the risk or the infection with deviance. The threat nonetheless comes from multiple sex partners, with heightened concern about sex with men, and somewhat implicitly sex with men who have sex with men. As Dunham said in an interview with *BUST* magazine, "in terms of HPV, I literally did not know one girl in college who hadn't thought she had it, heard she had it, or had to have some weird conversation with a guy who didn't think he had it. And I was like, Someone just needs to explain the basic facts of this on television so that guys will stop thinking that you're talking about HIV" (see Bean 2012).

Whenever HPV appears on television shows, in ads, on social media, or in professional meetings, it manages gendered and sexual scripts, narratives about who is at risk and how one might contain its threats to health. Dunham herself was born in 1986 and would have just turned twenty when Gardasil was released and approved for girls aged nine to twenty-six, and recommended for a lower age range of nine to twelve. It is likely that Dunham and the other girls on the show would have been vaccinated. The boys, however, would most likely not have been vaccinated, given the vaccine's original approvals and the CDC's Advisory Committee on Immunization Practice's (ACIP) recommendation only for girls. While studies were under way, Merck chose not to await additional clinical evidence on any direct benefit to boys and their own risk of developing HPV-associated disease that might sway the FDA, and went ahead with their original approval. They also chose not to lead their vaccine campaigns with a notion of community benefit, relying instead on appeals to a direct benefit for girls.

What unfolded with the prevention politics around HPV and HPV vaccines was a story not of the march of technological progress and public health inclusion, but of how tensions between "we" public health and "me" clinical medicine, and between collective and individual prevention, are navigated. These tensions are shaped by the organization and politics around health systems, health research, and political health agendas. They are also reflective of the ways health, risk, and illness are shaped along social categories—of gender, sexuality, and age, as well as vaccine status, insurance status, place, immigration status, and others—as pharmaceutical companies and the intermediary actors of health care research and public health entities negotiate the outcomes for inclusion and care, as well as their costs and profits.

In asking "What's in it for the boys?" this chapter shows how this question of whether a direct or indirect benefit to individual health guides vaccine agendas and uptake. It is a question about whose bodies matter and whether individual or community health matters most. It allows consideration of the *politics of inclusion* formed around this case of a virus and its prevention. The politics of inclusion references a concept developed by the sociologist Steven Epstein to draw attention to the ways categories of gender, race, and LGBTQ sexualities are incorporated within otherwise exclusionary frameworks to remedy health disparities.[3] A vaccine for boys was called for, at times for reasons of equity and at times as a way of including boys in the direct prevention of disease. While boys do not in and of themselves make up a monolithic population affected by any single specific health disparity and are more often the "standard" to which others are compared, boys came to be included in HPV vaccination in ways that suppressed both the ghosts and politics of gay men's health and any imaginings of queer health equity in the future.

My first indication that this was neither preordained, nor the result of pharmaceutical greed, came as I sat and listened to the technical presentations at scientific meetings. The question of genomic-type coverage was scientifically—and socially—complex.[4] The molecular processes used to develop the HPV vaccine allowed decisions regarding which precise virus-like particles, or VLPs, to include in the vaccine's structure. Would too many type inclusions compromise overall efficacy? Would they protect against all, or only some, risks, and in all or only some bodies and places? It was not well understood which HPVs would persist to cause disease, when, and for whom, or whether additional changes to the formula might deplete or enhance possibilities of reaching herd immunity—if this was even a goal at all.[5]

HPV talk clustered around the basic science and the social epidemiology of disease and death rates. A narrative took hold, about the people, places, and types of disease that shape diagnosis, suffering, and deaths. Concern about high rates of disease, especially cervical cancer, was joined with news of a "significant rise," an "alarming trend" or "coming epidemic" of rare HPV-associated diseases, including some cancers. As I sat and listened, another gendered HPV cancer risk narrative came to the fore, this time for boys and men who could benefit from a preventive approach. Framing the problem as one of "rare cancers" on the rise fit into the already palpable concerns of scientists and publics alike. Cancer is feared both individually and collectively; almost everyone knows someone who has been diagnosed with or died as a result of this broad constellation of disease, the "emperor of all maladies," as described by the historian of medicine Siddhartha Mukherjee in his Pulitzer Prize-winning book of the same title (2010). This alarm about cancer was evident at conferences, as experts came together to share and discuss scientific findings and build a case for funding, next steps in medical research, or a different shape for health care provision, among other goals. Depending on the particular focus of the conference—public health professionals, molecular biologists, AIDS researchers, cancer clinicians, or gynecologists—each were part of a larger scientific community with a shared purpose of understanding, addressing, and advocating for the knowledge and practice needs associated with rising rates of cancers. Because of this shared object of concern—rare cancers on the rise—they were able to come together and talk meaningfully about the mutual worry that was "HPV-associated" disease.

I listened to the array of specialized knowledge for distinctions in technical language, but also for nuances in the ways they spoke about risk, management, and containment of disease, and about how and for whom health could be protected. HPV-associated "rare" cancers were put to work to bring new experts and subjects of cancer risk and protection into the fold. When scientists and medical professional spoke of whether and when—not to mention why not sooner—to shift HPV vaccination from a gender-specific, girls-only approach to a gender-neutral one, I was primed to listen. Merck's pending application to the FDA was well known, a request to expand the patient base of girls ages nine to twenty-six to include boys and men of the same ages. The FDA approved this request in October 2009. The application by Merck the year before had been based on newly released evidence, known for years, and on the original clinical trial design (a decade before). It is an effective approach to preventing genital warts—a non-life-threatening, widely experienced STI, already addressed by the vaccine by virtue of its causal connection to viral types 6 and 11. Merck brought their evidence to the FDA in a request to expand the target population and consumer market of their vaccine product to boys.

The ACIP, as is customary, independently reviewed the new approval application to determine how the indication might fit into their national children's vaccine guidelines. Unable to come to a clear decision on its use, the committee included Gardasil in its recommendations for the Vaccines for Children Program (ensuring its coverage by insurance and Medicaid for males in the approved age range) but stopped short of recommending "routine use" of the vaccine in boys. The recommendation had no "teeth," so to speak. Instead, the group of experts chose to put professional discretion in the hands of doctors and their patients (and by extension, parents as well). Possibly recognizing the ambiguity of their stance, the panel noted that they might reconsider their decision and make the vaccine part of recommended guidelines if more data emerged proving the vaccine's effectiveness in protecting males against other diseases—in particular, cancers associated with HPV, including penile, anal, and certain rare cancers of the head and neck.

It was a surprising step: at scientific meetings it was cancer risk and fear of coming surges in these deadly diseases that was amplified; genital warts were indeed part of the conversation, yet the threat they posed was somehow always framed as a secondary or add-on concern. Were STIs somehow less worthy of broad protection by a vaccine? Or was this claim, and acknowledgment of the research focus on vaccines to prevent STIs more generally, a political risk that threatened the success (e.g., approval and subsequent adoption) vaccine proponents hoped for? Was this downplaying of genital warts indicative of the social attempt to contain sex, and desexualize HPV and HPV vaccination?

The ACIP recommendations concerning males were murky and underwhelming in their advice to doctors, parents, and patients, leaving these groups essentially uninformed—confused by the nebulousness of this "optional" choice and unclear about which actions to take. How can we account for this gendered discrepancy? Does it constitute what the sociologists Laura Carpenter and Monica Casper (2009b) identify as an omnipresent "double standard" in technology development when it comes to gender and sexuality? What were the gendered and sexual biopolitics swirling around and affecting ACIP's decision? Why would it take years for the US viewing public to lock eyes with a series of adolescent boys looking directly into cameras and expressing their own concern for the risk a virus posed to their health?

Gardasil for Him? What's the Benefit for Boys?

The "Gardasil for him" story is neither linear nor chronological. Gardasil's protection against genital warts was a basis of Merck's original vaccine design, which included variants 9 and 11, known to cause benign genital warts. While approval was given for girls, this proof of the first vaccine's preventive analog in males, of this benign STI, opened the door for an all-gender approach to vaccination.[6] Economically, the workings of patent markets made this an appealing if not essential market to pursue. What gradually unfolded, however, was an amplification by Merck (as well as several intermediary actors) of HPV's causative role in the later onset of cancer and the cancer-preventive qualities of Gardasil for boys. Teen boys and their parents, and later young adult males, would gradually become "aware" of their HPV risk and so would be driven to enroll in cancer prevention. These processes, like those for girls, variously ignited sexual politics—while simultaneously doing the work to push these aside.

Some boys and men, and their sexualities, would emerge as objects of prevention with visible attempts to either tame or render visible their gendered sexuality. For others, questions would be raised about whether they even needed protection at all. For teen boys and young men watching, their exclusion in these early years was clear; this was a girls' vaccine and part of the prevention of women's cancers. In 2009 it was by dint of narratives of "other diseases" that "on-label" protection was extended to boys. While it made sense for Merck to create an updated ad campaign aimed at boys' vaccination—Gardasil was indeed approved for "use in males"— teen boys (along with teen girls) were not and still largely are not widely encouraged to ask their doctors about genital warts. In the absence of an accepted, mobilized, and heeded claim of a cancer connection for boys and men, Merck as well as state and non-state organizations such as the CDC and other public health actors would be quiet when it came to promoting Gardasil to boys.

Little was said about the HPV vaccine's indication for genital warts in these, or anyone's, bodies; there was no outbreak narrative focused on girls' genital warts, despite this disease indication driving the vaccine's expansion. Gardasil had overwhelmingly emphasized cancer prevention when marketing to girls, with some additional mention of protection from what they referred to as "other diseases" (but not specifically warts or an STI). Even among girls, various publics (and some parents) opposed a vaccine explicitly targeting an STI in pre-sexually active teens. Many attributed their concerns not to safety, as is often the case with vaccine hesitancy, but instead to a fear and worry that it would promote sexual activity. Anticipating a biopolitical hornet's nest as Gardasil was introduced, Merck applied lessons learned from a wide swath of previous and ongoing debates, including school-based sexual education programs, birth control and abortion politics, and especially condom-use campaigns in the context of HIV and pregnancy prevention. They chose to manufacture and advertise a "quadrivalent" four-VLP vaccine to US markets as a "cancer vaccine" for girls (see note 6). At the same time, they continued studies into Gardasil's role in reducing incidence of what are clinically referred to as "anogenital warts" in young men. From 2004 to 2007 Merck conducted research in young men across five continents to prove the vaccine's effectiveness in the reduction of genital warts. When they presented the evidence to the FDA in 2009 and received approval to expand the vaccine's use to males for the indication of genital warts associated with HPV, ACIP did not enter the vaccine into its recommended childhood vaccine guidelines. Instead, they gave doctors the (confusing) *option* to talk with their patients.

In some communities and most high-resource countries such as the US and Australia, what followed was that HPV and HPV vaccination transformed from a cervical cancer prevention tool explicitly and exclusively for girls, to a novel tool in an all-gender risk-prevention for genital warts and "other cancers" of the anus, vulva, penis, and oropharynx—as well as cancers of the cervix. In other communities and mostly low-income countries across regions of Africa, Southeast Asia, and Latin America, HPV vaccination continued as a girls' cancer prevention strategy in the "war against cervical cancer." With each labeling change and new FDA approval, distinct dynamics emerged, some drawing boys and men into a disease prevention regime and others maintaining their place in the shadows. Various actors, debates, and governance strategies unfolded as HPV vaccination strategies expanded in what appeared to be a hope of Merck's to move from a single-sex "girls'" vaccine strategy to a dual-sex strategy in alignment with every other vaccine in the childhood vaccine program.

"PROTECTING THE HERD" IN A PUSH
FOR BOYS' INCLUSION

Vaccines play an outsized role in what is known in virology as "herd immunity," a vaccine approach to population-level health gained when a large enough portion of the population has immunity to a given disease to greatly limit future transmissions or prevent them altogether. Sometimes that immunity comes from antibodies resulting from "native" spread of disease, but more often it comes from vaccination. For some experts, vaccinating boys against HPV made the most scientific sense, as long as the goal was to get to herd immunity for genital warts and the cancers that were linked to HPV. For others, however, vaccinating boys as well as girls did not make sense economically, given the high cost and health care approaches needed to vaccinate boys along with girls. For yet others, the need to vaccinate boys was self-evident: bodies are not all that different, so it is presumed that boys and men are likely already at risk of HPV-associated cancers.

Despite early calls by academic researchers and health policymakers that vaccinating boys along with girls would provide optimal public health benefit given population goals, Gardasil was rolled out with a single-sex strategy.[7] Yet, when calls for expansion—specifically the inclusion of boys—were voiced, the reasons varied and were inconsistent: some emphasized augmented protection for girls, others a direct benefit to boys; still others emphasized "herd" immunity with its hopes for near total disruption. Of course, from a business perspective, a "gender neutral" (often referred to as "dual" sex) strategy would be as effective at expanding markets and maximizing profits as it would be in protecting community health. Merck's challenge appeared to be to find a way to broaden its strategy without bringing up sex or sexualizing their previous and future marketing efforts. With clinical evidence in hand, they could convince the FDA to give them the needed approval and request that ACIP expand its recommendation to boys, while concurrently highlighting an existing though relatively unknown boys' health problem—genital warts—that the vaccine already prevented.

Harald zur Hausen, the German virologist who is recognized as the first to isolate HPV-16 and HPV-18 DNA in cervical cancer, had always argued that the vaccine should be given to boys and girls, expressing a view shared by many scientists at that time: the real promise of prevention vaccines hinged on the potential to secure herd immunity. The "herd," practically speaking, can never be fully vaccinated (vaccination is often contraindicated for certain groups like pregnant women and those with certain allergies, for instance; others may have difficulty completing a vaccination course because of side effects), nor is universal exposure to a particular virus ever considered ideal (for many of the same individually-specific responses to disease course), but if about two-thirds of a population falls into one or both of these two groups, the uncontrolled spread of a contagious disease will generally be prevented. Because an infectious disease's transmissibility depends on its basic reproduction number—known as "R0" or "R naught" in epidemiology—there is no single certainty nor universally applied measure of herd immunity. The specificity and materiality of each pathogen creates its own complexities, driving uncertainty about the ratio of vaccinated or exposed to unvaccinated or unexposed that would be needed; at times the very logic of the concept of the "herd" raises questions, given differences in groups, practices, and communities (such as age distribution, social habits, movements in and out of the area, and more recently, the concept of "hard to reach" populations).[8]

While a public health imaginary requires estimating and aiming for the ideal ratio for full population protection, the goals and visions of pharmaceutical development are more varied. Medical technologies, including vaccine technologies, are developed not only to address (public) health need, but also to secure early adoption in high-income countries (or patients), to ensure a return on research and development (R&D) investment (even when public funding is part of the start-up basic and applied research costs). From the start, technologies are designed, tested, and built with uses as well as users in mind to secure this monetary return. While not averse to doubling their potential market for the vaccine and going after a dual-sex strategy and herd protection approach, Merck and GSK from the outset faced the hard task of convincing the FDA, as well as parents, that boys should be vaccinated for their own protection. Yet given the chosen strategy of promoting a "cervical cancer vaccine" to protect girls, it would be a challenge to configure boys as part of the vaccine market.

Galvanized by the prospect of herd immunity and widespread protection, many public health experts advocated for vaccinating boys as a way to provide an indirect benefit to girls and improve cervical cancer prevention. Given the sexual transmission route, protecting boys against HPV would protect their sexual partners from the infections caused by intimate relations; girls (as well as boys) would be protected from the possibility that their own antibody resistance might not stop the incoming infection and a virus might hide and persist, ultimately to form an "HPV-associated disease." With gender inclusion and a dual-sex strategy, this vaccine could and should follow traditional vaccine strategies from the previous century that relied on epidemiological theory as evidence for the level of immunity required to protect a community—rather than any single body—from the onset of disease. Would a population's health strategy of "we" medicine be able to overcome the reliance of the US on individual health and the benefits targeted to "me"?

Vaccine expansion relied on claims of unaddressed problems and a need for additional data to ready a market. Clinical trial evidence would ensure the product approvals needed to ultimately produce a return on any current or previous investment. Value accrues from several sources: product sales, which are determined in turn by dose size and frequency of administration; the exclusivity of the product and its secured intellectual rights and patent protections, which keep the competition at bay; and government investments and incentives as well as price-setting and negotiation. Value is also tied to continual expansion of use and patient populations. As girls were urged to know the link and to act to engage in responsible health prevention, investments were underway to prove that boys too were at risk of cancers associated with HPV.

A push and pull emerged between community benefit and individual well-being. HPV vaccines and becoming "One Less" was a distinct achievement for some even in contexts with minimal health care safety nets and no universal health care. A narrative of people making good choices overlaid realities of others left either in clinical ambiguity or outside medicine altogether—what anthropologists refer to as a "pharmaceutical nexus" (Busfield 2006, Petryna and Kleinman 2006, Biehl 2006, Whitemarsh 2008).[9] Merck was not alone in shaping the prevention apparatus that would proliferate unevenly around the world. In the US and elsewhere multiple actors would collectively mediate the junctions between technological producers, like Merck and GSK, and consumers, including researchers in academia and at the National Cancer Institute, cancer organizations such as the American Cancer Foundation, and sexual health organizations, advocates, and activists—not to mention the media and public relations and advertising companies.[10] In the case of HPV vaccines, these multi-actor sites of decision making existed before and during the time of the HPV vaccine's diffusion.[11]

Configuring Boys: Epidemiology Shapes a Market

Configuring boys as part of the HPV vaccine market began as early as 2004 when Merck envisioned Gardasil as protective against a non–life-threatening STI—genital warts—and built that prevention into its basis. Protecting against what was once referred to as an STD and now as an STI might attract young men (and their parents) by offering a direct benefit to boys.[12] With evidence of protection efficacy for girls, Merck could have advertised this additional indicator of an STI prevention in its awareness and vaccine product advertising campaigns, but the acronyms STD and STI ever appeared. Such advertising may have risked calling attention to issues of sex, sexuality, and sexual transmission in ways that explaining the link between a virus and cancer would not. Reference to an STD might conjure ghostly matters: earlier symbolic associations among gender, sex, and disease, specifically viruses, that explicitly hinge on gendered sexualization. STDs, especially prior to effective therapeutic treatments, came with a stigma. STDs had also been associated with a moral failure, and had long been an object of campaigns for virtue, rightness, and the establishment of codes of conduct, regulation, and containment (Friedman and Shepeard 2007, Hoppe 2017). Was Merck willing to associate boys with STIs in ways they would not want to do for girls? The possibilities for associations with these ghostly hauntings may explain why there were no collectives of adolescent girls or boys who stood empowered to assert their capacity to protect their own bodies against an STD associated with sex before or during

Gardasil's campaigns. Merck, along with public health actors and academic researchers, chose instead to align with previously configured markets of cancer risk and cancer prevention.

In forgoing a male market, at least for a while, Merck provided fuel not only for contestation around girls, but also for a quiet and growing set of politics formed around the exclusion of boys. A major concern with this approach among public health advocates as well as a variety of social activists and disease advocates was that not including boys would prevent the herd immunity needed to reach protection even for girls. This single-gender approach was also counter to the standard all-gender approach for other preventive vaccines administered on a mass scale, for whooping cough, measles, mumps, rubella, and others.

Many researchers thought the rollout specifically to girls was a public health failure, especially when it came to global health. Op-eds were published in many of the leading medical journals by experts in the relevant fields of medicine and public health who supported the viewpoint of my respondent. As early as March 2006, Robert Steinbrook, a professor of medicine at Yale University, wrote of "The Potential of Human Papillomavirus Vaccines" in the *New England Journal of Medicine*. He argued (presumably to the FDA licensing board that was considering Merck's request) that the four-strain vaccine administered in three doses over the course of six months should also be given to boys and men "to prevent them from transmitting HPV to women or to other men." This indirect benefit was good for the population's health and would reduce girls' risk of cervical cancer. In Europe, the leading medical journal, *The Lancet*, would also exert pressure to shape the coming market. Immediately following the FDA's approval of Gardasil for girls, *Lancet* editors published their opposition to the single-sex strategy ("Should HPV Vaccines Be Mandatory for All Adolescents?" 2006): "Contrary to the FDA's recommendations, there is growing support for the vaccination of both boys and girls." The editors' claims relied on modeling studies to demonstrate that "a single sex (female) approach would be 60–70% less effective at reducing HPV prevalence in women than strategies that target both sexes." They were making a case for boys' inclusion based on "other benefits" such as potential protection against genital warts and "malignancies including anal cancer, which affect both sexes." It was well known that previous attempts at gender-specific initiatives had not succeeded—the UK's rubella immunization program had tried to target girls only until 1995, when it modified its approach after a rise in the number of pregnant women contracting rubella. The single-sex vaccine approach failure in Europe had likely invigorated many virologists to advocate for an all-gender strategy. *The Lancet*'s editors argued that "for effective and long-term eradication of HPV, all adolescents must be immunized." In making their call they were advocating for more research to conduct the clinical trials they deemed necessary to support vaccinating boys ("Should HPV Vaccines Be Mandatory?" 2006).

By April 2008, researchers were providing evidence and arguments for an expansion efforts. In "The Case for a Gender-Neutral (Universal) Human Papillomavirus Vaccination Policy in the United States," published in *Cancer Epidemiology, Biomarkers, & Prevention*, a journal of the American Association for Cancer Research (Giuliano and Salmon 2008), the authors' argument for dual-sex vaccination rested on the claim that men were the source of HPV infection, emphasizing the transmission pathway and vector of HPV. With little drama or fearmongering, they framed their argument for expansion as "good sense." The good sense was economical as well: "Since HPV infection is common in men and is readily transmitted . . . vaccination strategies that include both sexes may be more cost-effective in reducing HPV female disease burden than gender-targeted strategies." While testing for efficacy in reducing infection and lesions caused by HPV was underway among young men internationally, the authors' case was balanced, yet it held a warning of its own: "Vaccination of males may become inevitable if and when vaccination of females fails to adequately control disease because of suboptimal vaccine uptake," they argued. A specter of medical failure was also possible, they added: "female only vaccination may work well for controlling cervical cancer, but the realities on the ground may force us to consider other strategies such as vaccinating males" (Giuliano and Salmon 2008). The claim was prognostic; given the vector of transmission, it would soon become clear that risks to health extended beyond the reach of the current strategy.

Entangling a Gendered Script

Effectively including boys required untangling the now gendered script shaping Gardasil as a "girls' vaccine" and configuring boys as outside the need for protection. Expansion would require a complicated messaging strategy aimed at boys and their parents to convince them that a vaccine previously aimed at girls and the possibility of their developing a woman's disease in the future (cervical cancer) was the right tool for boys as well. But messaging around which "job" the tool of vaccination was best for when it came to boys would be another matter altogether (Mamo and Pérez 2021). Messaging by Merck and their advertising and marketing firms was still unclear on a single, best use—there was no straightforward problem for boys that was, if not explicitly and imminently in need of being solved, then urgent enough to require this particular vaccine at this particular time. Merck juggled multiple questions at once: If the market were to expand to include boys, would calls for herd immunity supplant the previous emphasis of the need for girls and their proactive mothers to be self-aware and personally responsible? Would Merck convince boys and their parents that vaccinating boys was the best approach to protecting girls from cervical cancer? Might they convince boys of the need to protect themselves from the sexual risk of genital warts or, as would later be the case, from another cancer—this one rare and "unmentionable"? At issue was the absence of a life-threatening and highly contagious HPV-related illness from which boys needed protection. For girls, an already established fear and risk of cervical cancer and its high incidence and mortality burden around the world were "fact" enough to justify a vaccine approach to prevention for girls. But a problem for boys' health would have to be configured before the vaccine market could be expanded to include them. By the time Merck released clinical trial evidence proving a health benefit to boys in (at least partially) solving the problem of their "*ano*-genital warts," and then headed to the FDA to seek expanded approval, it was too late—the vaccine message had already been well established.[13]

Intervening in boys' and men's health, sexual and otherwise, was not generally acceptable, nor was it built into already established medical practices in the ways that girls' sexualities were (for example, through contraceptive counseling and routine gynecological care). In July 2009, prior to the FDA decision on expanded labeling, Karin B. Michels, an epidemiologist at Harvard University, and Harald zur Hausen published the commentary "HPV Vaccine for All" in *The Lancet*. The authors argued for a vaccine approach more akin to previous public health efforts launched to fight diseases that affect children regardless of gender, such as measles and whooping cough. The then current target of vaccination of girls and women ages eleven to twenty-six, they argued, was insufficient: "The only efficient way to stop the virus is to also vaccinate the other half of the sexually active population: boys and men" (Michels and zur Hausen 2009b). Michels and zur Hausen made their claims based on evidence from an HPV vaccine trial conducted by Jorma Paavonen of the University of Helsinski and collaborators (Paavonen et al. 2009), which they said supported their conclusion that men and boys, as well as women and girls, should be vaccinated. (They also asserted that it is not just preadolescents and adolescents who should be vaccinated, but that HPV vaccination should move up the life course to ensure that those who were not able to be vaccinated earlier would be eligible to receive the vaccine—a point that drew some contention given the likely high rates of exposure to HPV and thus the reduced effectiveness of the vaccine in this age group.)[14] Women, Michels and zur Hausen argued, "have shouldered responsibility for contraception since its inception. The goal to eradicate sexually transmitted carcinogenic viruses can be jointly carried by women and men, and could be accomplished within a few decades" (Michels and zur Hausen 2009b).

M. Michele Manos, a molecular virologist who led research into HPV's role in cancer, opposed an all-gender approach in the context of nations "where a vaccine is most needed," arguing that "restricting vaccinations to prepubescent girls might be particularly prudent" in low-income countries where cancer incidence is high due to structural health care limits (e.g., lack of cancer screening and care)." She added, "Young or old, a woman's previous infection risk can be difficult to ascertain, particularly in cases of unacknowledged rape or other sexual molestation." In conclusion, she said, "Although the global eradication of HPV infection is a noble goal, we currently have neither sufficient evidence nor the requisite understanding of the immunology of HPV infection to suggest HPV vaccination for all" (Manos 2009, 1328). In a response to arguments by Tsu and Wittet (2009) that cervical cancer is a public health problem, while HPV infections are not, Michels and zur Hausen asserted that HPV cervical lesions are a public health problem in and of themselves. "It would be short-sighted to disregard the large number of cervical lesions that develop after infections with high-risk HPV types requiring surgical interventions. Since cervical cancer is caused by HPV infections, the most effective strategy to prevent this cancer, its precursor lesions, and the associated pain and suffering is the prevention of infection." Furthermore, they stated, "inclusion of men and boys in the vaccination programme [launched in 2016] was more effective than inclusion of only girls and women" (Michels and zur Hausen 2009a). The authors appealed to the direct benefit to men, including the prevention of all HPV-linked cancers in men (e.g., anal, penile, and oropharyngeal cancers), concluding that an all-gender vaccine approach would be cost-effective. The population effect of an eventual eradication, or even a drastic reduction in the rate of HPV infections, requires vaccination of both sexes, they argued. In direct response to Manos's recommendations, Michels and zur Hausen urged: "Although Manos considers the eradication of HPV infections a 'noble goal,' the development of HPV vaccines was unnecessarily delayed by doubts about the causal role of HPV infections in cervical cancer. We do not have to wait for more detailed immunological studies before we start planning large-scale interventions, since these will be highly effective public health programmes" (Michels and zur Hausen 2009a, 1329).[15] The important argument here was that without a strategic vision, the most effective global program would not begin. A debate begun in the pages of *The Lancet* was always a matter of global health relevance; centering cost-effectiveness arguments and gender equity contentions, this particular debate would cascade into a wider conversation in the US, especially surrounding Merck's advertising.

Why did ACIP stop short of a policy decision with teeth by not offering clear guidance for boys' vaccination in 2009? Why did they instead give doctors the *option* to vaccinate boys? Did this decision (or lack thereof) reflect the ways Gardasil was promoted as a consumer product and personal choice more than as a public health effort? Apart from following doctors' recommendations, parents are often brought into health decisions through school health requirements. Merck did not forgo this avenue, participating in vaccine-day events with doctors' offices and clinics, and providing office posters and other promotional materials. Yet despite the back-to-school campaign strategies, it was not clear that Merck would look beyond children and their parents to include teenage and young adult men, as they did with women.

While ACIP effectively left the ultimate decision-making in the hands of medical professionals and publics, including parents—despite their having only limited information—Merck chose to tiptoe into the waters of education with a campaign aimed directly at parents of young and preteen children that I call "Both." In contrast to previous pharmaceutical marketing to girls, the campaign was small in scale, far from a media blitz. It was a quiet appeal to parents to bring them into awareness about their boys' potential risk. As ACIP left it, it would be up to providers to assess whether protecting girls is reason enough to begin to move toward universal vaccination recommendations that include boys.

Journalists, meanwhile, were picking up on the private hesitations and public debate around promoting the vaccine to boys. Data characteristics also drew attention, as Merck's submission for FDA approval lacked key information, both about the vaccine's duration and, relatedly, about its potential to protect against cancer in males. Doctors, meanwhile, were given additional pause. "I am not prepared to say all boys in that age group should get [the HPV vaccine] without question," said one doctor in an article with the headline, "Doctors Say 'Wait and See' before Prescribing Gardasil in Boys" (Chitale 2009).

What else was behind this hesitation? The limited FDA approval of Gardasil specifically for use in boys and men to prevent genital warts, coupled with general concerns from some vocal groups, posed a dilemma for Merck: how to enroll boys with an advertising approach for a vaccine against a woman's cancer without igniting the kind of gendered sexual politics they had previously encountered—and successfully tamed—around girls' vaccination. Advertising Gardasil as a vaccine to protect against an STI linked to genital warts could backfire and risk calling attention to issues of boys' sexuality and sexual transmission to girls as well as to other boys. Merck proceeded with caution, testing the waters with a public awareness campaign to bring boys to HPV vaccination.

Advertising content included on both the Merck & Co. website and the Gardasil.com companion website featured a video with the lead character gently appealing to boys: "You may have heard," a teen boy confides, "that only women can get human papillomavirus (HPV). *But did you know?* Both men and women can get HPV and pass it on without even realizing it." Using the non-threateningly curious slogan, "You've Heard, But Did You Know," the website unfurls a set of linked facts: HPV will affect an estimated 75 to 80 percent of males and females in their lifetime; for most, HPV clears on its own; for others, certain HPV-related diseases—genital warts and cervical, vaginal, and vulvar cancers—can develop. Finally, the visitor to the site is informed that there is no way to predict who will or won't clear the virus—it's up to boys to "know the link." "You need to know the facts of HPV. You can get it too and it can affect you," teen boys (and adult men) are told. Once the illness is defined and ascribed to gendered bodies—that is, once boys are made "aware" and informed of their risk— the vaccine and its need are introduced. *"But did you know*: GARDASIL was approved by the Food and Drug Administration (FDA) for use in boys and young men ages 9 to 26 to help protect against 90% of genital warts cases." A caveat is added: "[I]t is important to remember that GARDASIL may not fully protect everyone, nor will it protect against diseases caused by other HPV types or against diseases not caused by HPV. GARDASIL does not prevent all types of cervical cancer, so it's important for women to continue routine cervical cancer screenings. Also, keep in mind that GARDASIL does not treat cancer or genital warts."

Merck provides boys a *direct* benefit to their future health, a strategy that may have seemed an easier sell than enrolling boys in a public health solution to protect girls from cancer. Publics were experiencing this information, and some perhaps were wondering how Merck, along with all the intermediary actors in favor of looping boys into the vaccine's uptake, would be able to generate a sense of anticipatory risk and fear among boys and their parents similar to that conjured for girls and their mothers. Was the specter of a relatively unknown and non-life-threating harm to health via an STD enough to center boys and convince parents to vaccinate their sons—without drawing too much attention to sexuality?

The Ghostly Haunting of Men, Masculinity, and STDs

From syphilis to AIDS, sexually transmitted disease[16] and the infections that cause them (STIs) have endured symbolic associations with categories of gender, race, and sexuality, and are thereby gendered, racialized, and sexualized phenomena. Certain people were designated as engaging in "immoral behavior," as having congenital "contagion," or as succumbing to unbridled and excessive sexual practices. Certain bodies, lives, and communities have thus unevenly endured stigma, shame, and blame for STIs and their disease outcomes. VD (short for venereal disease) was coined for its presumption of the erotic, from the Latin *venereus*, pertaining to Venus and sexual love and desire, and it has also long been deeply entangled with scientific racism, xenophobia, sexism, and homophobia. Contagion has been sexualized, differently shaped by its intersectional and often racist dimensions. This haunting, I am arguing, is important for the ways HPV and its vaccine targets have downplayed—and desexualized—sexuality through their own intersectional framings. It is also significant for the ways HPV has variously been associated with cancer risk or STIs, and variously configured genders and sexualities as targets of prevention.

The indirect term used to describe adolescent vaccination—"prior to sexual onset"—is entangled in assumptions and fears about whose sexuality is in need of containment, and when in their life course. From early sexual hygiene movements focused on "VD" to later sanitized and rebranded sex education campaigns targeting STI prevention, much of the focus was on Black communities, specifically Black men and the threats their bodies and sexual behavior posed to health. This focus was fueled in part by inflated statistics that began with prevalence studies of venereal disease among African American (male) troops during and returning from the Second World War (Moran 2000, 114), and in part by the hypervisibility of Black masculinity for public consumption, with its racist construction as being in need of containment and regulation (Brandt 1985, Jones 1993).As biomedical and other institutions mostly neglected Black communities, when it came to sex, masculinity, and disease, claims that Black men presented a risk because they were "hypersexual people who suffered from venereal diseases because of their promiscuous sexual behavior" (Jones 1993, 48; and see Sharma 2010) were given outsize attention.

The gendered, sexualized discourses and practices under study here, which linger in their symbolic associations with sex and disease, are always already racialized: discourse and practice around VD, STDs, and today's STIs have been replete with moral stigma and fears of contagion that variously capture different bodies and groups in a web of meaning and power—as well as with real health effects and suffering. The archive and its analysis of race, gender, sex, and sexuality, and their entanglements with disease, are multiple and yet also like Swiss cheese, full of random holes. When the medical historian Allan Brandt, in his 1985 book *No Magic Bullet: A Social History of Venereal Disease in the United States since 1880*, chronicled the social and cultural anxieties around sexually transmitted disease, he was also making visible many of the symbolic associations that would be managed, and suppressed, and that would linger across history and through medicine.

The historian Keith Wailoo showed how "virtue" and the campaigns to address STDs were racialized and shaped along a color line: the "bad blood" of venereal disease (VD) was given meaning through an already present racist logic of difference. As VD was racialized, the meaning shaped public health practice. It was said that to be fit and healthy was to be engaged in "good" health behaviors reflective of a form of white acceptability. Eventually, as Wailoo shows, cancer and STDs would come to echo mid-twentieth-century segregation, with whites part of cancer prevention and Blacks relegated to the world of STIs. Constructing bodies and lives as raced, gendered, and with sexualities that are variously biologized and made into identities, practices, and communities is deeply entangled with science and medicine, as well as with ideas and realities of "health" and disease (Brandt 1985, Jones 1993, Sharma 2010).[17]

Siobhan Somerville's groundbreaking book, *Queering the Color Line*, highlighted the ways that turn-of-the-century scientific discourses on race "provided a logic through which sexologists and other medical 'experts' articulated emergent models of homosexuality in the United States" (Somerville 2000), showing that the ways we think of race and sexuality are intertwined. The naturalization of heterosexuality and reproductive sex has been a racist, homophobic project in which prostitution and receptive anal sex are pathologized. Regulation of nonwhite gender and sexual practices have long been part of "vice commissions, residential segregation and immigration exclusion" (Ferguson 2003, 69).

Scientific ideas, clinical trial design, and the technologies of prevention are shaped in white supremacy and its logics, which combine to allow for the political justification of oppression and discrimination. Gendered, racialized sexualities from mythical scientific claims of Black masculinity as conferring risk and threat (to self and others) arose in slavery and linger into the present (Sharma 2010). Black queerness was produced in the white imaginary as having excessive and unbridled sexual desire (Ferber 2007), beliefs formed in (white) cultural associations of Blackness with deviance, delinquency, and dangerousness. The cultural critic and Black feminist scholar bell hooks (2004, 67) attributed this construction to "the convergence of racist sexist thinking about the black body, which has always projected onto the black body a hypersexuality," and argued that the "idea of the black male rapist" was produced as a white fantasy to justify state-sanctioned violence as a tool of political oppression and discrimination.

Throughout the twentieth century, medical science and public health projects incorporated these racial ideologies into their research and practice (Brandt 1978, Hickey 2006), studying "racial" differences, especially between Black and white people, and accepting at face value these so-called scientific beliefs of "natural" difference (Roberts 1997, Hammonds and Herzig 2009, McKittrick 2021). The mid-twentieth-century Tuskegee Trial for the Study of Syphilis exemplifies the racist logic. Power and racism intertwined, as they always do, to allow scientists to not see Black men's humanity, thereby rendering their bodies and lives available for a study to understand the progression of disease. The Black men of Macon County enrolled were harmed not by a lack of informed consent, but by the logic and working of power resulting in a seemingly acceptable denial of effective medical treatment (both the earlier heavy metals, and then penicillin after it was shown to work), and thereby also allowing the continued transmission of syphilis in communities (to their wives through sex, and to children through prenatal transmission). The decades-long public health study is one example of this enduring legacy.[18] These are some of the ghostly matters that shape the meaning of risk and of disease.

Viral infectious diseases, from hepatitis B in the 1970s and 1980s to HIV in the 1980s and 1990s, hold unique and overlapping histories that include processes of gendering, sexualizing, and racializing disease; they also reflect their own outbreak narratives (Wald 2008), forged in population "risk groups" with "risk behaviors" clinging to those already stained by prior stigma and associations of shame and blame (Preda 2005) that often followed racism, sexism, and homophobia. What kind of person "got" the disease and what they were (presumably) doing to get it were early questions in the histories of HIV, landing first on drug users and then on homosexual men, as people blamed and stigmatized each grouping for their particular deviance. Drug users and Haitians were quietly pushed aside (Epstein 1996, 49) in favor of a homosexual risk group that was often racialized as white. Hemophiliacs who contracted the disease through blood transfusions, and somewhat later, children born to HIV+ mothers, were granted "victim" status, with its cloak of innocence, thus exempting many of them from the sort of causal links that cast behavioral blame on a "particular kind of person" (Treichler 1999, 361) who engages in "particular" kinds of behaviors. "Two taboos"—against promiscuity and against homosexuality—were forged in disease (Altman 1986, 143).[19]

Some Boys More than Others: Implicating Pre-Gay Men, Gay Men, and Men Who Have Sex with Men in Cancer Prevention

In 1990, Joel Palefsky, a professor of medicine and an infectious disease specialist at University of California, San Francisco who served as chair of the HPV working group of the National Cancer Institute AIDS Malignancy Consortium, released results from a clinical study of ninety-seven gay, HIV+ men which showed that 50 percent were infected with HPV (Palefsky et al. 1990); 15 percent of those with HPV also had abnormal cellular growths in the epithelial (skin) cells around the anal area. The findings indicated that high-risk or oncogenic viral HPV could also cause cancer in this bodily region, at least for men with HIV. With this research, more than a decade before the public was introduced to Gardasil, an entirely new association between HPV and disease started to take shape—one framing male-to-male sex as a risky practice and gay men as a risk group. These identities and sexual behaviors would become highly entangled in what was developing into a clearly gendered sexual dynamic of HPV and HPV prevention. Given that the research was conducted with men with HIV, and the subjects' immunosuppressive status was hypothesized as a possible culprit for the development of abnormal cells, the research could say little about the extent to which boys were at risk of cancer. The data pointed to at least some risk for some boys, to be sure, but were parents ready to see their boys in the study subjects: as gay, or at risk of a virus that could or would be transmitted to their anal areas? Could they consider them "pre-gay" if it meant doing what was best for their long-term health?

Palefsky's research was part of a decade of new evidence of correlative associations between anal sex and anal cancers that presumptively brought "homosexual men"—and their precursors, "pre-gay" boys—and anal cancer into symbolic association. As the sociologist Steven Epstein argued, prior to this research and the formal link of HPV with anal dysplasia or the abnormal cellular changes associated with precancers, a body of research had slowly created a new conceptual framework for thinking about the issue of anal cancer. This framework, as Epstein describes, created "a certain level of confusion, which lingered, about how to define the (pre)population at risk." "Was this (anal cancer) then a 'gay health threat?' and one that adhered to gay identity and the property of a 'gay community?'" he asked (Epstein 2010, 64). Just how much of a health concern *was* anal cancer, and for whom? These questions, along with the identities, cultures, and sexual practices influencing their very construction, remained largely invisible in the HPV vaccine trajectory, even as the vaccine labeling and approvals expanded to include boys and men.

By around 2007, with cancer associations—however uncertain—now established for boys and men with HPV (and with HIV), appeals for Gardasil not as prevention against a concerning STI, but as a protection from the danger of cancer for boys, found firmer footing. In a *New York Times* article titled "New Vaccine for Cervical Cancer Could Prove Useful in Men, Too," David Tuller (2007) suggested that Merck might have the opportunity to expand the market for its new vaccine after all. The article raised the specter of an HPV-associated men's cancer, and with it the potential new configuration of a market for the HPV vaccine as a vaccine against anal cancer for a subset of boys and men. This "new" cancer prevention tool was linked to the hope that it would prevent a less well-known, but potentially fatal disease in gay men: anal cancer. Tuller informed the public that cervical cancer and anal cancer are caused by the same strains of HPV, and warned that "anal cancer can affect anyone." Yet, as the article continues, we are told that anal cancer "is most common among men with histories of receptive anal intercourse—an annual rate of about 35 cases per 100,000, and perhaps twice that for those infected with H.I.V., which weakens the immune system." Within the space of a few words, the problem shifted from that of a cancer that affects anyone with an anus—man or woman—to one for which those at most risk are men who have sex with men (MSM) and people with HIV—a decidedly more specific population. Tuller then quoted Palefsky making an aspirational, not yet FDA-approved case for the potential use of Gardasil for protection against anal cancer, and by extension, a case for the vaccine's use in boys: "The cervix is similar biologically to the anus, so there's plenty of hope that it [Gardasil] will work there also."

Health care and public policy experts would wonder if parents were ready to vaccinate their teen and preteen sons to protect them against a cancer associated with anal sex. Gay health advocates would forge ahead, seeing the vaccine as a tool for their own community health and hoping to find ways to normalize the vaccine as a tool for boys and men regardless of sexual identities and practices. To do so effectively, they knew, it was essential to either create distance from stigmatized sexual practices and identities or to destigmatize those sexual practices and identities; potentially even more effective would be to symbolically dissociate anal sex from men and men's bodies. After all, receptive anal sex was likely a frequent practice among many women, and all genders have anuses. But the data tell a more complicated story: men who have sex with men have higher proportions of anal cancer causally linked to HPV, but in terms of absolute numbers, women carry the larger burden of disease. It is estimated that 9,090 adults—6,070 women and 3,020 men—will be diagnosed with anal cancer in the US in 2021, and 879 women and 560 men will die from it (American Cancer Society 2021). Although the absolute numbers are relatively small, by comparison it is estimated that in the same period 14,480 people will be diagnosed with cervical cancer, and 4,290 will die from it. The incidence of anal cancer in HIV-infected MSM appeared to be shaping the debate around HPV vaccination for both boys and young MSM. Anal sex practices—among both men and women—continue to be suppressed in popular discourse, and remain the "great undiscussable" in public discussion of HPV vaccines (Epstein 2010).

Despite the evidence of the vaccine's protection against an STI, and its approval for boys to prevent genital warts, the inclusion of boys was neither fully realized nor demanded until it was shown to confer protection against a cancer. This causal association, between HPV and anal cancer, would carry its own gendered sexual associations in need of taming if the public was going to agree to have their sons vaccinated. In 2010, almost twenty years after his initial research into the HPV-anal cancer connection, Palefsky published interim findings of a clinical trial in the *Journal of Adolescent Health*, reporting that the quadrivalent HPV vaccine is highly effective in reducing external genital lesions (and precancers) in young men, making the case that "there may be a strong rationale for vaccinating boys" (Palefsky 2010, S12). These data, which Merck used in their FDA application for expanded labeling for boys, provided evidence of a link between HPV and "other diseases," as well as a scientific basis for a dual-sex vaccine strategy. HPV is "Not Just a Women's Issue," the title of Palefsky's 2010 paper stated. The case was made that "male HPV infection is also an important concern [along with female HPV], both for the disease burden in men and for the risk of transmission to women" (Palefsky 2010, S12). Boys and men were therefore being summoned into a politics of vaccine inclusion—not only as actors responsible for their own health, but also as the source of HPV infection in women and other men. Anal warts had been the most common STD in gay men prior to the HIV epidemic; studying HPV in HIV+ gay men and developing health care programs to ensure their health made good sense.[20]

A Report to the Nation: Epidemiology and the Case to Vaccinate Boys

The American Cancer Society (ACS) published their *Annual Report to the Nation on the Status of Cancer* in 2013, based on their analysis of US cancer surveillance data. The report was a collaboration with the CDC and the National Cancer Institute of the NIH. It would shape a picture and establish a narrative about the population risk of HPV-associated cancers.[21] At the time of the release, I was near the ACS headquarters in Atlanta, attending another meeting. I contacted the lead author of the report, the epidemiologist Jemal Ahmedin, then director of the Surveillance Research Program, asking if he might have some time to be interviewed for my research while I was still in town. I was grateful to receive an immediate and affirmative response to my request, along with an invitation. We scheduled a time for the next day at his ACS office. That evening I read the report carefully in my hotel room. This cancer report to the nation felt different from others I was familiar with. It moved beyond general cancer statistics and took up a focus on claims-making I had not found in earlier reports. Its focus for 2013 included, along with the usual epidemiological data reporting on morbidity and mortality of all cancers, a featured section on "the burden and trends in Human Papillomavirus (HPV)-associated cancers and HPV vaccination coverage levels." To my knowledge, there had yet to be a comprehensive cancer surveillance review of HPV-cancer associations, with the exception of those done by epidemiologists for cervical cancer. What particularly got my attention, though, was the ways HPV vaccination rates were linked to other cancers and other population groups aside from "women." The report to the nation emphasized a key finding of its epidemiological analysis of available surveillance data in the US: "Although death rates were declining for all cancers for men and women of all major racial and ethnic groups, and for most major cancer sites; a decrease of 1.5% per year over the last decade 2000–2009; *incidence rates increased for two HPV-associated cancers*" (Jemal et al. 2013, 1, emphasis mine). Surprisingly, the report found that it was two little-known cancers—anal and oropharyngeal—that were increasing among Americans. I was reading this report at a conference on cervical cancer prevention, where the role of HPV vaccination in this cancer's prevention was the major concern. This report, in contrast, brought forward two HPV-associated cancers that were on the rise, as reported by the ACS. Because the vast majority of people—of any gender—have the biological sites affected by anal and oropharyngeal cancer, the report's findings configured HPV as an *all-gender* health concern, and recommended a "dual-sex strategy" for HPV vaccination.

The following day I headed to the ACS headquarters and sat down with the report's lead authors, Ahmedin and Edgar Simard, both epidemiologists. I was interested in finding out about the choices they had made in constructing the report. Specifically, I wondered how they understood the gender and sexual dynamics of HPV-associated cancer rates and prevention, and the role those understandings played in producing a narrative. I sketched out some questions for the authors and arrived at the ACS headquarters around lunchtime. I asked questions about the metrics and understandings the team chose to assess who was at risk of HPV-associated cancers, and therefore in need of a prevention effort. Which factors (e.g., behavioral, social, biological) and whose bodies came to matter and were rendered visible, or silenced, in the epidemiological research? And ultimately, how might the claims-making of the 2013 report render boys and men increasingly visible in the politics of cancer prevention? This report, of course, was not the first instance of boys and men being called into discussions about HPV-associated cancers and other diseases, nor was this the first time that an advocacy organization called for their inclusion in the then 4-genomic-type vaccine, Gardasil. Yet, by making these claims in the report, the ACS was acting in their capacity as an intermediary organizational actor in the politics of inclusion and the commodification of markets for health technologies—in this case, HPV vaccination expansion to boys and men.

Simard, the epidemiologist who worked on the report with a team of other epidemiologists under the leadership of Ahmedin, was usually the one to respond to my questions. He was eager to share his views, and seemed to get my sociological inquiry. He began, "We decided to focus on HPV in the *Annual Report* because it's timely and relevant. A lot of advances have been made, such as vaccines, but also anal and oropharyngeal cancer rates are increasing. We focus on HPV in order to stimulate further research and to inform the public . . . of this and the available means of prevention in the vaccine." The publication of the report, as well as communications in this and a subsequent interview discussed later in this chapter, demonstrated that despite the newly strategized, aggressive advertising by Merck, the pharmaceutical company was not alone in making appeals to the public. The ACS aligned with pediatricians, gynecologists, infectious disease and cancer researchers, and state and non-state public health entities to shape the markets and users of this new cancer prevention. ACS's attention to the increasing *incidence of two HPV-associated cancers*—anal and oropharyngeal—and their call for increased HPV vaccination for girls *and boys* helped configure the uneven and multidirectional politics of vaccine expansion by highlighting the plurality of HPVs and of HPV-associated cancers. It takes hindsight to understand what ensued in the years between when the public was first informed of what researchers had suspected for centuries—that a sexually transmitted infection was associated with the development of cancer—and when Merck began marketing its product directly to consumers to configure its intended market. Ghostly matters punctuate the unfolding of conceptual understandings and approaches to sex and disease.

The ACS claims were different in nature from those advanced in the early years of the transformation in cancer prevention. While ACS and Merck shared a frame of HPV-associated cancer as a preventable disease, the particular diseases that each foregrounded and the bodies they presented as being at risk differed. The 2013 *Report to the Nation* did not exclusively center the girls and girlhoods that had previously dominated commercial advertising and public health messaging for HPV, cervical cancer, and Gardasil. Instead, it was boys and their likelihood of developing rare cancers largely unknown to the public that emerged as important at-risk bodies. And it was HPV vaccine rates among girls and boys that were documented in an effort to show both current trends and needed areas of renewed emphasis. What accounted for the divergence? Was the focus on boys in contrast to Merck's approach, or was it in alignment with, or even driving, the social trajectory of the HPV vaccine? Was ACS one of the various intermediary organizational actors working to configure a new market of prevention? The ACS researchers, especially Simard, were intentional in how they approached the new analysis and especially how it was written up in the report to the nation. As Simard explained, they purposely sidestepped talking about HPV's association with sex. Rather, they chose to emphasize the connection between HPV vaccine and cervical cancer, stating that while they recognize a "big elephant in the room," the way the ACS addresses sex and sexuality is to sidestep this transmission route. The approach of the ACS "from the cancer prevention and control standpoint is to go around it," Simard explained, and to deliberately craft a message for HPV vaccination as "an anti-cancer vaccine." How one is exposed and what one does "behind closed doors" is not important, he told me. "The important thing is to give them these 3 doses and they'll be prevented from ever getting cervical cancer for the rest of their lives."

Merck too had been careful not to risk calling attention to issues of sexuality and sexual transmission when addressing disease indication for boys. As Simard added in our interview, we all "go around it"—we acknowledge it, and say "that's there." After all, "no one wants to think about what their 13-year-old daughter might be doing once they are a freshman in high school. And that's not important really."

Then Simard paused, and chose to render visible the risk groups and practices often hidden behind the strategic construction of an anti-cervical cancer vaccine. "[I]t's very interesting," he told me, "the intersection between anal cancer and HPV." And then he added, "The rates are going up in men and women. But for men it's really driven by HIV. In the absence of HIV, the risk for anal cancer among men is not very great. Not very clear. But in the presence of HIV it's an important co-factor . . . in women it's kind of a different message in terms of what's causing the increasing trend." In making this claim, Simard conjured the ghosts of exclusionary politics and the struggles of gay men for a politics of inclusion in biomedical research and the advancement of "gay men's health" and LGBTQ health as objects of concern. By sexualizing the domain of HPV cancer prevention, and thereby infusing the virus and its transmission with sex and sexualities, he was doing important work guiding medicine and public health where it was needed.

In the ACS report's conclusion, the authors made a compelling case for "additional prevention efforts for HPV-associated cancers, including efforts to increase vaccination coverage." They cite the scientific evidence: First, studies have shown that persistent infection with oncogenic HPV types is etiologically linked to cervical cancer, as well as cancers of the oropharynx, anus, vagina, vulva, and penis. Second, data from clinical trials of HPV vaccines have shown efficacy in preventing vaginal, vulvar, and anal precancers. While no data had yet shown efficacy in preventing lesions of the oropharynx, the authors stated, we can nevertheless assume that the HPV vaccines will prevent these cancers, given their efficacy in preventing HPV 16.[22]

The ACS report to the nation, and Simard's words, were making visible a risk and constructing a narrative—one that HIV doctors and gynecological oncologists already knew to be routine: While overall numbers were and had always been relatively small, anal cancers were "on the rise" in both men and women (American Cancer Society 2014, National Cancer Institute 2014). With this increased emphasis, however, a concern was raised around the estimated incidence of anal cancer in men who have sex with men living with HIV. This population group, they argued, held the "greatest" proportionate incidence: approximately 100 cases per 100,000 person-years (American Cancer Society 2014, National Cancer Institute 2014). ACS was presenting an epidemiological picture of the risk and incidence of cancers in adolescent boys and young men. Simard emphasized to me the importance of HPV vaccination for boys, as well as the use of anal screening as secondary prevention for HIV+ men and women in the US. He wondered whether such screening should be further extended to all MSM.

Desexualizing Boys' Risk, Promoting
a Gender-Neutral Vaccine

In an update to the "One Less" advertising campaign for girls, in late 2011 Merck began a campaign for boys. The ads, which I refer to as the "Both" campaign (I never learned the official name, if there was one), portray young teens using a binary gender logic: boys and girls are pictured separately, on either side of the page, each "character" individually enclosed in its own frame, thereby conveying a symbolic separation or even the suggestion of (sibling) kinship. The relationship between the characters is decidedly differentiated and certainly not sexual. These were the first advertisements to include images of boys as protagonists. In one Both ad, male and female are designated with the pictograms for male ($\male$) and female ($\female$), and the gendered normative colors blue and red are used to collectively and clearly demarcate their difference. Boys appear with a blue circle drawn around their heads; girls appear with a red-hued (or is it hot pink? you might wonder) circle. The words "boys" and "sons" are in blue, and the words "girls" and "daughters" are in red. The glyphs for man and woman are combined but bisected by color. The presumed audience for the ad is not peers of the young people depicted; instead, parents are urged to learn about the ways their children are "affected by HPV." The carefully selected words of this new campaign preserve an ambiguity as to what the precise "effect" is of vaccinating one's child with Gardasil. What protection the vaccine might convey and to whom is not made clear.

Nonetheless, boys and their parents looking at this ad were likely already well-schooled in the cancer protection Gardasil provided for girls, given the multimedia and pervasive advertising that had already appeared. In 2011, the vaccination completion rate (all three doses) for adolescent girls was about 35 percent (Curtis et al. 2014). Now, it seemed, pharma was once again attempting to sidestep sexual matters and desexualize the now known risks of genital warts and penile and anal cancers that HPV posed for all genders. More specifically, the ads divert attention from any potential homo(sexualization) of cancer prevention a campaign against anal cancer might pose. Sexual politics continued to shape vaccination processes as boys struggled for inclusion in vaccination; the terms of this inclusion remained somewhat shaky. Were boys being offered the chance to protect themselves against genital warts (a known STI) and a future related cancer, or the opportunity to contribute to herd immunity and thereby participate in cancer prevention more broadly?

With the message that "Both" could become "One Less" (person with cancer), Merck built on its existing message to parents—especially mothers—to be "aware," "know the link" between HPV and disease, and do the responsible thing: get their children vaccinated for their direct benefit. Mothers were told both their daughters *and* sons share a risk of disease associated with HPV. While girls' sexual risk was largely suppressed within the messaging—even as ideas about sexuality were hard to fully tame, given the conversations about age of sexual onset and the fears of sexual promiscuity that were sparked in the early years—it was unclear if gender and sexuality (which are always already intersecting) would remain masked as HPV and Gardasil expanded to include all genders. Would Merck convince boys and their parents of the need to protect themselves from a sexual risk of genital warts or from the threat of another cancer and their own cancer risk? Perhaps Merck might even convince boys and their parents that vaccinating boys is not only the best approach to protect men's health, but the right approach to protect girls from the risk of cervical cancer via herd immunity.

Media reacted to the ambiguity and lack of clear direction in the new messaging: "What's in it for boys?" asked the *New York Times* science journalist Roni Caryn Rabin, in her 2011 article, "A Vaccine May Shield Boys Too." In her coverage of FDA news, Rabin directly posed an important set of questions: Should boys be included in vaccination to help prevent the spread of HPV to girls? Should they be included based on the protection of their bodies from a cancer risk, or based on protection against the risks associated with an otherwise non-deadly but generally troublesome STI, genital warts? Up to this point, the *New York Times* had emphasized that Gardasil ostensibly offered little to boys aside from what Rabin described as "a selfless opportunity to curb the sexual transmission of HPV to future sexual partners." While a common health threat, "genital warts aren't cancer." Yet, a growing body of evidence linking HPV to cancers in men would eventually emerge to provide the evidence needed to encourage pediatricians and parents to find something "in it for the boys" (Rabin 2011).

Evidence came from Merck's own clinical studies: for men who have sex with men the vaccine protects against anal cancer, and possibly other cancers as well. The trial included several hundred MSM serving as an exposure group and receiving HPV vaccination; three years later this group was significantly less likely than an unvaccinated group to have developed early signs of disease. Rabin (2011) asked in the *New York Times* why experts had dismissed the idea of a vaccination campaign aimed at these young gay men, or addressing anal cancer risk in women.

The answer can be found with the CDC and others who advocated for careful avoidance of anything sexual. In 2012 they asked doctors to navigate away from mentions of STIs in advocating vaccination, thereby de-sexualizing the domain of cancer prevention. These hesitancies have stakes for health care and public health, as they affect vaccine information, tar-get groups, and uptake. In 2013, vaccine completion rates reported based on NIS (National Immunization Survey)-Teen data had only inched up for US girls, to 37.6 percent; boys' completion rates (over a shorter time frame) were lower, at 13.9 percent (Stokley et al. 2014), with rates vary-ing by state (Alabama had a 9 percent completion rate among boys in 2014—Reagan-Steiner et al. 2015). (In comparison, it is estimated that 31.1 percent of girls and women aged ten to twenty in Europe had com-pleted an HPV vaccine series by October 2014—Bruni et al. 2016). These low rates were despite the vaccine's endorsement by the CDC, the Ameri-can Cancer Society, the American Academy of Pediatrics, leading cancer centers, and others. As risks of cancer began to emerge, later another "rare cancer" of the head and neck would also be shown to be on the rise, prompting renewed calls for inclusion of boys that did not include stigma-tized sexual identities and practices.

Calling All Boys! To "Know HPV"

In late 2015, the FDA approved the use of a nine-variant HPV vaccine, HPV9, for males ages sixteen to twenty-six (it was approved for use in girls in 2014). The nine-variant vaccine would immediately become the only vaccine available on the US market.[23] Gardasil 9 would be administered in two doses instead of three when started "before the 15th birthday," at a cost of US$238.50 per dose, not including office visit or administration fees (Merck & Co. Inc. 2021c). This cost had been negotiated by Gavi, the Vac-cine Alliance (GAVI), down to as low as US$4.50 per dose when purchased in bulk by the lowest-income countries (GAVI 2021).[24] By 2016, with evi-dence of the HPV-cancer link mounting steadily, and especially in light of the vaccine's new approval, health experts would be asked to deploy a new strategy for vaccine adoption—"don't talk about sex" (McKay 2016). In October of that year, the US Centers for Disease Control and Preven-tion called on doctors to quiet the talk of STD prevention. Doctors, they argued, should talk up the vaccines' ability to prevent deadly cancers as a way to persuade skeptical parents to protect their kids (Sagonowsky 2016). Bringing boys ages nine to seventeen, and then young men ages eighteen to twenty-six, into this health message would follow a path that was dif-ferent from, yet no less choppy than, for the message aimed at teen girls and young women. In 2016, with an updated "One Less" campaign produced by Merck, boys would stare into cameras asking, "Mom, Dad . . . Did you know?."

In June 2016 Merck launched the awareness ad "Know HPV." This ad began a major shift when it placed parents of "sons" and gendered boys as central actors in HPV risk and prevention. Masculine-presenting young people appeared on their own and relationally alongside girls. The new media blitz, developed with media partner BBDO Worldwide, was shaped by and constitutive of a twenty-first-century digitization of health. The ads, which stopped short of naming the newly approved-for-boys vaccine, transmitted a fresh take on the One Less message across Facebook, Twitter, and YouTube feeds, as well as through various television and cable channels during family viewing hours, including during major sports events such as the 2016 Rio Olympics.

While reminiscent of the earlier non-branded information ads from 2005 that told girls to "know the link," these ads spoke directly to parents about their boys. As the *Washington Post* interpreted it, these ads aimed at "a tender spot: parents' worries about doing right by their kids" (McGinley 2016). With vaccine rates as low as they were, these ads relied not on outright promotion but on what psychologists refer to as "anticipatory regret," or a sense of feeling the negative consequence *before* one makes a choice, as if the choice is already the wrong one. Advertising, including the Know HPV campaign, has relied on a similar formula of provoking a feeling among consumers of a potential negative outcome and sense of regret if they make the wrong decision, an approach that activates consumer behavior based on a fear of missing out on health.

Appealing to parents, again with youth speaking directly to the camera—and ostensibly into their parents' eyes—this campaign began the work needed to convince parents that their preteen sons should receive the HPV vaccine along with girls. In the US, three commercial spots, in three contiguous and escalating narratives, were designed to fill in knowledge gaps and bring cancer risk forward as a well-known risk to the bodies and lives of girls and women that is *also* shared by boys. iSpot.tv, an advertising metrics company that documents the titles, descriptions, viewership, and other data on television and streaming ads, included the ads for Gardasil in their research archive, which is available to the public (https://www.ispot .tv/ad/Ap1V/merck-hpv-vaccination).

Three spots made up the Know HPV video campaign: "It's Personal: What Will You Say?"; "I Knew"; and "Who Knew: Cancer." Collectively they galvanize fear and worry about cancer—rather than about an STI. The first spot (ID:1358469/2016), a sixty-second video titled "It's Personal: What Will You Say," first aired in June 2016 and ran through most of 2019.

It begins with a still image of a young boy that quickly shifts to video of an adult woman who looks directly into the camera and says, "I have cervical cancer." This (presumably white) woman pauses momentarily and adds: ". . . from the HPV virus." The focus at first seems to be on the girl protagonist with its message of the link between adulthood and adolescence, and between risk and disease. The majority of the commercial focuses on the woman and her younger self as a girl, but by the end the story shifts to a boy—the same boy who was featured in a later 2019 advertisement for "I Knew."[25]

The images of the woman travel backward in time along her life course: her time as a young adult woman as she shows off her college dorm room, then as a teenager off to the prom and symbolically on the brink of hetero-womanhood, then back further as an active adolescent in a soccer uniform tossing the ball on a field, and finally as a preteen eating ice cream in a car and blowing out the candles on a birthday cake. She smiles throughout. The adult narrator returns to say that there is a vaccine that "could have" protected her "way before" she was exposed to HPV. As the woman reports her cancer diagnosis, it's a dire warning for those who are eligible to get vaccinated, to avoid being diagnosed later in life. The last image is the preteen birthday girl, presumably around eleven years old, looking directly into the camera: "Mom, Dad," she says with a sense of importance, asking what they have to say now. "Did you know?"

White text scrolls across a red screen, as if urging viewers to recognize the emergency and to stop and take notice. The bold white letters inform: "Who knew HPV could cause cancer and certain diseases in Girls?" What happens next is significant: the white text on this same red screen shifts to "and boys. . . ." It is here in the very last seconds of the TV spot that boys' inclusion is introduced. This ad evokes the early (2005–2006) campaigns for HPV and Gardasil featuring an adolescent can-do girl playing soccer. Here, in contrast, the musical overlay does not suggest active defiance, with chants reminiscent of collective organizing or team sports; rather, it conjures a sense of danger as slow piano music plays ominously in the background. As the video slows to the ending birthday scene, some viewers may recognize the trope used in cancer prevention messaging more generally of a finite number of candles and birthdays.

The next two TV spots use a similar reverse time convention, but begin the story with a male protagonist. Spot 2 (ID1358469), "I Knew," begins with a young (presumably white) man. He looks into the camera, telling the audience: "I was infected with HPV—maybe my parents didn't know how widespread HPV is," he says with a puzzled expression.

"Maybe they didn't know I would end up with cancer because of HPV."

"Maybe my parents just didn't know."

As he speaks, the ad shows a flashback sequence, from high school graduation to a kid doing homework in his bedroom, to a very young boy riding in a car. The flash ends with a preteen boy (the age of vaccine eligibility) standing outside school with a backpack slung over his shoulders. "Maybe they didn't know. . . . Maybe they didn't know there was a vaccine to protect. . . . Maybe they didn't know I would end up with cancer. . . ." He speaks into the camera, asking his parents directly, "Right, Mom? Dad?" The three-part campaign concluded with spot 3 (ID: 1535751), which ran from spring 2017 through 2018. This video's protagonist is a young (presumably Black) woman. The backward composition begins with an image of a young girl that flips to herself as an adult: "I have cervical cancer." She reflects on how many people don't know about the link between HPV and certain cancers as images wind back through her life, ending again with a preteen, the age of HPV vaccination, standing in a kitchen alone, looking somber and staring directly into the camera, asking, "Mom? Dad? Did you know?" In thirty seconds, she evolves from an adult woman with cancer to a brooding preteen, active not in preventing cancer but in enrolling adults as guilty and negligent parties whose lack of knowledge led to their child's cancer. White text on a red screen asks parents, "What will you say?" The three-part series brings adult viewers into responsibility, and some blame. A question from children to adults prompts adult viewers to imagine a response, and children to confront their own aging parents as they ask if *they* had known what could have been prevented.

The final narration is the same in all three ads: "Talk to your child's doctor today," and "Learn more at HPV.com."

Each clip ends with the introduction of "and boys" as Merck urges parents (the generation who is at risk of cancer and may in fact have already been diagnosed) to get their children vaccinated. If parents don't heed this warning, perhaps they will have to say something more dire once their children become adults diagnosed with what was a preventable disease. "What will you say? Don't wait!" At best, this approach can be read as a means to enroll parents in the will-to-health of their children; at worst, it can be seen as a form of shaming parents (Pflanzer 2016). Many did not welcome the personal attacks they perceived to be leveled at parents, and particularly mothers, in the advertisements. Laurie McGinley (2016), for example, in the *Washington Post*, accused the company of guilt-tripping mothers by using familiar tropes of mother-blame. Twitter was abuzz with similar assertions, and as McGinley reported, many others opposed the approach of these direct-to-consumer ads.

The informational ads never mention Gardasil. They subvert any potential sexualization, and especially homosexualization, of boys and men, mirroring the cancer prevention narrative of previous campaigns. Boys are carefully curated as independent, as they too speak to the camera and place the responsibility for their health squarely on their parents. Merck had, indeed, set its sights beyond these early rollouts to adolescents and their parents, and looked toward young adult men in the same way they had with women. As early as 2009, in a company statement, Merck was reported as "firmly committed to achieving greater vaccination rates in the 19-to-26 age group" (Staton 2009). And they were still hoping for approval for new indications—for boys and for women up to age forty-five—from the FDA. This first step would be achieved with Gardasil 9.

With Age Expansion, There Is Something In It for the Boys

What was a weak and optional suggestion to vaccinate boys in 2011 was followed in 2015 with a clear message. The CDC advisory committee, ACIP, this time recommended routine vaccination of boys aged eleven to twelve and included a "catch up" recommendation for boys up to age twenty-one. Further, they added a recommendation of vaccination up to age twenty-six for men who have sex with men (MSM) and for any immunocompromised persons. These age cutoffs persisted until June 2019, when ACIP harmonized recommendations so that catch-up vaccination is recommended for all through age twenty-six following Merck's application to the FDA for approvals of Gardasil 9. Age had always been a consideration in protection, and one that illustrated the surveillance of sexuality along with disease risk. Age of sexual onset and thus risk of transmission differed by geography, gender, and familial expectations. HPV incidence, evidence showed, was high among young people within the first few years after initiating sexual activity; delaying HPV vaccine initiation as people become sexually active, we are told, leaves individuals vulnerable to HPV infection, and specifically to HPV-genomic type infection and persistence, and the threat of later disease. Following approval of Gardasil 9 (in late 2018) as a vaccine for "all people" ages nine to forty-five, a target group that was gender-neutral the most inclusive yet emerged as responsible for their health. In *New York Times* reporting (Grady and Hoffman 2018), Dr. Peter Marks, director of the FDA's Center for Biologics Evaluation and Research, was interviewed and asserted that this is "an important opportunity" in the prevention of all HPV-related diseases and cancers, especially in a "broader age range."

Behind the scenes the celebrations were not focused just on age. It was the fight for "gay" inclusion that helped fuel this age expansion. Research had shown that vaccinating HIV+ MSM aged twenty-seven and older following diagnosis and treatment for anal lesions proved to be effective in reducing cancer incidence (squamous cell carcinoma of the anus, or SCCA) and saving costs (Deshmukh et al. 2015). The scientists conducting the study had called for age expansion specifically to protect these men. Evidence showed that vaccinating individuals who have already been diagnosed with "pre-cancer" could also decrease the risk of cancer's return and/or progression after treatment. Once again, anal cancer was in the spotlight: post-treatment HPV vaccination was recognized as having the potential to decrease the lifetime risk of anal cancer, lower health care costs of treating patients for recurrence and cancer, and improve their life expectancy and quality of life (see Deshmukh et al. 2017).

Anticipating the approvals and new market expansion, Merck's Gardasil website incorporated a new campaign, titled "Get Versed" or "Versed on HPV," which also ran on Instagram and Snapchat in April 2018. (A YouTube video series followed, but was taken down before we could capture its content.)[26] The Versed messaging, launched two years after the 2016 updated "Know the Link" campaign, established boys not as implicated actors or companion figures in adolescent vaccinations, but as lead protagonists, fully informed and ready for action. Here, Merck and its public relations firm, Klick Health, brought a collective of teens and young adults together with their own will to knowledge.[27] These young people were in the know, asking their peers to also "Get Versed on HPV." The campaign included its own website,[28] depicting young models wearing fashionable hoodies among a group of musically "versed" friends striking various poses along a white backdrop or captured in action hanging out with friends and playing music. The campaign made full use of the increased digitization of biomedicalization, which firmly established social media as a key channel in the promotion and distribution of disease awareness and pharmaceutical product campaigns. This included everything from patient-led calls for inclusion on YouTube to crowdfunding: the digital media sphere further collapsed distinctions among corporate and public entities (even as corporate power and reach far outweighed that of any individual, organization, or patient group). As reported in *FiercePharma*, an online industry coverage publication, "'Versed' went beyond social media, too, but in keeping with its street-raised brand aims, the campaign stayed off mainstream media. Instead, it went to college campuses and music festivals and rode the subways. It even showed up in a pop-up stunt at the end of New York Fashion Week" (Bulik 2019).

Yet, as Klick sought to configure a market for its HPV vaccine campaign that included all genders, silence somehow continued to linger around

LGBTQ and diverse sexual practices; and this silence continued to influence the ways gender, sex, and disease are entangled in a politics of health and illness. Sex and sexuality were proven yet again to be hard to tame in the context of a sexually transmitted virus—even as the virus was the object of a now well-known and effective vaccine solution. Extending the age range for vaccine recommendations allowed boys and men to walk side by side with girls in reducing cancer risk associated with HPV.

At first glance, "Get Versed" reflects a "politics of inclusion," as it establishes boys and young men as fully versed in the need to get vaccinated. "HPV doesn't discriminate. It can affect someone of any gender or sexual orientation," the ad states, asking them to "Get VERSED on HPV." Images depict pairs and groups of young people who appear as gender- and racially diverse, a contrast to previous campaigns with young boys alone with cameras. They deserve credit for embracing youth and parents alike who are trying to make sense of vaccination and the ways that their bodies and lives include sexual and other health negotiations.

"Get Versed" (no longer running) was designed to inform and thereby configure a market that includes young men. The task then was to degender Gardasil and HPV from a girl's vaccine aimed at addressing a concern for cervical cancer to one that includes boys. The campaign, however, was somewhat silent about LGBTQ sexual lives specifically, although it includes gender and sexual ambiguity. *FiercePharma* described the campaign as young adults outfitted "in fashion-forward hoodies, hats and T-shirts branded with a modern 'Versed' logo" who showed up where young people already are: on social media platforms such as Instagram and Snapchat, and in digital channels like YouTube. They did not go to mainstream media, instead asking young adults to "speak for themselves" (Bulik 2019) and get vaccinated.[29] Friends are intimately connected in what appears to be four heterosexual pairs. The campaign does endeavor, however obliquely, to enroll diverse sexual risks, practices, and identities. The Versed website's quiz asks users to click on "I am not the type of person who has to worry about HPV," where they learn that "HPV can affect people of any gender or sexual orientation. HPV can be transmitted through any type of sexual activity with someone who has HPV." Speaking to its audience, one actor states, "I always use condoms, All good then?"

This is the first time that a Gardasil ad makes explicit reference to or offers information on sex and sexual transmission: "Condoms only cover so much. HPV can affect areas that aren't covered. So while condoms might lower the risk of getting HPV if used all the time and correctly, they don't fully protect you against the virus. There are other ways to protect yourself, like abstinence, limiting the number of sexual partners you have, and, for women, routine cervical cancer screenings." When ACIP convened following the FDA's approval of Gardasil 9 in 2019, they updated vaccine recommendations using the language of "shared clinical decision-making" for those aged twenty-seven to forty-five years. The American Cancer Society disagreed. On July 9, 2020, the ACS rejected ACIP recommendations for shared clinical decision making (and lowering the recommended age for HPV vaccination to include nine- to twelve--year-olds), citing lack of data supporting the claim of its effectiveness (Saslow et al. 2020). ACS was endorsing an equality approach and one that explicitly addresses sex: boys and girls should be vaccinated between nine and twelve to increase the number of cancers prevented; as Saslow at the ACS stated, this early age parity is recommended to ensure that vaccination takes place before young people become sexually active (what is often referred to as sexual onset).

There are few alternative tools for HPV prevention available. Unlike the case of STIs more generally, including HIV, very little research or public promotion has been done to answer the question of whether condom use or other "safe sex" practices could reduce the risk of transmission. The "Get Smart about HPV" (no longer available for viewing) part of "Versed" was based on small clips of young men and women producing a documentary or perhaps an Instagram clip. They travel the streets, asking young people if they know what HPV stands for and that it can cause cancer and other disease. A young woman provides the facts, as a group of young men, teenage boys, laugh awkwardly at their own ignorance. These two-minute videos with young people are designed to assess their knowledge and expose boys' information deficits. "NOPE" is spelled out in large letters across one young man's face—a young man who waspart of the group that had previously struggled to answer the question "What is HPV?" Did you know "you can be infected and pass it on to someone else without even knowing?" asks the interviewer, explaining that HPV is a symptomless disease and one they, as sexual beings, are responsible for transmitting.

This symptomless disease centers genital warts. "How much do you know about genital warts?" asks the interviewer—explaining that these warts are contagious and chronic. The campaign concludes by recommending: "Ask your doctor for ways to prevent HPV, including screening and vaccination." As shown in episode 2, another young man's image is overlaid with the bold-type statement "What You Don't Know Could Surprise You" as he enters a room of peers creating a photo shoot. "We Are Creating a Movement," the tagline asserts. Data are presented—"thousands already have it"—shifting adolescents from being in the dark about HPV to seeing the light about HPV and their own and their peers' risk. It is in this campaign that safe sex makes its debut as an approach to prevention, but it is presented as only potentially partially effective: "Condoms Only Cover So Much," the video states, warning that "Tens of Thousands Will Get HPV-Related Cancers This Year." "Are you versed?" they ask.[30] Then, in the fourth and final segment, heterosexuality and men and genital warts (theirs and their partners') become the primary objects of the messaging. A smiling young woman is the first character to appear, accompanied by ominous music. The tagline reads: "What Do You Know About HPV?" With a woman as the lead, the audience assumes she knows *something*, but in this case the question alludes to a risk not of cancer, but of genital warts. Yes, she tells the audience, HPV can cause cervical cancer, but she didn't know it could cause genital warts. A text-only screen documents: "HPV can also cause cancer in men." It then flashes to two young men, one with a baseball cap on backwards, both looking befuddled and a bit concerned. The tagline switches to: "What you don't know could surprise you." The final scene, a group of young—and ostensibly recently informed—people stand together and vow, "Let's Be the Ones . . . Who Refuse to Stay in the Dark." It is young men who join young women in making a vow and a difference. This time sex and sexuality are allowed to land on masculinity and heterosexuality, as boys and men consider the usefulness of condoms.

There is something in it for the boys, we come to realize. Over time, increased attention to HPV as a causal agent in cancers of the anus and oropharynx shifted attention from a girls-only approach, bringing renewed attention to the ways sex and sexuality play out in technology development and diffusion. These efforts demonstrate the volatility of the politics of sexuality, as well as the difficulties Merck and its allies confronted in their attempts to keep sex under wraps. The persistent appearance of sexuality and aggressive attempts to banish sex from view—efforts characterized less by simple repression of sexuality than by a proliferation of discourses and practices relating to sexuality, health, and the body—continued to be aimed at managing populations in the service of social ends (Foucault 1980, Rose 2007). While girls and cervical cancers were the primary objects of HPV vaccines that shaped girls as "pre-sexual" and innocent actors, a quiet story of gender and sexual "inclusion" appeared to ignite and then tame boys' sexualities, as boys took action to "get versed" as young adults.

[CHAPTER THREE]

The Cancer That Dare Not
Speak Its Name

When a new professional society dedicated to the study and treatment of a rare cancer held its inaugural scientific meeting, I made sure to attend. The cancer, once associated mostly with elderly women, and otherwise not very well known, was said to be on the rise.[1] If the public was paying attention to Merck's advertisements for Gardasil and the growing evidence they highlighted around HPV's role in various diseases, they may already have been aware of the "new" cancer risk presented, especially to certain subgroups. Not only had cases of the cancer that was drawing novel interest, anal cancer, quadrupled between the 1990s and 2013; its incidence was also strongly correlated with HIV infection, which was shown to have reached epidemic proportions in the US only a few years earlier (Jemal et al. 2013).

At the scientific meeting of the International Anal Neoplasia Society (IANS), I sat in an audience gathered for three days of information exchange, collaboration, and training activities. I listened to the opening remarks and presentations, paying careful attention to the talk of risk and prevention. A leading address referred to "the beginning of a 'major discussion,'" of what was called, emphatically, "the cancer that dare not speak its name."

The speaker's choice of words was intentional, signaling an end to a discursive silence—and silencing—that he hoped the professional membership before him would join him in breaking. It was "time to tell the world" about this cancer, he said, emphasizing the assembled group's collective responsibility to "reduce stigma," "fight taboo," and ultimately bring this cancer into the open. "This is our coming out event," the speaker proclaimed.

With these remarks, the speaker was drawing attention to another, related concern also once shrouded in silence: homosexuality. Here, however, he was referring to the cancer's oft-clinging association with the anus and with anal sex. He did so with a bit of fun, calling on providers to indeed "dare" to go where one has been told not to: in clinical terms, the acronym "DARE" refers to the digital anal rectal examination used to check for anal abnormalities. For this speaker, anything to do with the anus (e.g., anal health, anal cancer, and anal sex) had been made to dare not speak its name in the same way any and all sex and physical intimacy between men had been tacitly suppressed; now "coming out" could refer not just to one's sexual identity, but to anyone affected by anal cancer—be they patients, medical researchers, or other professionals.

"Coming out," in the well-known historiography of the term, refers to several things at once. First, it is an act of proclaiming same-sex desire and sexual practice, an identity as lesbian, gay, bisexual, transgender, or queer (LGBTQ), and thus of demanding to be seen and recognized. Second, it is also a sign that you are part of a broader community, a gender- and sexuality-inclusive LGBTQ+ or otherwise expansive gender and sexual community. It indicates coming out *from* secrecy (and its metaphorical closet and silence) *into* social visibility. Coming out had taken on its political meaning in the context of the 1970s "post-Stonewall" liberation movements and then the spate of highly publicized celebrity "outings" of the 1980s. Initially associated closely with political struggles to destigmatize—and fight for political rights, social visibility, and inclusion of—LGBTQ people, coming out traditionally told the outside world of what had previously been hidden from (their) sight, in order to mitigate and counter stigma and discrimination. It has since spread to more individualized and common use as a way to share information and tell others of one's previously undisclosed identities, communities, behaviors, and desires.[2]

But to be gay and in the closet throughout the twentieth century was also, for many, a way of life as much about protection from overt stigma and shame as about pursuing or enacting freedom in the formation of community. "Coming out" referred to a practice of acknowledging identity or desire to oneself, and then communicating that identity to others who share in your identity and with whom you could create a vibrant life. Only later in political struggles around rights to employment, health care, and marriage, for example, did the shift congeal around a specific experience of some individuals who were "in" by virtue of passing and secrecy and now could "come out" for celebration, politics, and/or to gain belonging in familial and social communities.

When the conference speaker at this inaugural meeting announced a coming-out party, they drew attention to a shared understanding as an outward call, invoking the political gay liberation movement's rallying cry to come out of the secrecy of the closet. Indeed, the meeting featured a jubilant drag performance not just as entertainment, but as a counternarrative to the legitimacy of sociocultural and political stigmatization and discrimination around queer gender and sexuality. The concept had an elasticity that was used to generate and amplify discourse around a cancer and a body part that had each been variously suppressed, and when put into discourse often carried stigma or shame. The meeting marked the first convening of a group of about a hundred clinicians, researchers, health advocates, and patient groups dedicated to the prevention and treatment of anal cancer; it was also the formation of a new community of researchers, clinicians, advocates, and activists who called upon mainstream medicine to recognize their place in medical prevention and care.

The latest figures (from 2021) estimate that approximately 9,090 adults—twice as many women as men—will be diagnosed each year with anal cancer in the US, and of those, about 1,430 will die. These predicted annual diagnoses are over 60 percent (to be precise, 62.77 percent) higher, and deaths almost a third greater, than those estimated for cervical cancer (American Cancer Society 2021). Officially designated a "rare cancer," it is in fact a rising cancer concern, as shown by epidemiological evidence that anal cancer incidence is increasing at a significant rate of about 2.2 percent per year, with death rates increasing an average of 3.1 percent each year in the US (Surveillance Research Program 2019). Numerical reports of findings obscure material uncertainties and important symbolic politics. What is amplified by and what lingers below the surface of these demographic fact-making processes is that a disease, one largely associated with HIV, is on the rise. The demographic story amplifies a gendered and sexual association attributable largely to men who have sex with men (MSM), and for bodies and lives who are HIV positive. Several obfuscations are at work in the ways gender and sexuality come to shape anal cancer research, prevention, and care needs. First, the behavioral risk for all genders and sexualities of the cancer's primary mode of transmission, penile penetrative sex, is obscured when women are not seen as receptive anal sex partners, be it in heterosexual relations or queer ones. Second, the epidemiological narrative obfuscates the ambiguity of the roughly half of HIV-positive MSM who have been diagnosed with what clinicians term high-grade squamous intraepithelial lesions (HSILs), a broad diagnostic category used to describe many cellular abnormalities associated with HPV. This designation, clinically referred to as a "precursor" to cancer, is now estimated to be 80 times more prevalent in HIV-positive MSM than in the general male population (Silverberg et al. 2012). This coming-out party was bringing into visibility cisgender and trans women's bodies and sexual lives, which had been rendered invisible by the gendered sexualization of both HIV and HPV. The speaker acknowledged these ghostly matters as they called for a collective refusal to allow anal cancer to be rendered the province of any one group, or a risk to the "general population." Particularities of bodies and lives cannot be sanitized or erased when the goal is to provide equitable prevention and good care.

Speakers were also careful to broaden the associative links between sexuality and disease from the co-infection of HIV and HPV among gay and MSM as they acknowledged and thanked the speakers as well as conference sponsors in attendance, among them the pharmaceutical and biotechnology companies Merck, Hologic, and QIAGEN. Two leading advocacy organizations were there: the Anal Cancer Foundation (ACF) and the Farrah Fawcett Foundation, whose representatives would speak eloquently of their own organizations' founding and commitments.[3] Web-based research would confirm that the ACF was launched by three siblings whose mother died of anal cancer and who sought to establish an organization dedicated to the disease's eradication. The other organization was established to recognize the renowned actress Farrah Fawcett, who died in 2009. Speakers included children, doctors, and caregivers who emphasized the ongoing and pervasive burden of anal cancer among women as well as the cancer's associated stigma as a disease that provokes speculation about taboo sexual practices. We must "remove stigma and the association with sex," said one speaker.

Speakers sought to "find common ground" by rendering visible women's anal cancer and destigmatizing prior associations of this cancer with sex. These women and their deaths, we were told, were also shrouded in stigma, contributing to a lack of information, research, and care. HPV and HPV vaccination provided a shared object and set of concerns: to prevent this disease through vaccination of our youth and screening for adults, and to address the anus, anal sex, and anal cancer with the open and forthright attention they deserve. The ACF and the Farrah Fawcett Foundation were somewhat typical of many research foundations and health nonprofits that sprang up in the 2000s in response to a lack of scientific and public attention, and to honor those diagnosed with, living with, or having died from a cancer. These advocacy- and education-focused groups were formed to raise funds (and awareness) that could be funneled to social support, research efforts, and education (as well as to support the organizations themselves); to partner with (and make demands of) government, scientists, and clinicians; and to forge community. Yet they were also a departure from the health and social movement organizing for structural change of previous eras, which had emerged largely from political struggles to demand basic data collection and research on diseases of unknown etiology or insufficient medical attention—around HIV, or the role of DES (diethylstilbestrol, a synthetic form of estrogen—Bell 2009) and other toxins in breast and other cancers (Brenner 2016, Klawiter 2008), or environmental injustices such as pesticides affecting farm workers and Superfund sites exposing poor communities to unknown chemicals.

The newer brand of activist organization reflected more fully the twenty-first-century social advocacy born in celebrity-suffused social media than it did the grassroots activism of the twentieth century. It was a culmination of patient movements, now with corporate tie-ins beyond pink ribbons and disease-awareness walks, to include patients in clinical trial recruitment as advocates and patient board members (Klawiter 2008, Sulik 2010, King 2008, Epstein 2007b). As I listened, I heard the speakers convey clearly—despite never putting it into words—that this disease was personal: anal cancer had claimed the lives of people who mattered to the speakers, and the private pain of their families and social circles merited public exposure. Their approach reflected what the sociologist C. Wright Mills (1959) meant when he said that personal struggles were public issues that needed to be brought into the light to forge connection, support, and change. Yet something about this cancer made its presence less conspicuous—quieter, and more quietened—than that of other cancers; and this quieting was driven by its symbolic association with the perception of anal sexual practices as taboo. More specifically, the ways these sexual matters have adhered to gay men and MSM—through not just a homosexualization, but also a lingering homophobic and misogynistic linking of receptivity with subordination—played a role in how anal cancer was talked about or not talked about. It was these attributions around which the speakers appealed to "common ground," to a shared goal of quashing stigma around certain sex practices and the people who engage in them.

The cancer meeting called for inclusion of seemingly excluded subsets of people who were epidemiologically significant due to their designation as being at high risk for the onset of this cancer. These subsets included people living with HIV regardless of their gender and sexuality, as well as gay and bisexually-identifying or active men who are HIV negative. Given their ages and, for many, their genders, these subgroups of adults had not been configured as explicit targets of the mass-scale screening protocols of cervical cancers—none of them were "girls of Gardasil." Instead, they were left outside the HPV vaccine's preventive bounds, lingering in its gaps. They signified what the sociologist Steven Epstein (2010) described as a "dialectic of inclusions and exclusions" that shaped the early years of the Gardasil campaigns: the ways some groups are configured as users of a new technology and others remain in the shadows of exclusion. Specifically, it was these populations' HIV status and their adult ages that located them as the already sexually active patients living with another viral disease, and conferred on them the familiar social label of having "at-risk" sexual practices or identities. The women in honor of whom the new philanthropic organizations were founded, however, were not part of this designation. Their sexual risk, if they ever even had any, was shaped by altogether different threats.

At this meeting, as at others, despite the presence of women and diverse genders, and the organizational actors who came to support further research, training, and awareness of anal cancer and its link to HPV, it was mostly MSM and people with HIV/AIDS—whose bodies were already subject to ongoing surveillance due to their disease risk—who were centered in discussions of how to ensure the best prevention and care. Importantly, these individuals were also the patients and clinical trial subjects, as well as the activists and patient advocates, who served as advisory board members for clinical research studies. Their experiences and advocacy shaped the contours of the clinical debates that unfolded over the next three days of meetings about how to prevent anal cancer, what groups to include, and what professional experts and expertise were most appropriate for its jurisdiction.

While vaccination program aims were mired in negotiation over whether to highlight or shroud HPV as an STI prevention, there was an important discursive shift. "Lots of people said an STI vaccine just can't work," said one of the keynote speakers, John T. Schiller, the deputy chief of the Center for Cancer Research at the National Institutes for Health (NIH) and co-principal investigator, with Douglas Lowy, of the scientific research that led to the initial development and characterization of the human papillomavirus prophylactic vaccines in the 1990s.[4] During Schiller's technically focused presentation, he told the audience "I am going to go virologic on you" as he explained why HPV vaccines work so well compared with "other STD vaccines." He spoke of the double-stranded DNA genome, the ways virus-like particles produce antibody response, and the differences in anal and cervical epithelial cells. The two cancers were "basically the same disease biologically," Schiller stated as he made his case in support of the HPV vaccine as a preventive tool for an STI that can lead to cancer. Suddenly it seemed that here—at a cancer meeting—cancer itself was being sidelined, at least for the moment.

A reconfiguration of the meaning of cancer was taking hold, as a virus (specifically an STI) was becoming recognized as central to the shape of this disease. A politics of inclusion and a call for equity underscored Schiller's concern that a vast majority of people remain at risk for developing anal cancer so long as they are unvaccinated. Schiller's claims produced and included new at-risk subjects who were caught in a biomedical failure of their own: with no parallel cancer screening guidelines (to the Pap test) that would reduce their cancer risk and possibly prevent their developing cancer. There were no accepted and scientifically agreed upon guidelines for anal cancer screening, and limited agreement on the best approach to prevention. Schiller had come before this audience to ask what could be done to protect these other groups of at-risk bodies. Specifically, which of our "population groups," he asked, are at risk for developing anal cancer? What are their degrees of risk? And is there a preventive screening tool equivalent to the Pap test that can be used to protect anal health and reduce anal cancer risk?

HPV-anal cancer associations compelled drug companies to deploy a politics of prevention and associated inclusion in biomedical offerings that differed from the one which had emerged in the early promotion of a new vaccine aimed at girls. In this evolving case, a politics of prevention would take hold that was marked by debates around how best, and whom, to enroll not in vaccination, but in HPV-associated disease screening as a prevention tool for cancer. Scientists, practitioners, and patients were collectively asking how to "make the Pap smear work" for the prevention of anal cancer in the same way it has worked for the prevention of cervical cancer. They were drawing on the well-known "women's health" preventive practice of the Pap test, a cytology approach used to identify lesions and cellular abnormalities in another "epithelial zone" [skin] of the body. When abnormalities are found, referral to colposcopy and biopsy of "early" clinical findings can prevent invasive cancer. The Pap test's use is limited to the cervix and, for the most part, to the professionals who hold jurisdiction over "women's health." There was no analogous screening standard for its use in and on the anus, nor for expanded use beyond cis women, trans men, or gender queer people with cervices. If an anal Pap was going to be included in preventive medicine guidelines, as the cervical Pap test had been decades before, both vocal transparent debate, as well as more quiet negotiations, would be needed (Clarke and Casper 1996). In 2013, there was neither scientific consensus on the best approach nor useful scientific evidence to bring an anal cancer screening tool into the prevention apparatus. The only thing that was clear was the growing concern that anal cancer was on the rise, with its own particularities (albeit also with ambiguities) over who was at risk. Starting that year, and continuing in the years since, the IANS meetings have taken on the technical, social, and cultural work needed to make the anal Pap test the right tool in the prevention of this HPV-associated cancer.

Screening tools are most often developed from prior diagnostic approaches that follow symptom reports in patients, with a renewed goal of developing a standard for early detection. In anal cancer diagnoses, the high-resolution anoscopy (HRA) was in place as an approach to visualize and assess disease presence and stage, followed by biopsy of cellular abnormalities. Could this diagnostic tool be incorporated into a preventive approach in the same way the cervical colposcopy is used in cervical cancer screening, following an "abnormal" Pap test? Many clinicians were already relying on HRA, acting on their professional judgment and the best interest of their patients. Adding any new tool to a preventive regime on a mass scale requires the development of a well-articulated and targeted protocol that has been clinically proven effective and has gained professional consensus. Making the anal Pap the preventive tool of choice would require not only scientific evidence, but also careful navigation of the complex ways gender and sexuality intersect with health politics.

When the inaugural meeting of the IANS was referred to as a coming-out party, the speaker rendered visible gay and bisexual men and MSM, and their health care needs. An implication was made that while queer sexual practices and lives are, in many places, no longer pathologized, stigmatized, or medicalized, a silence persists around the anus, anal sex, and anal cancer. While sex practices involving the anus are not the exclusive province of any one group, they nonetheless often symbolically cling to the bodies, identities, and lives of one or more groups, but not those of others. "The anus is a body part we all have." It is this body part, audiences would be told, that must be discussed. How might a proliferation of discourse about this body part, this cancer, and their association with sex in light of the transmission route of HPV follow Foucault's (1980) assertion that it is not the repression of sexuality, but a proliferation of sexual discourse aimed at managing populations in the service of social goals, that matters? Would this appearance of various sexualities linked with disease provoke aggressive attempts to banish it from view?[5]

The attendees at IANS were not primarily trained cancer specialists (as far as I could discern), but gynecologists and infectious disease clinicians, many with clinical specialization in HIV/AIDS. All were finding themselves increasingly caring for HPV-associated health concerns of their patient populations, which consisted of cis women, trans men, and MSM, each and all too old for the HPV vaccine. And importantly, most of those specialists in attendance had joined to receive continuing medical education (CME) training in HRA.

Aside from older adults, the "unvaccinated"—at this time 60 percent of girls and 79 percent of vaccine-eligible boys, as well as pockets among religious opt-outs, migrants and refugees from countries without vaccination or access to vaccination, the underinsured or uninsured or under-medicalized, etcetera—are the potential subjects for cancer screening for

HPV-associated disease. Through what claims-making would some be included while others remained outside its bounds? Until "[a]ll our children are vaccinated," as the Deputy Director from the NIH exclaimed, cancer prevention for these groups would remain limited to secondary screening practices such as cervical Pap tests, anal screening, and penile and oral cancer checks. Consequently, those most excluded from biomedical protection would likely remain in a state of precarity. Thus, the questions pervading this scientific meeting were: What kinds of screening tools are possible? At what frequency might they be the "right tool" for prevention? And for whose bodies and lives?

Politics of Cancer Screening: Categories of Risk and the Ghostly Hauntings of HIV/AIDS

Social categories such as race, gender, and sexuality, as well as medical and social categories like "underinsured," "unvaccinated," or those with clinical "biomarkers" of disease, are embedded in the ways cancer "risk" is understood and acted upon. Who and what is included and excluded in scientific and medical practice—specifically, in this case, in the screening technologies and professional and policy guidelines in place to assess risk of and prevent anal cancer are epistemic politics (Hess 2004).[6] Questions about whom to include, using which claims, and how to implement their inclusion in biomedicine reflect struggles around knowledge and practice as various "expert" actors and their organizations attempt to minimize uncertainties and maximize categories of significance for intervention or non-intervention.

With the HPV-anal cancer prevention link, epistemic politics cluster around evidence of who and what constitutes "high" risk; claims of commensurate biologies and thus commensurate practices; and finally, the arena of clinical trial development. Separately, and at times together, these politics temper uncertainty and produce claims to support inclusion. Claims pivot on inequitable treatment and, by extension, demand for biomedical equity as they seek to stabilize preventive politics and a consensus approach to HPV-associated anal cancer prevention. Such claims rest on an assertion that screening for lesions and "pre-disease" risk in alignment with the practices of cervical cancer prevention is the needed approach.

Questions lingered about how best to stabilize uncertainties associated with whom to include as subjects of anal cancer prevention and what behaviors or bodily attributes to designate as a "risk." The biological marker for anal cancer is an unstable category: in technical terms a "precursor" to cancer is a "high-grade squamous intraepithelial lesion" (HSIL) or "anal intraepithelial neoplasia" (AIN), both measured on a scale of 1 to 3 designating the depth of the skin in which the cellular abnormalities are located ("1/3" equals one-third thickness; "3/3" equals full skin thickness). HSIL usually corresponds with AIN2/3. These are cancer risk categories as analogous to those used in Pap testing of cells collected from the cervix.

Yet, like HPV itself, these designations are also made without a standard approach, with no stated consensus on best practices for follow-up and/ or treatment of any abnormalities identified. The absence of this medical recommendation is driven by inherent uncertainties: some cases will "regress" or clear on their own without any intervention. As HPVs enter the body, the immune system produces antibodies to resist infection and shed the viral infection. Yet even with strong immune responses, the virus can find shelter in small and hidden crevices of the body (the cervix or anus, or deep in the back of the throat) and persist there to cause later cellular abnormalities. HSIL or AIN are classifications that indicate these changes, yet they also operate much like HPV itself; their presence may be necessary, but they are also insufficient to cause the later onset of cancer (that is, like HPV itself they may regress and clear on their own).

This classification, then, is socially significant as a risk designation for several reasons. Epidemiologically speaking, HSIL is a "diagnosis" often received by HIV+ gay and bisexual men or MSM whose bodies are more likely to undergo screening tests related to those health statuses. As a result of this more frequent screening, these bodies are more likely to be situated on a continuum of risk requiring more frequent surveillance and more invasive diagnostic procedures (Aronowitz 2009); a vast number of otherwise healthy individuals with HSIL are thus transformed from healthy to "at risk," and through constant surveillance their experience and identities resemble more closely those of people with chronic conditions than those of people at risk for disease. Thus, the epistemic politics of anal cancer prevention reveal themselves as struggles for the production of, and inclusion in, biomedicine's infrastructures of the surveillance and treatment of chronicity.

Disease screening tools and approaches are social and cultural: Their evidence, promotional claims, recommended guidelines, and organization actors are materially and symbolically significant for monitoring and surveilling the body politic. They have the "capacity to define who matters and who does not, who is disposable and who is not" (Mbembe 2003). They convince healthy, asymptomatic people to submit their bodies to routine surveillance for early signs of disease, as well as for ongoing disease surveillance or management. Promoted as diagnostic tools for not only early-stage disease, but also "pre-"disease states, cancer screening tools have brought people variously into risk regimes, as well as making them responsible health actors, population health targets, or both.[7] They can be part of a public health strategy that values community health or a privatized regime that protects individuals. They can align with capital and with power, as some bodies, lives, and communities are over-provided for and others under-cared for or left outside care altogether. With HPV-cancer knowledge came the possibility for expanded and new preventive approaches, including cancer screening tools. The Pap test would undergo rethinking and retooling (as shown in chapters 7 and 8), and so too would the protocols for its inclusion. Despite uncertainties surrounding HPV's clearance and progression, the assumption that if you find cancer early in its progression, and excise it, then a patient has the best chance for survival would endure.

ESTABLISHING "HIGH-RISK" FOR ANAL CANCER

Until the 1990s, anal cancer was thought to be a rare disease mainly affecting elderly women. These cancers among older women had not been a major concern, going largely unnoticed, that is, until a generation of people with HIV began showing up at routine health checks with this disease. A health care infrastructure for HIV/AIDS care and long-established research programs focused on AIDS began to track an unsettling increased incidence of this cancer among people, mostly in their fifties and sixties, living with HIV. Anal cancer was designated a "non-AIDS-defining" illness due to research showing it was more likely to occur in people who are infected with HIV than in people who are not infected, and because it is not part of the symptomology of AIDS itself.

Yet something peculiar happened as this cancer became more well-known due to its causal association with HPV. As the vaccine was introduced to the public, anal cancer remained somewhat hidden, especially for women, even as some men's risk and disease were brought into the light. The medical attention to this rare cancer, now on the rise, rendered men's lives and their suffering more visible, while women's anal cancer, as well as women's risk, remained stigmatized. In 2020, the Society for Women's Health Research (SWHR) held a symposium, "Assessing Gaps and Unmet Needs in HPV-Related Disease," in which they convened experts and patients alike to understand how to improve health outcomes for women with "pre-disease." Anal cancer's gendered and sexualized symbolic association as an "AIDS-defining cancer," and by association as a gay men's health threat, is a ghostly haunting of this cancer and its stakes for prevention and care. The timeline—specifically, the linkage between identity and disease that preceded HPV knowledge and the rollout of the vaccine in the early 2000s, particularly in the emergence of HIV/AIDS in the 1980s—sheds light on the ways sex and disease are often and variously entangled. The connotative meanings that ossified around gay men's lives, risk, and disease were already established given the homophobic linkage of "deviant" sexual practices and presumed sexual excess prior to HIV. The gendering of some gay men and some queer sexualities as feminine because of their receptive anal sex practice (or what is commonly referred to as being the bottom) is steeped in misogyny and belief that receptive sex is the passive position, associated with stereotypes of women and their prescribed roles. These social ideas were embedded in the ways risky behaviors and risky people became synonymous with the health threat of HIV (Patton 1994). The cultural associations drawn in "the earliest period of the HIV epidemic of the 1980s," in which gay men, MSM more broadly, and people diagnosed with HIV came to be associated with disease risk, was forged in stereotypes from earlier decades. Then, these same "risk groups" coalesced into a social movement demanding nondiscriminatory health care. These, I am arguing, shape the contours of anal cancer and anal cancer preventive politics that have unfolded in the decades since.

By 2020, when the SWHR held their symposium on women's anal cancer, the rising incidence of anal cancer was evolving as an epidemiological story with specific gendered, sexual contours: this cancer had increased 2.7 percent each year from 2001 to 2020 (Deshmukh et al. 2020); yet while a greater number of women were diagnosed each year than men, it is subgroups of gay, bisexual, MSM who are shown to be "the most at risk," proportionately speaking, given the significantly higher prevalence of anal cancer among this group as well as among People Living With HIV (PLWHIV) of all genders and sexualities, people with prior anogenital cancers, and people with immunosuppression disorders (Thrift and Chiao 2018). Emily Ortman reported on the meeting held by SWHR, stating that HPV-associated cancers, especially anal cancer, are associated with widespread stigma. When women share their diagnoses, most are met with either silence or the question "How did you catch that?" (Ortman 2020).

The invisibilities and visibilities around health and illness and around anal cancer risk were in part produced before and during the early 1990s. The narrative that "anyone having homosexual sex" had done something excessive with their bodies lingers—an idea forged in biases toward monogamy and narrow and normative sexual regulations suggesting that anything over or outside prescribed ideas of (hetero) gendered sexuality and identity were seen as pathological excess, deviant, and in some cases criminal. This rendering has at times included gay, bisexual, and men who have sex with men as presumptively hyper-visible in ways that placed other lives in the shadows and largely invisible. The stakes for women were also high during the early HIV/AIDS epidemic—women with HIV presented with something amiss in their bodies, yet they were unseen as people with HIV. This similar ghostly haunting played out in the epidemiological narrative and clinical practices clustered around anal cancer prevention, at least until recently.

To see anal cancer, and to render it visible in biopolitics and social hauntings, is to look through a historical context of medical research and the now established requirements for the inclusion of "women and minorities" in health research. It is to see a burgeoning field of health disparities research that incorporates LGBTQ and "sexual minority health" in calls for targeted efforts to understand cancer and other health disparities and to work toward health equity where needed.[8] Research into HIV and research into HPV conjoined in ways that have both reshaped and reignited the cultural politics of AIDS-related stigma, discrimination, and social activist and advocacy demands, many of which were forged inside biomedicine and by medical experts. Anal cancer's preventive politics in the twenty-first century reflect another gendered sexualized dynamic in the ways some are rendered invisible or viewed through stigma and shame. Women's sexual risk, for example, has long been shaped by the discriminatory claims of promiscuity, and especially by the precarity of the lives of poor women, whose sexual bodies have been stigmatized and associated with prostitution, hypersexuality, unwanted pregnancies, and other claims to render them in need of social containment and regulation of their presumptive excess sexuality and risk of disease.

Women had always been significant actors in the patient and activist community around HIV/AIDS—it was the early gendering of HIV as associated with homosexuality and men's bodies that rendered them invisible. Yet women's presence as patients, and more so as activists and health care providers, pushed for a definitional broadening of AIDS itself. It is this haunting that I suspect was felt by the members of the foundation as they appealed to the IANS audience for "common ground" in bringing women's bodies and lives into the calls for guidance in anal cancer research and care, and equity in prevention practices. These ideas are viral, in the social imaginaries that connect sexual transmission with identities, practices, and cultures; they are able to disrupt the ghostly hauntings of invisibility as well as hypervisibility from the past.

The politics around understanding and intervening in HPV-anal cancer grew out of the now professionalized expertise in infectious disease and the umbrella of LGBTQ health, and HIV care in particular. In the 1980s, research found that anal carcinoma was more common in MSM than in the general population (Daling et al. 1987, Daling et al. 1982). Research followed showing that 54 percent of a group of ninety-seven gay men with HIV were also infected with HPV, thereby positing the first link between the HPV virus and a higher risk of anal cancer in men who have sex with men (Palefsky et al. 1990). The epidemiological narrative brought a concomitant sense of urgency: although the number of anal cancer cases is greatest in heterosexual cisgender women in the US, the relative population rates are highest among HIV+ MSM. This latter group—those with higher in-group prevalence—is already subject to ongoing screening and disease surveillance, thereby constituting a population base for ongoing human-subject study about anal cancer and its care and prevention. The statistical claim provoked questioning: would HIV-negative gay men and MSM men, or HPV+ women, be not only at increased risk, but also the subjects in need of preventive care? The metric—a hoped-for analog to the Pap screening tool—of 35 per 100,000 women (Bosman 2019) became the target number to support a screening claim. The cervical Pap test and its screening programs have led to overall cervical cancer reductions of up to 70 percent; could a comparable screening tool for the anus—and the men who were ostensibly most at risk for anal cancer—lead to a similar success? A politics of inclusion in cancer prevention rested on claims of high-risk designations and commensurate biologies and practices—that anal cancer risk and anal cancers hold "facts" analogous to cervical cancer risk and prevention, and therefore can be prevented in much the same way.

This was far from the cancer referenced in the July 1981 headline of the *New York Times* alerting the world to a "Rare Cancer" seen in "Homosexuals." That "cancer" referenced Kaposi's sarcoma (KS), the purple blotches of which had begun to appear on the skin of young gay men in New York and California. The disease was part of a constellation of other conditions not normally found in that population, like pneumocystis pneumonia (PCP), that indicated that something troubling was afoot (Epstein 1996). Given the ways that trouble was discursively associated with a prior construction of a dangerous sexuality, the early virus-cancer associations (of HHV-8 and Kaposi's Sarcoma) led to the designation "gay cancer," briefly standing in for what later became AIDS. This narrative linkage rendered some bodies and lives sources of disease, and thus blameworthy, and others outside of visibility altogether, drawing on associations that preceded AIDS. Stereotypes of gay sexuality as somehow perverse, of Black men's sexuality as somehow suspect, and of (white) children as innocent each and all took root in the early decades of the epidemic. These shaped social activist responses to STOP AIDS and to bring into visibility the rhetorical claims that rendered these lives visible and others invisible. Yet narratives linger shaping the struggles for inclusion in clinical and biomedical infrastructures that would lead to large and globalized forms of HIV exceptionalism (Benton 2015).[9]

Women with HIV were subject to a different disease regime with its own distinctly gendered and sexual contours—part of "reproductive health and medicine" and "cancers of the reproductive tract" that shaped their bodies. While researchers and clinicians took note of the high rates of HIV infection in women's bodies as early as 1983, activists would fight to shift the narrative of a gay men's and largely white disease to reveal the stakes for diagnosis and care for women and for Black, indigenous, and other communities. Racial health disparities were also epidemiologically known as early as 1983, as the heaviest burden of HIV in the US began to fall on Black women (Holmes, Karon, and Kreiss 1990). A gendered and racialized lens that rendered these bodies less visible, and less in need of care, has been aptly named *injuries of inequality* (Watkins-Hayes 2019). The symbolic association between gay sex and white men rendered invisible the overlapping and mutually reinforcing epidemics of violence, drug addiction, and HIV that shaped the health effects and disparities of HIV (Singer and Clair 2003). The story of women's epidemiological "risk" of HIV transmission is unlike that of the gay white men who dominate the popular imaginary; this discrimination productive of risk too often, but not always, includes sexual trauma and violence, as well as proximity to sex work and (sexualized) drug economies (Watkins-Hayes 2019, Cohen 1999, Brier 2009, Hammonds 1997, Hammonds 1990). These power dynamics and inequalities were shaped by the health precarities prior to and during the early HIV/AIDS epidemic, and they would follow these groups into the social imaginary of sexual transmission and its signification, including the ways HIV and HPV became entangled in anal cancer research and prevention politics from gynecology to oncology.

The political contestation around the disease classification for AIDS before there was a standard epidemiological story is found in the early moniker "Women Don't Get AIDS, They Just Die From It," the sarcastic title of a campaign slogan from the Women's Caucus of ACT UP (see Alexis Shotwell's analysis of the ACT UP Oral History Project—Shotwell 2014). Gay men became the standard for AIDS diagnosis, while symptoms women with HIV experienced such as vaginal thrush, pelvic inflammatory disease, bacterial infections, and others were omitted from what became the disease classification for AIDS. As a result, countless women were invisible in the official classification, and subsequently from the infrastructures that count and care for the lives (Shotwell 2014). Yet activists in the Women's

Caucus saw the omission and fought for inclusion of these symptomologies, as well as for a different rendering of risk and disease to ensure a more just provision of care.

Reflective of the ways cis- and transgender women alike struggled to have their embodied experience of disease included in the AIDS response, the politics of prevention around anal cancer brings forward struggles for inclusion among LGBTQ and women's health. HPV-anal cancer associations are unable to shake these symbolic hauntings and present ghosts: women presenting with the distinctive disease symptomology of anal cancer are less likely to be asked about anal sex, and more likely to be excluded from anal screening, even as a politics of inclusion is underway. To bring this to the contemporary epistemic politics and in terms of understanding "high-risk designations," a gynecologist collaborating on a white paper as part of the IANS meeting on high-risk groups told me in an interview: "[W]e don't even know who those women are who have anal cancer. I mean, if you look at anal cancers, we know who are 'high-risk women' [referencing prior anogenital cancers and HIV]. But, if you look at those who have anal cancer, most do not have any high risk. . . . [I]t's really healthy women [referring to women who are HIV negative and otherwise cancer-free] who get anal cancer, but we can't figure out why. And that's the majority of anal cancers—of those with anal cancer—that predominantly are assumed to be healthy heterosexual women."

When classification systems work well, they become infrastructures, making it impossible to see the ways struggles and politics have shaped category formation (Bowker and Star 1999, 2000). People living with HIV and/or diagnosed with AIDS are mostly accustomed to being subjected to a variety of chronic disease surveillance systems, treatment protocols, and risk models to measure "viral loads" and CD4 counts—the measurement of T-cells that indicate the robustness of the immune system—and to assess symptom presentations associated with immunosuppression or medication effects. Some people in some places have access to an "AIDS safety net" medical care and research infrastructure, mostly embedded in sexual health, which exists to provide knowledge and care. A significant and ongoing biomedical infrastructure is found in the Multicenter AIDS Cohort Study (MACS), a thirty-plus-year study of HIV infection in gay and bisexual men that began in 1984. Funded by the US NIH, the study had a first enrollment of nearly 5,000 men, with four medical centers participating in the US. This knowledge source of aging with HIV has enrolled men int the research study in 1987, 2001, and 2014, with data analyzed by thousands of researchers. The structural presence of the population-based cohort has been a factor in the production of the gendered sexualization of

HPV-associated anal cancer, given the capacity to "see" anal cancer in this population group with a higher relative risk than others.[10] The history of AIDS and the research conducted by its many advocates and researchers may have produced the epidemiological categories, but it has also done a great deal to redefine sexual diversities and acts as ordinary. As a result, while the domain of research is sexualized, research has done much to "demoralize" and thereby normalize sex.

While cisgender, heterosexual women are represented in anal cancer rates and risks, the social imaginary and infrastructural practices amplify the gay, bisexual, and other MSM designated as most at risk for anal cancer. As a result of this gendered sexualization, many working within and outside of sexual health organizations, including LGBTQ activists and advocates, have become key actors in the politics of HPV-cancer associations and their prevention practices. It is these voices that are most clearly audible in "fact-making," as professional associations, clinical trial researchers, and patient advisory boards seek to stabilize uncertainties and call for equity and inclusion in HPV-associated cancer prevention regimes. A quieter call for "common ground" is also being voiced by philanthropic organizations formed around women's disease.

Screening as Prevention: Building a Case for Anal Pap Plus HRA

In both the teach-in spirit of AIDS activism and the ways medical professionals were part of the activism and advocacy demanding knowledge and care, appeals among advocates and activists inside and outside biomedicine have been made to "make the Pap smear work" for the prevention of anal cancer in the same way it has long worked for the prevention of cervical cancer. A search for lesions is an obvious next step when symptoms are present; yet Pap tests were made part of a mass-screening approach for cervical cancer prevention starting in the 1960s *regardless*—and mostly in the *absence*—of symptom presentation. The Pap test, as the sociologists Adele Clarke and Monica Casper (1996) argue, was never inherently the "right tool" for cervical cancer prevention, but it was made into the right tool over the course of the latter part of the twentieth century. Through tinkering and negotiations, technical advances as well as social ones, the Pap test became an accepted mass-screening tool. To make the anal Pap the "right tool" for anal cancer prevention would require similar work strategies and negotiations.

The "cervical cancer paradigm" and claims to commensurate biologies and practices drive clinical arguments in favor of anal Pap testing as a secondary screening tool for anal dysplasia and/or its precursors (Summers 2019, Chiao et al. 2006). Given the professional training required to administer the test, it was gynecologists who were the first to train in and deliver anal cancer preventive care to their patient groups. For some of these medical professionals, those groups include gender and sexual minorities and transgender people. The current clinical approach to anal cancer screening comprises two companion technologies: anal ("Pap") cytology and high-resolution anoscopy (HRA) (UCSF Medical Center 2008, MedLine Plus 2012). In the anal Pap, a moistened swab is inserted into the anal canal (unlike for the cervical Pap test, no speculum is needed). Once in contact with the anal surface, the swab is swirled around the canal walls to collect cells, which are then stored and transported—usually in a liquid-based collection vial—for cytology "reading" by a pathologist or cytologist.[11] The cytologist smears the biomaterial (cells collected) onto a slide, applies a stain for visibility, and then places the slide under a microscope for visual reading. The examination identifies the presence or absence of abnormalities based on an accepted protocol depicting a range of cellular compositions, from "healthy" to "pre-diseased" tissue, noting tissue of uncertain composition in the latter category. If cellular uncertainty or abnormality is indicated, clinical referral is made for HRA.

In contrast to the anal swab or Pap, HRA is a relatively new procedure used in the prevention of anal cancer. It was designed and first used in the context of gastroenterology in the 1980s, and was soon thereafter adopted by cancer specialists in the context of oncological gynecology to monitor the anal tissue of women with prior "reproductive" or "anogenital" cancers, as well as for women with HIV who were shown to have specific anogenital abnormalities now known to be associated with HPV co-infection. The technology was then introduced into cancer screening as a gendered tool for the prevention of women's cancers. HRA technology offers the ability to remove cellular areas deemed precancerous or cancerous, or otherwise a risk to health, for biopsy. It uses the same "advanced colposcopic skills," training, and techniques as cervical cancer screening to identify abnormal cells of the anus. In contrast to cervical colposcopy, though, HRA is said to be considerably more complex, and consequently very challenging to execute.[12] Obstetricians and gynecologists, with their expertise in colposcopy (as well as their extensive experience in managing HPV-associated diseases of the cervix, vagina, and vulva), are well situated to learn these advanced techniques and perform HRA; to date they have accounted for the vast majority of clinicians training in HRA skills.

Regardless of who performs the procedure, insurance reimbursements for HRA are only provided upon the report of an abnormality (such as a cytological finding of HSIL or AINS), a history of disease or other abnormalities, or results from a digital rectal examination, which strictly constrains the technology's availability. When abnormalities are identified in an initial anal Pap test, if reimbursement for the follow-up HRA needed to assess the abnormality cannot be secured, it becomes difficult to convince patients, doctors, and especially health care institutions seeking payments, to pay for or otherwise cover the procedure. This means that anal Pap, or cytology, defaults to remaining the first—and sometimes only—step in anal cancer screening. A resulting question emerges: is anal cytology via Pap sufficient as an anal cancer prevention tool, or is the vastly more complicated, costly, and heretofore inaccessible HRA the "right tool" in the same way that the colposcopy following an abnormal Pap smear is for cervical cancer?

While the cervical Pap test in the US has undergone its own debate and modifications to recommended guidelines over the years, as long as no abnormalities are presented or identified, it is generally accepted as a routine procedure for cancer prevention for women and other people with a cervix at age twenty-one and older, and at various progressive intervals throughout the life course (such as every three years). In contrast, there are no official guidelines for screening for anal cancer on a mass scale: the state of New York is alone in recommending anal Pap screening at all, and it is recommended only for HIV+ men. As of 2019, no consensus exists about anal cancer screening, but some doctors advocate for guidelines and recommend and offer anal Pap tests to those in "at-risk" or "high-risk" categories, including HIV+ individuals and MSM.

Questions of whether to screen this body part are permeated with uncertainties, specifically around whether identifying and removing abnormal cells will indeed prevent the future development of anal cancer. HPV is a necessary though insufficient cause of anal cancer; it is not known whether HPV high-risk cancer genotypes will clear on their own, or when they might persist over decades to eventually result in the formation of cancerous tissues or lesions. This uncertainty shapes the regime of cancer prevention practices and processes for all HPV-associated cancers.

While the CDC does not recommend routine an anal Pap test as part of preventive cancer screening, it—along with a few others, such as (once again) New York—does recommend "anal cytology screening of HIV-infected men who have sex with men" as a useful preventive measure, while also citing its uncertainty and the ongoing need for further evidence (that is, clinical evidence that is not from a singular practice group or case report, but includes the "gold standard" in evidence-based medicine, the randomized clinical trial—Masur, Kaplan, and Holmes 2002). In 2007, the New York State Department of Public Health AIDS Institute was the first to make a subgroup recommendation stating that "screening for cellular dysplasia is prudent and recommended, particularly in persons at high risk for infection with papilloma viruses" (Medical Care Criteria Committee 2007). Its guidelines recommend that, as part of a comprehensive annual exam for all HIV+ adults, regardless of age, clinicians should perform a digital anal rectal exam (DARE) and anal cytology at baseline and annually in three HIV-infected populations: MSM, people with prior cancers of the anogenital region, and women with abnormal cervical and/or vulvar results (New York State Department of Health AIDS Institute 2007). While no other guidelines have been widely approved (at least by the end of 2021), regular clinical screening for anal cancer has been adopted by some providers who see gay men living with HIV (Nathan et al. 2010, Pantanowitz and Dezube 2010).

In 2002, Joel Palefsky and another UCSF infectious disease specialist, Peter Chin-Hong, joined the state of New York and the US Veterans Health Administration to advocate for anal cytology annually for all HIV+ individuals, basing their recommendation on the prevalence and size of lesions[13] and the rising rates of anal cancers. These specialists were raising separate questions, yet they shared a concern: they wanted to determine whether and when to remove an anal lesion. Based on clinical experience, it is larger lesions that most often accompany the symptoms that bring a patient to a clinical appointment for examination and diagnosis. Large lesions should always be removed. Smaller, less defined lesions, however, can also be "found" when screening asymptomatic but otherwise "healthy" people. Yet, despite this knowledge, the United States Preventive Services Task Force (USPSTF), the American Cancer Society (ACS), and the Infectious Diseases Society of America (IDSA) do not support routine screening. There is also no approved clinical test to find HPV DNA outside of the cervix in the context of preventive medicine. In December 2022, however, the USPSTF signaled they would begin to study the question of whether to recommend anal cancer screening for "high-risk" groups.

The cervical Pap test is firmly ensconced as part of routine screening guidelines, its efficacy (it reduces invasive cervical cancers by a striking 70–80 percent) a direct result of the triage of precancerous lesions to colposcopy, subsequent monitoring, and/or treatment to remove cellular abnormalities when they meet certain criteria (Dehn, Torkko, and Shroyer 2007, 2). Despite often being characterized as a poor technology due to its weak sensitivity and specificity, the annual Pap test was accepted as a "good enough," and therefore best, tool for the job of cancer prevention in the domain of "women's health." It was the test's frequent repetition at annual exams, though, that was key to its success in reducing cervical cancers— from being the leading killer of women in the 1940s and before to being the fourth most common cancer in women worldwide in 2020 (Arbyn et al. 2020).[14] As a researcher explained, and as was oft repeated in my field-work, anal cancer rates are said to be "as high as the pre–Pap testing cervical cancer rates," and therefore warrant a similar (public) health response. The claim is based on the epidemiological evidence showing that cervical cancer rates have dropped from about 80 per 100,000 (the current rate of HIV+ MSM's anal cancer) to the much lower rate of approximately 2 per 100,000 since the beginning of Pap testing. This was the evidence upon which in 2008 a nurse health educator, Mark Cichocki, called anal cancer "the silent killer in men with HIV," referencing the phrase often used to describe cervical cancer in women (Cichocki 2008).

There has now been a decade of meetings and trainings held by the International Anal Neoplasia Society (IANS). The organization and its many members constitute an important preventive advocacy organization in configuring the infrastructure for the prevention and care demands around anal cancer.[15] Questions for prevention, however, remained, including for whom, when, and at what intervals to perform this Pap test if it were to become a widespread tool in the prevention of anal cancer. For individuals already deemed "high-risk" for this cancer, IANS's priorities include building knowledge and expertise to create prevention and treatment guidelines for best practices, and establishing the protocols needed to ensure reimbursable procedures. Its mission states: "Advocacy is needed to encourage insurers to cover the cost of anal cancer prevention programs; increasingly insurers are denying coverage." To do so, IANS works in partnership with the HPV and Anal Cancer Foundation, the Farrah Fawcett Foundation, and other nonprofit advocacy organizations. They set their sights on training, based on the fact that few specialists were available who had been trained in anal Pap tests plus HRA—a clinical care workforce needed to provide care and to ensure that this approach could also become a tool in prevention.

(In)Equality and (In)Equity Claims for Inclusion

Prior to HPV vaccines, activists for gay men's health argued that the inaccessibility of the combined anal Pap test and HRA procedures—or more precisely, the limitations of the infrastructure needed to ensure their use— reflected structural discrimination and LGBTQ inequity. These structures of inequality are often hardwired into medicine, shaped as it has been by social and cultural stigma and discrimination. Proving the existence of inequality relies on claims to "sameness," specifically similarities of biologies, and on the willingness of individuals and groups to fight for equal treatment based on that sameness. To put resources where they are needed most based on different profiles, be they embodied, behavioral, or structural, is to ensure equity and justice in what is an otherwise pervasively unbalanced and thus unfair system. In the case of anal cancer prevention, as an infectious disease specialist indicated to me in an interview, "we accept that it [the cellular changes in the cervix] is the same surrogate marker [as changes in the anus] . . . so why not use the same procedure to locate a similar biomarker?" The presumed unsuitability of the anal Pap smear is the result of the smear having been produced as a tool for the cervix and not the anus, and thus as a tool not only aligned with femininity, but meant exclusively for "women."[16]

In my interview with Jeff Taylor, a cancer survivor and long-term HIV activist, he stated: "The tests that work in the cervix also work in the anus." Further, he said that anal cancer "is identical to cervical cancer. It is the same virus, it is the same mucous, just in a different geographical location of the body . . . and it could have been prevented if I had access to the Pap smear." He paused and said rhetorically, "You're killing people, that is what frustrates me." Many scientists, practitioners, and patients alike argue that given these commensurate biologies and the "success" of cervical cancer prevention, withholding or not offering anal cancer screening is simply unjust. Specifically, as one of my anonymous interviewees stated, "there is an appropriate model in place . . . that the same kind of screening and treatment should happen for anal cancer prevention."

With HPV-cancer associations came knowledge questions in the domain of gender and health: for instance, why did "women's health" persist in being the main focus of HPV prevention? Several problems of knowledge as well as cultural associations would need to be overcome if anal Pap and HRA were to become routinely and universally used prevention tools. As a medical provider who chose to remain anonymous explained, "It is a disease of HIV and in particular gay men, so it is highly stigmatized. When it is gay sex and gay men it is worse." As if anticipating my next question, he then said of cancer screening, "When gay men come to me and say can I get a Pap smear, I have to say 'No.' I could do it and send it to the lab, but the lab won't process it. Just because it is a man. The lab won't process it [the specimen]." In explaining the difference, this provider told me this inequity is structural, built into biomedicine's infrastructure and largely invisible. He then added that recently, however, more men have been requesting the Pap test, and given the infrastructure of medicine, these men are paying out of pocket for care that takes place exclusively in their provider's office. To make this exclusion visible, he stated, would require evidence that "a lab won't process a sample and an insurance company won't reimburse the cost." Without hesitation he said, "If it were another population group, we would not just leave a cancer in place. We would remove it."[17]

Gendered Technologies, (De)Gendering Practices

Reframing the Pap as a prevention tool for bodies and identities different from those of women and people with a cervix—specifically for "women's health"—would require social finesse. Convincing people living with HIV to subject their bodies to an additional surveillance tool might not have been a hard sell, given the ways their bodies and lives were already constantly monitored and medically managed, often with life-saving results. And, perhaps, getting anally sexually active people to "get swabbed" for infectious disease would also be an easy path to acceptance. Yet, convincing men (gay, bisexual, and MSM) that they might have a risk for anal cancer based on their sexual identities and practices would require negotiations concerning the technologies of screening, the meaning of those technologies, and the preventive approach available. Screening for an HPV-associated cancer might conflict with the gendered contours of HPV, or with the operation of masculinity that relegates anal health to queer boys and men; it was also clearly aligned with the goals of activists and advocates fighting for gay men's health.

Throughout the 1990s and early 2000s, activists for gay men's health organized health summits and documented unique as well as unmet health care needs. Many previous AIDS activists were broadening their health focus "beyond AIDS" to include addressing systemic bias in health care, advocating for an explicit designation for gay men's health, ameliorating safe sex education deficits, and de-stigmatizing sexuality more generally. By 1999, a new iteration of the gay men's health movement was in place, partially made up of AIDS activists, but also including queer cultural critics and sex advocates (Scarce 1999, 4). As AIDS prevalence in San Francisco shifted away from being a crisis and toward being a chronic illness, room was made for other "sexual health" priorities of gay men. (Black MSM, meanwhile, were facing a crisis of infection marked not so much by infectious disease itself as by structural discrimination increasing their risk and decreasing their access to medical care, including HIV testing and treatment.)

Throughout the 1990s, the sociologist Michael Scarce (1999), now a writer for the *New Yorker*, advocated for the "tush Pap," a swab and micro-scopic analysis for monitoring potential illness. Contending that the medi-cal establishment "inscribes gay male bodies within a renewed context of perversion and sexual pathologies," Scarce documented the pre-AIDS la-bel of "Gay Bowel Syndrome" found in medical literatures in 1976, and later taken up in news media and sex manuals in the context of HIV (Scarce 1999, 4). Scarce called for structural accountability in his 1999 book, arguing that federal agencies and medical professional organizations had failed to create a medical protocol for effective screening and insurance reimbursement for anal health. In much the same way that Susan Sontag (1989) set out to free AIDS, its patients, and the public from the tyranny of the disease's symbolic meaning as "plague," Scarce aimed to destigmatize anal health and anal cancer from earlier disease associations with risky practices, risky bodies, and HIV/AIDS.[18]

With HPV's causative role and the rising rates of anal cancer—rates that, epidemiologically speaking, are reported as especially high among HIV+ MSM—this *other* cancer, distinct from KS, was emerging as symbolically and materially attached to gay men's bodies and their presumed sexual lives. Defined as an "HIV-associated cancer" but a "non-AIDS-defining cancer," as well as a "human papillomavirus–associated malignancy,"[19] anal cancer's close association with HIV comes with implications both negative and positive in terms of gendering and sexualizing the disease. The alignment further entrenched a gendered sexual politics that equated anal cancer with MSM and not with women, and specifically with MSM's symbolic associations with anal sex. While this sexual practice is for many an important part of their identities and lives, the ways in which one ac-tivity clings in less positive ways to the bodies and lives of gay, bisexual, and other MSM—despite its practice and value among other identities and sexual subjects—is illustrative. Although KS may have been the canary in the coal mine flagging an increased risk or propensity of malignancies in people with HIV infection, it was brought about not by the virus, HIV, but by the immunocompromised body. Importantly, while the incidence of AIDS-defining illnesses has gone down with anti-retroviral therapy for HIV, the incidence of cancers associated with non-AIDS-defining illnesses has increased (Deeken and Pantanowitz 2019).

Injuries of Omission: Erasures Produced by HPV Vaccination

When HPV vaccination hit the market, gay men's health organizations were well established in some areas of the US, having gained their footing decades earlier around HIV prevention, treatment, and care, in addition to HIV+ sociality and activism. Already established as "at-risk" for STIs and well-versed in a critical stance toward medicine and its normative practices, the construction of the girls of Gardasil as the population most in need of protection from cancer was of particular and personal concern to them. While boys' bodies and lives were implicated in early rollouts of awareness campaigns to know the link, they were not yet configured as part of the HPV vaccine's product market. MSM and PLWHIV who were already accustomed to medical classification as high-risk were the objects of comparatively frequent and robust biomedical surveillance and monitoring, and were often no strangers to clinical trial research; they were also already produced as actors likely to demand inclusion. Many of the people in the audience at meetings dedicated to anal cancer's prevention and care, as well as at some other meetings I attended throughout the decade, had been part of earlier demands around HIV, and were now fighting for another kind of epistemic and material inclusion, this time in biomedicine's preventive approaches to HPV-disease associations.

It was the clinical indication of HPV and its linkage to genital warts that first brought boys into vaccine inclusion, yet it would be HPV's association with anal cancer that shaped the developing entangled politics of prevention around vaccination and screening tools. In 2007, the San Francisco Stop AIDS Project convened "Hole Health: A forum for gay men on the HPV vaccine, anorectal cancer, and anal health," which brought together gay, bisexual, and other MSM with health care providers to discuss whether these men should seek the newly available HPV vaccine "off label" for the prevention of anal cancer and to ensure their anal health while they awaited scientific evidence supporting the idea.

The infectious disease specialist Joel Palefsky was invited to provide advice on how to advocate for greater resources for what the forum considered to be a "critical area in gay men's health." At the time, Palefsky was the principal investigator of a sub-study that was part of the double-blind randomized clinical trial administered and funded by Merck (2004–2017) and designed to show Gardasil's efficacy in reducing the incidence of anogenital warts in young men (regardless of sexuality, sex practices, or history). The sub-study enrolled 602 "healthy" MSM aged sixteen to twenty-six years old without evidence of genital warts to evaluate precancerous anal lesions. It would be on the basis of a larger ongoing study that included 4,065 men, with evidence from this smaller sub-study as supplementary support, that Gardasil would in 2009 be approved for an additional indication: the prevention of anogenital cancers in men and women (Palefsky et al. 2011).

In 2009, GMHC—started as Gay Men's Health Crisis in 1981 in New

York—reported in its newsletter that HIV+ MSM are forty times more likely to be diagnosed with anal cancer than HIV-negative people. Anal cancer, the article stated, is caused by the same strains of HPV that cause cervical cancer in women. Newly published research from the Fred Hutchinson Cancer Research Center in Seattle, Washington had found that HPV lesions make the surface epithelial tissue thinner and more susceptible to another viral infection, HIV. This finding was commensurate with what had been known about cervical cancer for some time: that HPV increases risk for HIV, and vice versa (Margolies and Goeren 2009). Further, the immune cells activated by HPV infection were now known to be more vulnerable to HIV infection than uninfected cells. This was the first time this evidence for a virus-anal cancer association was shown. Non-treatment, or leaving a questionable cellular cluster (considered benign by some, potentially risky by others) in place, was shown to increase risk for anal cancer as well as for HIV.

Though anal cancer prevention has yet to claim its "right tool(s)," by establishing and disseminating the evidence, and no doubt through lobbying as well, for the mass use of the anal Pap test and HRA, classifications of risk and categorizations of bodies were brought together into this domain as *pre-symptomatic* bodies and risky subjects in need of prevention. Many professional associations, activists, and advocacy organizations, as well as a growing number of clinicians, currently recommend that many men and transgender people who have anal sex with men, and especially those who are HIV+, receive anal cancer screening.

The National LGBTQ Cancer Network (LGBTQ-CN) was founded by New York City activist Liz Margolis to address the needs of LGBT people with and at risk for cancer. In 2014 LGBTQ-CN launched a social media campaign to "expose" anal cancer and involve people in the movement (National LGBT Cancer Network 2021). Reflective of biomedicalization and its consumer-engaged and -generated content, yet also shaped by LGBTQ and feminist health activism, the LGBTQ-CN launched their own efforts to bring awareness to this health concern with an accompanying site to raise awareness about anal cancer among gay, bisexual, and MSM. With direct and playful appeal, they used the slogan "Behind Closed Drawers," a discursive reference to queerness and the closet, and especially the ways coming out in large part created a movement for social change. This multimedia campaign aimed to create a directory of free and low-cost LGBT-friendly anal cancer screening facilities throughout the nation; organizers encouraged donation via texting of the word "UNDIES," and encouraged people to spread the word about this initiative by posting a photo of their underwear on social media with the

hashtag #BehindClosedDrawers. The campaign, and the organization behind it, was decidedly queer, with both a distinct focus on LGBTQ and/
or HIV health and a refusal to shroud this cancer prevention message in
acceptability politics that render sex and sexuality invisible.[20]

In a January 2015 piece in *The Body: The HIV/AIDS Resource*, Margolis
explained the impetus behind the campaign:

> No one else really cares about this population and I feel like we are the
> organization that should be taking this on. Rather than beating on doors
> to try to get money, I thought we could, with Behind Closed Drawers,
> have a double-edged campaign that tries to raise money that we could
> use without government interference but, at the same time, alerting
> people to anal cancer. And we do it in a way that reaches our community
> by making it fun. We put the *fun* in fun̲draising. And making it sexy—
> because gay men like nothing more than something sexy.

When I sat down and talked with Margolis in her apartment in lower Man-
hattan, she told me she started the network after losing many friends to
cancer.[21] While mainstream organizations raise awareness of one's risk, encouraging people into an expectation to act upon that riskiness (or at least
to acknowledge that one should act on it), here in the awareness of anal
cancer there were not yet ways to become enterprising actors in disease
risk reduction. While people across all genders and sexualities responded
enthusiastically, donating money to create the resource guide produced by
the LGBTQ cancer network and posting photos, the message of seeking
medical attention was tempered by the fact that there was very little to actually offer this cadre of health consumers-in-waiting.

"Now, it's time to shed our anxieties (and our pants) to face anal cancer
head on," the campaign declared. "What you think is a hemorrhoid, get
it checked," was a message of the campaign, and "get a colonoscopy too
for early signs of that cancer and the removal of polyps." Margolis and the
campaign drew on medical research to support the need for anal cancer
screening. "A growing number of physicians and health activists recommend that all men who have sex with men, especially those who are HIV+,
be tested every 1–3 years depending on their immunological well-being
and CD4 count," organizers said in a statement. They continued by raising the specter of additional "high-risk" groups and the expectation to act:
"[Doctors] suggest that HIV negative individuals be tested every 3 years.
This work is important, because most people know little about anal cancer,
have never been tested for it, and don't know that screening tests exist"
(Nichols 2014).

HPV knowledge and HPV vaccination set in motion a transformation of cancer prevention as two disease regimes converged—one linked to cancer itself, the "emperor of all maladies" associated with "bad luck"; and the other linked to sex and the transmission of infectious agents. The transformation was shaped not by biomedicine alone, but by the ways biomedicine and society are mutually shaped by historical social and cultural ideas that linger and haunt contemporary practices.

CHAPTER FOUR

A Tale of Two Trials

Settling Debate through Evidence-Based Medicine

Preventive medicine is not neutral nor universally provided. Clinicians and health care organizations may offer certain services, but these are governed by multiple organizations—from the professional associations that convene advisory groups to organizations that provide guideline recommendations, and, in the US, including the decisions of insurance corporations and the semi-governmental body of the US Preventive Services Task Force (USPSTF). Given this fragmentation, many physicians and patients struggle with which are the "right" and "best" guidelines to follow. The USPSTF is significant for its review of the evidence and its weight as a preventive guide for insurance reimbursement.[1]

Clinicians expressed frustrations with US insurance companies' refusal to cover via reimbursement the cost of an anal cancer screening technique many were offering patients, seeing it as good care. They were being trained in the procedure, and they understood its role in effectively preventing anal cancers. Evidence-based medicine, with its reliance on the randomized clinical trial, is considered the gold standard in medical decision-making. As a research practice it is relied upon to overcome uncertainty, guide clinical care, and provide the basis for evaluating whether and how to move procedures and approaches into clinical care with reimbursable codes. In the US and other high-resource countries with LGBT rights and especially an infrastructure for HIV/AIDS care, many providers were already screening their gay and MSM patients for any signs of early anal disease. Gynecological oncologists providing care to women and people with a cervix who had a prior cancer were also often offering this screening approach to their patients.

Clinicians were left with a puzzle. They knew that many of their patients, like all of us, were exposed and likely constantly re-exposed to HPVs; and especially for their patients with HIV, they wondered whether this posed an urgent or additional risk to their health. Researchers and clinicians who focus on HIV were accustomed to thinking about their patients' risk for

AIDS-defining and non-AIDS-related malignancies as a way of monitoring and understanding cancer risk among people with HIV. In 2013, when this research began, I attended the National Institutes of Health's International Conference on Malignancies in AIDS and Other Acquired Immunodeficiencies (ICMAOI).[2] The conference introduced me to the advocates, activists, and researchers and clinicians dedicated to ensuring that people with HIV receive the best care that "evidence-based" and clinical medicine can provide. I followed their subsequent annual meeting virtually as they focused on the entanglement of (non-HIV) infectious agents and HIV infection, and the way these interact to cause cancers, with a focus on causation, treatment, and care. The meeting would report the latest evidence as well as research underway.

ICMAOI led me to understand another puzzle and frustration: how best to provide early screening of what is now known to be HPV-associated anal cancer, and more importantly, what population- or risk-groups should be provided this care to achieve the best and most needed results. The problem was not the lack of a validated screening tool or an approach. Research was still needed to understand the groups poised to benefit most from a screening tool. Yet as one researcher told me, the real problem is reimbursement, and the "real solution to the problem [of insurance coverage] is to provide the data that people [e.g., companies and governmental entities] say they want." From the standpoint of evidence-based medicine, a multi-million-dollar clinical trial would be needed to provide the amount, type, and strength of data showing health outcomes improved enough to influence health care and insurance policy and practice. In the case of the anal Pap test, if the evidence reflects disease reduction as a result of its use (along with its associated technologies), then the door would be opened to establishing new protocols and standards. As one interviewee explained, we need to show that removing high-grade lesions in the anus provides results in cancer reduction similar to those obtained by removing high-grade lesions in the cervix:

> [There] is clearly an at-risk population. But, the one thing that's missing is obviously, if we screen and we treat, are we preventing anal cancers? If I treat this lesion will I actually prevent this person from getting anal cancer? That's the controversy and why no one wants to put these technologies [anal Pap with HRA] in firm [prevention] guidelines, because we don't have evidence.

Distinct knowledge politics would unfold as social categories and processes—often gendered and sexualized—shaped the ideas attached to, and adoption of, the anal Pap test as the right tool for cancer prevention.

Merck and the American diagnostics company Hologic, a major player in cervical cancer cytology and HPV DNA testing markets, were frequent sponsors of the meetings I attended. These multi-billion-dollar international corporations hoped to shape the implementation and standardization of cancer screening tools, including those for anal cancer—for which such an approach was not yet nationally governed. Settling uncertainty about whether and how to implement anal cancer prevention on a mass scale and incorporate it into clinical health care guidelines could and would only come in the form of randomized clinical trial evidence.

During a conference I attended in 2013 organized around HPV-associated cancer, one focus of the meetings was assessing the current evidence. When conference attendees asked whether men should be screened for anal high-grade squamous intraepithelial lesions (HSIL), it was Richard Hillman, the clinical lead of Australia's "Study of the Prevention of Anal Cancer" (SPANC) clinical trial, who responded with a "we don't know." Uncertainty underscored the need to find the best approach. At the same time, clinicians and researchers alike had different hunches and ideas about the risk and approach. Hillman added that HSIL does not cause symptoms and never causes death by itself.[3] HSIL is the precursor and often the outcome benchmark for anal cancer risk, yet whether or not it is sufficient to cause cancer is unsettled. His words were in stark contrast to the other speakers'. He said, "The cervix is not the anus," and argued that given "sufficient differences between the cervix and anus, there is a lack of evidence to suggest that the same approach to prevention—what is referred to as the cervical cancer paradigm—applies." Hillman then reiterated the uncertainty upon which these claims rest: "HPV is insufficient [as the cause of cancer], and HSIL is insufficient in causing cancer." I was left to wonder (as you may be) why Hillman's take was so different.

There was another "side" to the debate, and one that was included in the conversation to make a point. This was the soon to be funded ANCHOR study (Anal Cancer HSIL Outcomes Research), a clinical trial designed and led with a different claim: "the anus is just like the cervix," and since "we [already] have the cervical cancer model," it makes good sense that a similar screening approach would work for anal cancer. ANCHOR would be funded that year by the NIH NCI's AIDS Malignancy Consortium, with a grant award of US$89 million for a multi-site, eight-year clinical trial based at UCSF. The research goal would be to "establish standard of care guidelines for the prevention of anal cancer." The study would recruit HIV+ people to understand whether anal cytology (Pap) and HRA would reduce the incidence of anal cancer. The discussion among panelists began by invoking the public health transition that had followed population-based cervical Pap smear screening guidelines for women; a similarly better world would be possible with anal cancer screening guidelines. Audiences were told, "We know the three risk groups. . . . We can see the lesions (using HRA)," and "since we can see the pre-cancer, we can identify it, and remove it." A clear difference emerged in which claims of evidence were being asserted. Even more evident, though, was a difference in politics. "How much cancer is acceptable?" was the question, emphasizing that we don't know when, or in whom, cancer will develop, and arguing, "Waiting for cancer to develop is a poor option."

A speaker representing the "other side" (and other clinical trial) asserted the position that until we have a treatment, we should provide routine health care with annual digital rectal exams (DRE or DARE) and triage as needed. Presumably, we should not embrace an approach that would drive more unnecessary and invasive High-Resolution Anoscopy. Many others, like the attendee voices heard before, were firm in their belief that this approach, which assumed that a person should wait to "feel a lesion" or "for symptoms" to present, would delay action until it was "too late." In contrast, the direction deemed best would be to perform Pap test cytology screening, followed by HRA on those deemed to be at "high risk," comprising mostly HIV+ MSM. When pressed on why this approach, I would often hear: "Because it is the ethical and moral thing to do."

The somewhat contrived two-sided discussion was nonetheless informative in the ways it mobilized traditional ethical claims that weigh harms and benefits—the risks associated with doing or not doing the procedure, and the benefits incurred if the procedure is performed. While ethics in medicine begin with a "do no harm" axiom, in many cases the question becomes whether or not there is harm in not doing something, and intervening is presumed to be the best course of action. This is part of the sociological critique of medicalization: medicine defines problems in ways that presume a needed intervention (or vice versa). Ethical questions become whether it is better to do something than to risk the potential harm of doing nothing—that is, whether the risk of doing does or does not outweigh the harm of not-doing. Here it was especially unclear whether a diagnosis of "not-cancer" (what clinicians at times refer to as "pre-cancer") might create psychological harm, or a pathway to ongoing and unneeded surveillance and intervention, or both.

While knowledge is beneficial, so too can be uncertainty, when it comes to cellular changes that might never become full-blown disease. HPV-associated anal cancers are considered "the most common non-AIDS-defining cancers in HIV-infected individuals" (Robbins et al. 2015; Shiels et al. 2011; Pantanowitz, Schlecht, and Dezube 2006), and thus HIV+

people have a "high-risk" designation. It is often stated that about half of HIV+ MSM have anal HSIL, or precancerous lesions, and that at least 1 in 10 may develop anal cancer (Wang, Sparano, and Palefsky 2017). Yet there is embedded within these scientific claims also a great amount of *uncertainty* surrounding the actual risk associated with this categorization. Like HPV itself, HSILs might clear on their own or remain as they are, never developing into cancer.[4] Nonetheless, given that precancerous lesions are not always symptomatic, by the time symptoms are noticed cancer may have already developed. Gathering the evidence to understand when and whether HSIL will progress or regress and when it is best to identify its cellular presence may result in a diagnosis that is "too late" for many people's health outcomes. Answering these questions is the focus of both the ANCHOR trial and the SPANC study. The uncertainties over whether disease will occur are joined by ambiguity over when a precancer is indeed a precancer and when it is nothing at all, as well as over what preventive tool is the best approach. The answers to questions of whether and when to intervene, I have argued, are shaped by the processes of constructing risk, always already gendered and sexualized.

There is also a significant ethical contour to this question—an equity- and justice-based argument for who ought to be screened and when, based on establishing where the need is greatest and the vulnerable are least protected. The activism strategy of teach-ins and disruption embraced by ACT UP was invoked in debate, with the imagery of attending multiple funerals and deaths from anal cancers mirroring similar uses of imagery from the height of the AIDS epidemic in the 1980s and early 1990s. ACT UP and other AIDS activists' claims for inclusion in medical care and research rested on claims of social injustice and pervasive structural neglect, including in biomedical funding and care.

Gay men, while configured as *the* "risk group" for HIV, a sexually transmitted viral infection, were implicated yet absent actors in the narratives, and thus the care, established around the prevention of HPV that unfolded in an HPV vaccine approach. Over time, with gay health advocates and others recommending vaccination for men and boys, this already constituted group (as singular as it may have been) was called forward into HPV-cancer associations. It turns out, however, that ethics-driven calls for inclusion had not only pre-dated the girls of Gardasil, but (given the dictates of evidence-based medicine) were already part of the Randomized Clinical Trials (RCTs), and were part of activist and advocate struggles (many led by those aging with HIV) for inclusion in an evolving regime of cancer prevention now clustered around multiple HPV-associated cancers.

The question being asked was no longer "to screen or not to screen," but whether the gay community would accept (additional) surveillance, and if they wouldn't, how many gay deaths would result if surveillance was not increased? An audience member asked a speaker as he stood at the podium: "How many funerals do you want to go to? How many deaths do you want to watch?" "That standard has never been acceptable for women," they added, emphasizing what many in the audience were wondering: did what they were seeing amount to discrimination against PLWHIV and MSM? While I was struck by the rhetorical claim and embedded assumption that women have and continue to receive good care based on good science, I put my wish to historicize and contextualize this claim aside and tuned back in to the debate.

"Why would we want to discriminate against people who are HIV+ who are 'sexual minorities'?" another person asked. The response, and I paraphrase from my fieldnotes, was "we protect those individuals with good health care and until there is an effective treatment, we leave it at that" (referring to the ethical standards of do no harm, yet also advocating for good and regular health care).

A speaker who advocates for HRA technology and removing precancerous lesions as a treatment aligns with the methodology of the ANCHOR study design, which was the first to create treatment and non-treatment arms for HSIL identification and removal and ongoing surveillance. The two sides of the debate were artificial, but the US stance, at least as transmitted through the ANCHOR trial, seemed to align with a phrase heard at scientific meetings: "There is no other place in the body that we are okay having a lesion and not doing anything about it . . . so until we know we shouldn't do this, we should actively intervene."

When I spoke with Hillman months later at another conference, we discussed the US context of reimbursement for health care and his belief that this context is driving much of the research underway in the US. He added his opinion that in Australia, the cost of Pap plus HRA for screening all MSM would never be approved, at least not with the evidence available. This was also the sentiment shared by Christopher Fairley, Director of the Melbourne Sexual Health Center at Monash University, when he said: "People make large sums of money out of doing things that are not recommended. In this specific example [of anal cancer screening], there was no evidence that despite these similarities, that anal cancer, cytology, or HPV testing, or high-resolution endoscopy and treatment of abnormalities prevents anal cancer. It's not like cervical disease where you treat it and it stays away. You treat this, it all comes back." He then added, "even if you were sure that it works, It's hundreds and hundreds of thousands of dollars. There's lots of other competing health care costs that deserve the money."

Fairley was concerned in the short run about how best to provide preventive care, but as a public health leader his sights were set on the long term. For him, if vaccination is done right, with Gardasil 9, there won't be much need for screening at all, for any of these HPV cancers. I felt myself agreeing and wondering, why don't we just vaccinate everyone we can? Australia is a national and publicly funded (rather than insurance-based) health care system driven by population prevention and cost concerns. If a screening approach is expensive and unproven, from prostate cancer to anal cancer screening, it would not be the approach to take. Yet Fairley, like many I spoke with, agreed that when and if needed, the best approach is to go where disease, or infection, is highest and target prevention to those groups who might need it most—and to do so as quickly as possible to reach community protection.

Finding out whether or not screening would "pay off" in terms of preventing later disease in those populations that need it most was the aim of both the ANCHOR clinical trial in the US and the SPANC clinical trial in Australia. An examination of these studies makes clear that these groups were respectful of, and a part of, ensuring good care for the LGBTQ patients they see. The recruitment materials for ANCHOR and SPANC reflect not only the high-risk subject-making practiced by clinical trial recruitment, but a refusal to stigmatize sex and sexuality. The ANCHOR study was expressly launched to provide the clinical evidence needed to settle the anal screening debate, and to degender HPV technologies and destigmatize the anus and anal disease more generally (Anchor Study 2021). The on-the-ground message was simple: now that living with HIV is easier, it is time to give your butt attention. The promotional materials used for enrolling participants reflect what Epstein calls "recruitmentology"—the new science of enrolling underrepresented groups in clinical research, which emerged with NIH requirements to include "women and ethnic minorities" in clinical trials (Epstein 2008). In this case, the focus was on enrolling HIV+ MSM in clinical research they were confident would also provide health care and potentially reduce cancer risk. In well-tested marketing materials, the website and recruitment featured animated images of dancing humans—masculine and feminine—with two conjoined symbolic associations: a plus sign indicating HIV+ and placed on the right cheek of a well-defined buttock. By situating the plus signs on the butts of these characters as they face away from the camera, a gaze on their rear is encouraged; employing a seemingly gay aesthetic, HIV+ bodies and their butts are made the objects of biomedicine. Prior to these clinical trial study designs, the sociologist Steven Epstein (2010, 61) had argued: "In order for the promise of medicine to reach this constituency, a largely invisible disease must be brought into the open, and medical technologies that have been associated with women's bodies must be recoded as usable in men." The text of the recruitment ads for ANCHOR read: "Living with HIV has gotten a lot easier. With longer lifespans, however, we face a new set of challenges." The accompanying imagery brought HIV status and the butt into close association and risk construction; the spot ended with a plea: "Making the case to MSM: Just call 1–844-HIV-BUTT."

Recruitment materials for the ANCHOR trial asserted that "While deaths from AIDS are way down, anal cancer among people living with HIV is on the rise. We think that anal cancer can be prevented by routine screening and removal of precancerous cells." Invoking the cervical cancer paradigm, the recruitment materials state: "This strategy has reduced cervical cancer rates by 80 percent. But to get the insurance companies to cover routine anal cancer screening and preventative treatment, we need to prove that this strategy actually prevents cancer. The best way to show that is to recruit people with High Grade Squamous Intraepithelial Lesions (or HSIL for short) into a study and assign them randomly to a treatment arm or a monitoring arm. We then follow everyone for five years to compare the rates of cancer in both study arms. At the end of the study we'll know whether screening and treatment of HSIL are effective strategies in preventing anal cancer."[5]

Attention is captured, and urgency invoked, with numerical evidence of rising rates, measurable difference, and health inequities. Debate claims hinged on the data: Estimates of the rates of cancer for HIV+ MSM are "highest"; anal cancer incidence among HIV+ MSM is "even higher" than that of a cancer that is routinely screened for in the general population. That cancer is cervical cancer, and the screening approach is Pap tests at regular intervals. Making a case for an inequity—that women had long been screened when rates of cervical cancer were lower proportionately than those of HIV+ people with anal cancer—was the key claim upon which the ANCHOR trial entered evidence-based medicine. The home page for the study made the argument—"No one knew that cervical cancer was preventable before the use of Pap smears became widespread in the 1960s and cut the incidence of the disease by 80 percent"—asserting that this study could be just as important in reducing cancers. For already established patients given HIV management, media would run headlines that include phrases such as "The Pap Smear That's Not Just for Women" in an effort to degender the technology and, by extension, influence how health care providers offering and performing screening tests, laboratories processing results, and especially men (with HIV) perceive the Pap tests (Marcus 2015).

The SPANC trial launched in 2010 as the project of a university HIV epidemiology and research center in Melbourne, Australia, with sites in Sydney and Melbourne. The dedicated website (see https://kirby.unsw .edu.au/project/spanc) similarly raised concern about an "increase in the number of anal cancer cases . . . that affect certain groups significantly more than the general population." They explain that the risk factor is not identity or behavior, but rather "anal exposure to HPV," and then make the link that gay and bisexual men are at particularly high risk, experiencing rates of anal cancer that the recruitment website states are at least twenty times higher than the general population. People living with HIV were said to have even higher, "30-fold increased rates." The numbers skyrocket for one particular group: the "combination of immunodeficiency and HPV exposure means HIV+ gay and bisexual men are the most affected group, with rates of up to 100 times that of heterosexual men."

Both studies, designed as RCTs, built their research on the available research data indicating HIV+ MSM as the highest (by far) risk group for anal cancer. SPANC's very name alludes to this focus; it is a play on words simultaneously invoking butts and gay-associated BDSM play. The study's imagery confirms this production: a man's ass centered in the frame surrounded by peeks of jacked thighs, back, and arms; a graphic rendering of an oversized, playful "X marks the spot" indicates the location of the anus, bisecting yet discreetly obscuring the cleft of his butt. While nothing about a male-appearing body explicitly says gay, bisexual, or MSM, both the spectacle of the muscular, buff body and the presumable gaze settling on its backside conjure same-sex male desire.

Sexual Health at the Cancer Meetings

The annual congress of the European Research Organization on Genital Infection and Neoplasia (EUROGIN[6]) was held in southern Spain in 2015. While conducting observation, I interviewed several clinical and research experts. The first day, feeling a bit out of place as a social scientist at a meeting for clinical researchers and basic scientists, I made eye contact with two scholars who seemed approachable. They sat at a round table in the cafeteria area with laptops open and papers spread about, and they seemed to be having a good time. I quickly said "Hello," and was delighted when they responded with an invitation to join them. They were young and dressed casually compared with the majority of attendees, who mostly wore suits and ties. As usually takes place at professional meetings, we opened our conversation by exchanging our professional titles and expertise. I was relieved to hear that while they were both MDs, they were also epidemiologists and health researchers; this made me think we might share some vocabulary and perspective as PhDs. When I told them I was a medical sociologist attending the conference as part of my fieldwork to understand the social and sexual aspects of viral-cancer associations—my noncommittally vague go-to description—I was surprised when their eyes lit up with curiosity. They exchanged glances and the man said, "Oh! That's the elephant in the room," corroborating what I had long observed: sex and sexuality are not discussed at these meetings.

"These researchers are very conservative and scientific," he said, and with a smile added, "we are sexual health researchers, we talk about sex all the time." They asked if I had watched the then-recent episode of *Girls*. I was delighted, as I had captured its contours in my notes, and my mind raced back to the episode and my thoughts about how it dramatized HPV as an STI one could "catch" and trace to a previous partner as the source. As we spoke, I told them that the characters reminded me of the college-aged girl-identified students I teach in San Francisco who often speak of being afraid of sex—not because of unintended pregnancy or HIV, issues that concerned my friends when we were in high school and college, but because of HPV. We talked about the idea of finger-pointing and the ways questions of "who I got it from"—so similar to the partner notifications of the HIV/AIDS epidemic—were the focus. I was delighted to be brought into a cultural conversation and replied with my own take on the episode and the ways the showrunners had depicted HPV as a catchable STI akin to chlamydia or gonorrhea and something these girls should be aware of transmitting and catching.

To my surprise, these two pop culture enthusiasts turned out to be Mary Poynten and David Templeton, medical providers and investigators working on the SPANC trial launched in 2011 for which Hillman is the clinical lead (and Andrew Grulich the principal investigator). Poynten is a senior lecturer and project leader of SPANC, which was by that time underway in Australia (in Sydney and Melbourne). They told me generally about the study's methodology and how it was progressing in terms of recruitment, given that findings were not yet available. Recruitment was the challenge at that time, and they were promoting their new study on Facebook, on websites directed at HIV+ people, and by tabling at community events. The study was producing newsletters that were sent to those enrolled in the hope that it would drive "word of mouth" enrollment. I was able to follow up with interviews over the next weeks, some in person at the meeting and others over What's App. The website listed many of their community partners—LGBTQ- and HIV-focused organizations, as well as hospital groups and health care organizations more generally. Like ANCHOR,

SPANC hoped to inform about the potential development of anal cancer screening guidelines for HIV+ and HIV-negative gay, bisexual, and MSM. These men would not have received HPV vaccination, having been too old to qualify for the vaccine when it was approved.

By my last communication with Templeton, I had already learned quite a bit about SPANC—about the uncertainties the SPANC trial hoped to resolve and about the controversy and debates underway between the team in Australia and their American counterparts running the ANCHOR study. I had also heard other official presentations on SPANC's design, methods, and preliminary results by other team members.[7] But my intention to stay in touch with Templeton and Poynten was cemented after I read an update on the study reported in an AIDS magazine, *AIDS MAP*, distributed by a UK charity. The article announced that SPANC results were beginning to roll out with big news: "clearance" of HSIL—or the rate at which abnormal cells *revert back* to normal or to a less severe grade of abnormality— was proving to be quite high among those enrolled. The implications for screening guidelines, therefore, could be that *not screening at all* is the "best tool" in the fight against anal cancer (Poynten et al. 2020). The authors speculated that preventive screening and the sharing of "abnormal results" may cause psychological distress and impact quality of life, including sustained intrusive thoughts, increased cancer worry, and heightened perception of cancer risk. They joined others, especially their principal investigator, Richard Hillman, who had all along warned that the potential for psychological harm needs to be considered when implementing anal cancer screening programs (Cvejic et al. 2019).

Questions about implementing screening programs without definitive evidence of their effects on physical and mental health had come up regularly as I traveled from conference to conference listening to the latest "talk" and research. Should we routinely screen HIV+ people, especially MSM, for anal cancer? Some asked whether "we," meaning clinicians, might perform unnecessary HRAs following anal Pap screening. Some described the procedure as "easily performed" and "quite well tolerated," while others viewed the procedure as "invasive" and "uncomfortable." While different people experience screening technologies differently, and some find that knowledge—even when uncertain—helps to quell anxiety, others consider any invasive tool unsettling and, in the absence of clear guidance on next steps, unnecessary. Medically, as well as sociologically, tests that found precancerous cells were said to potentially lead to unnecessary and meaningless diagnostics, as well as disease identities of having precancer, the ambiguous diagnosis of "not-cancer." Most significantly for my focus and the results now rolling out from the SPANC trial, some people were arguing vocally for equity: leaving MSM and HIV+ people out of screening regimes would be akin to the "silence = death" ethos that infused the early years of AIDS mortality. It would also be inequitable—i.e., "less than" what is provided for women, who are included in a routine cervical cancer screening paradigm with protocols, insurance reimbursements, and clinical expertise. Before SPANC, clinical knowledge confirmed that persistent infection with high-risk—or oncogenic—HPV *might* lead to cancerous lesions. However, given that cellular abnormalities associated with HPV may never become full-blown disease, resolving and stabilizing this uncertainty became a priority of researchers (and a goal of both ANCHOR and SPANC trials).

From a clinical perspective, the results showing a high degree of "spontaneous resolution" or self-clearance meant that what researchers had posited about how a disease progresses from precancerous to cancerous needed to be revisited—especially the decision to treat (i.e., remove) HSILs. As described above in the debate at IANS, one aspect of the contestation concerns whether to "just leave it there," as Templeton reminded me, adding, "the thing is, we can. Now that we know that some HSIL regresses." Templeton felt that the SPANC results would mean "we can no longer disagree," and "no longer say [regression] can't happen."

When I previously spoke to an ANCHOR trial researcher, they explained that the one important need for the RCT was the issue of self-clearance: "Since there's no evidence from a randomized controlled trial [referring to whether anal Pap plus HRA reduced cancers], we have to go through this process of doing a trial and establishing standard-of-care guidelines." Unfortunately, "it will take 8 to 10 years and cost $89 million," they added, referencing the cost and timeline of the ANCHOR trial. Most of my US interviewees welcomed the ANCHOR study and the NIH support behind it. Prior to these trials, and over the years since, these researchers—largely gynecologists and/or sexual health researchers—met at various HIV, HPV, and other clinical conferences aimed at viruses and disease. In the US context, they shared a hope that evidence would exert pressure on insurance companies to cover screening costs, which are still largely paid out of pocket. ANCHOR's website states this goal clearly:

> We know [HRA followed by colposcopy] prevents cervical cancer, but the research funders, insurers and health care professionals need evidence that we can also prevent anal cancer this way. The only way to do this is to randomly assign participants to one of two groups, one treated and the other monitored, to see which group has the most cases

of cancer. The ANCHOR study is designed to provide this evidence and to establish the standards of care to prevent anal cancer.

The cervical cancer model became the lead indicator for claims for equity and inclusion for patients and providers alike. I would repeatedly hear that there are few physicians trained to provide HRA; that providers are restricted in what they can do; and that no standard of care (and thus insurance reimbursement) exists for prevention, rendering the exam inaccessible.

The politics of evidence—specifically, what counts and what doesn't—was a frequent topic at various conferences. As one researcher explained: "A quarter of the HIV- MSM had high grade lesions. If it was a population of women and we knew a priori that 25% of them had high grade CIN [cervical intra-epithelial neoplasia] we would have said to just colposcope everybody."[8] They added, "There are other high-risk groups: HIV+ women. . . . Part of this whole story is the incidence of anal cancer is unacceptably high in those groups. But much of the risk is concentrated in these smaller groups. So that means we can focus our prevention efforts in them." Later this researcher emphasized a strong need for clinical trial evidence—not for the purpose of adding to the knowledge base, but to justify insurance coverage—lamenting "the difficulty in getting reimbursed for what we do; constant fighting with insurance companies, etc. And so the real solution to this problem is to provide the data that people say they want in order to approve this as standard of care."

Most other US clinicians working in this space also feel they are having to overcome HIV stigma as they struggle to care for patients. "It's a disease of HIV and in particular gay men. It is also highly stigmatized, you know, it's associated with gay sex," one researcher told me. HPV transmission, he pointed out, is associated with anal receptive sex, but it is transmitted through other routes as well. "Within the HIV community . . . we often don't want to recognize it. Gay men have trouble talking about it with a provider and even if they do, I remember in my experience saying, 'Well, I've heard you can get Pap smears' and the doctor said, 'We only do that on women.' It would be rejected." He then said, "We were forced to spend all this time and money on all these other things just to prove a point that we already know. The alternative is that people don't get it [screening] and die. . . . Gay men and especially gay sex has always been kind of a taboo topic."

But there are differences of opinion on this very point which are often pegged to different health care contexts. When I spoke to Christopher

Fairley in 2015, we talked about the clinical trials underway to assess anal cancer screening protocols. His strong opinion about the indication for mass screening differed markedly from that of others: "It's a whole lot of other different people who make large sums of money out of doing things that are not recommended. And clearly, what they're doing is doing it for money. . . . It's not like cervical disease where you treat it and it stays away. You treat [anal lesions], it all comes back." "The clearance rate is terrific," he enthused. "You get 90 percent of the same effect if you just let them be."

Degendering the Pap smear and reducing stigma about the anus and anal cancer are goals already being pursued as clinical trials gather evidence to support a new preventive approach, one that in the US will hopefully come with a needed reimbursement code. Once a protocol is in place, an infrastructure must also be established for the technology to be accepted at a meaningful level. In the push to establish the evidence to guide an anal cancer prevention regime, these processes are being undertaken simultaneously. In an interview, one of the ANCHOR team members pointed to the stigma of the anus and problems with naming a procedure the "anal Pap." "The first challenge is that this is a part of the body that people generally just don't want to think about . . . just a lot of taboo around it. I think that for women there's a clear kind of pathway. They understand Pap smears." He continued to bring a gendered focus into relief: "For men I think it's another issue in that Pap holds a feminized–associated with women and the vagina that I think it's going to take a lot of effort to convince them that this is something that men should get screened for. Maybe calling it a Pap smear would probably be not the best thing for men."

This idea is often repeated as contributing not only to recruitment challenges to ANCHOR but also to an absence of conversations around women and anal sex. As ANCHOR's well-tested recruitment materials attempted to demystify the butt while still evading sexualization, many lay advocacy groups and experts seeking to "expose" anal cancer joined their cause. The Behind Closed Drawers campaign of the LGBT Cancer Network is the most vocal example to date, doing the cultural work needed to degender and even, in this case, proudly sexualize a prevention approach as gay and as a degendered and male-inclusive Pap test.

While news from both trials broke in late 2021, before the close of ANCHOR and following the end of SPANC, the results of the trials were not aligned. SPANC found HSIL regression, and ANCHOR found that removing high-grade squamous intraepithelial lesions (HSIL) significantly reduced chances of progression to anal cancer (Fernandez 2021). The "public health importance of the findings" led the ANCHOR investigators to release their results early. The information will be used to develop standard of care guidelines "for people at high risk of anal cancer, including screening for and treatment of anal HSIL" and to prove that, "like cervical cancer, anal cancer can be prevented even in high-risk populations, such as people living with HIV." ANCHOR's results also suggested that anal cancer prevention could be similarly possible in other groups known to be at increased risk of anal cancer, including MSM who are HIV negative, women with a history of vulvar or cervical cancer, and men and women who have immunosuppression for reasons other than HIV infection. The evidence now supported a claim long made: the cervical cancer paradigm should be applied to anal cancer prevention.

In October 2021, UCSF announced that the ANCHOR trial would be stopped early due to evidence suggesting that removing high-grade squamous intraepithelial lesions (HSILs) significantly reduced the chances of later progression to anal cancer. In June the findings and an announcement were published in preview on the website of the preeminent *New England Journal of Medicine*. Research findings from the ANCHOR trial showed that treating anal precancer in people at high risk, particularly those living with HIV, reduced cancer risk. The study also showed that prevalence was higher than originally thought among women living with HIV. The study revealed that of the 4,446 people enrolled, nine of the people in the "treatment arm" who rigorously followed the regime of anal Pap tests plus HRA over two years were diagnosed with biopsy-proven HSIL, compared with twenty-one people in the "active-monitoring" (control) group, demonstrating a lower rate of progression to cancer in the treatment group than in the active-monitoring group (Palefsky et al. 2022).

The findings provided the clinical trial evidence that treating anal precancer reduces progression to cancer, making the case for early detection (much like screening for other cancers through colposcopy, mammography, and cervical screening tools). The phase 3 RCT was based on the claim for needed evidence and the hypothesis of biological similarity and techno-scientific equivalents. "Treatment for cervical HSIL reduces progression to cervical cancer; however, data from prospective studies of treatment for anal HSIL to prevent anal cancer are lacking" (Palefsky et al. 2022, 1). Following the release of the evidence and the good news, on August 22, 2022 the International Papilloma Virus Society (IPVS) held a free webinar titled "Prevention of Anal Cancer: Will the ANCHOR Study Be Sufficient to Start Screening Programs?" Press releases and email notifications followed reporting the "groundbreaking" news that anal cancer can be prevented by routine screening and the removal of precancerous cells (Anal Cancer Foundation email issued on June 16, 2022), and major medical organizations issued emails of congratulations. In December 2022, the USPSTF signaled they would begin to study the question of whether to recommend anal cancer screening for "high-risk" groups, likely as a result of the evidence from the ANCHOR Trial.

Despite all the evidence apparently indicating a new direction, all is not (yet) settled. Templeton of the SPANC trial acknowledged that there is still much to understand, postulating that cytology co-tests with HPV may be the future direction of prevention tools. That is, the next step for anal cancer screening may be to bring together HPV tests and a biomarker, such as HSIL, and then decide how to monitor (but again, not necessarily treat) disease. He speculated, "There is likely a huge amount of over-treatment." Now that we have some evidence of clearance, this is likely to have been the case "at that time [when studies were developed] and at that point in our knowledge," he said. "The incidence had been going up and had peaked. It seemed to be very high among HIV+. So people were treating, but they were doing so without evidence." He indicated that there had also not been any results from cohort studies. And while he acknowledged that questions remained to be addressed before we can consider the debate settled, it was clear that from the perspective of SPANC and its researchers treatment should be limited to those with disease and not used as a cancer-preventive screening tool.

By way of conclusion, I return to the sense of excitement evoked when a conference speaker at a major cancer meeting affirmed, "This is the beginning of a major discussion . . . [of] the cancer that dare not speak its name." An inequality and medical omission was invoked that was in need of change. It was a previously quiet conversation among a sub-population of researchers and health care providers, as well as patients already construed as being at risk due to their HIV status and/or sexualities, who were central yet not exclusive actors. The work of the meeting was "finding common ground" among the women with and without HIV diagnoses, in need of treatment and care, and in many cases dying of this cancer. Speakers, nonprofit disease-awareness organizations, and audience members alike were also troubling the framing of high risk as linked to HIV and MSM. Women with prior cancers, with HIV, and many without a co-infection or disease indication were carrying a heavy burden of anal cancer, an associated stigma and "taboo" of their own, as well as a need for prevention, treatment, and care.

Many in the US are familiar with Farrah Fawcett's death from anal cancer. Fawcett held a special place in 1970s US pop culture, playing a private investigator alongside the actresses Kate Jackson and Jaclyn Smith, on *Charlie's Angels*, a popular weekly TV show watched in millions of

American living rooms from 1976 to 1981. Fawcett had appeared in many other shows and commercials, including alongside her then husband, Lee Majors, in the *Six Million Dollar Man*. With thick long blond hair and a thin body, Fawcett posed in a red bathing suit for an iconic image that was reproduced as a poster that sold 6 million prints in its first year, and decorated the bedrooms of countless adolescents (the suit is part of the Smithsonian Institution collection in Washington, DC—Gresko 2011). Fawcett was a heartthrob for a large segment of teen boys (and quite a few teen girls, possibly expressing their pre-queer and lesbian selves). She remained a popular figure in the 1980s and 1990s, winning several Golden Globe awards for her part in iconic films such as *The Burning Bed*, which depicted intimate partner violence. Her diagnosis with anal cancer in 2003 at the age of sixty-two, and the documentary film she would co-produce chronicling her illness and treatment leading up to her death, *Farrah's Story*, drew attention as she neared the end of her life. In my interpretation, the film reflected a general cultural push by the pharmaceutical company Merck, as well as many health care organizations and actors, to desexualize and destigmatize anal cancer, although HPV was never given explicit attention. The film was likely viewed by most of the people who made up the audience at the inaugural meeting of IANS, members of a generation most at risk of cancer due to their age (in their fifties and sixties).

ACF and the Fawcett Foundation, along with LGBTQ activists, worked to overcome the symbolic association and taboo of anal sex and anal cancer, while refusing to suppress sex altogether. At the same time and with shared goals, many researchers and clinicians embraced the gay or transgender cultures of their patients and hoped to use playfulness to draw attention to the butt and anal sex. "We all have an anus" is often said somewhat gleefully, using words such as tush, butt, backside, and bum and often calling attention to the ways HPV-associated diseases "affect your junk," which adds a bit of fun to the seriousness of infectious disease and cancer. Unlike the cancer foundations, which were new to raising awareness of an STI-related cancer, these other researchers and practitioners were part of a now thirty-year history of HIV care, funding, and research infrastructure. They were accustomed to a gendered, sexual politics surrounding HIV. Yet, surprisingly, there are no celebrity men who are the public face of this cancer. Instead, it is Farrah Fawcett and, more recently, the actress Marcia Cross from *Desperate Housewives*, who are the well-known women and public-presenting faces of this HPV-associated cancer. In 2018, Cross revealed in a series of photos she posted to Instagram that she had been diagnosed with anal cancer. She was choosing to speak openly about her cancer, and especially to "destigmatize" the disease. At fifty-seven, the actress told CNN media she is "not ashamed of her cancer," reflecting her own attempt to destigmatize the cancer and refute what she perceived as the continued blame that hung over this cancer (France 2019). Cross told the world that it is important to be aware that this disease is caused by HPV. Social media websites devoted to cancer took note: SurvivorNet, a website that provides curated cancer information from experts, reported that phrases such as "taboo sex act" and "HPV-linked cancers"—including anal cancer—are not only stigmatizing, but inaccurate. Seeming to obscure the role of anal sex in transmission, the media focused on the inaccuracy over lingering sexual stigma: while the human papillomavirus, or HPV, can indeed spread during sexual activity—including anal or oral sex, which some people label "taboo"—sex doesn't have to occur for the infection to spread. In fact, the article quoted a New York City–based head and neck oncologist who said, "The vast majority of humans in the U.S., both men and woman, will eventually get infected with human papillomavirus." Marcia Cross was now dedicated to eliminating the stigma surrounding HPV-linked anal cancer, as she stated during several public interviews. "I care deeply about saving lives," Cross told CNN. "To that end, the important thing to do is educate the public about HPV. It is so common that nearly every person who is sexually active will get it at some point in their lifetime."

Echoing this information in the same news segment, the executive director of ACF, Justine Almada, destigmatized the infectious agent by stating that "HPV is ubiquitous. . . . The primary risk factor for getting it is being a human being." When a "high-risk" strain of HPV lingers, as we were told was the case for Cross, it can cause cancer: "Over time, meaning decades after we were first exposed, the virus gets into our DNA, and likes to settle in the tissues of the cervix or the back of the throat [or anus], and can ultimately cause changes that form cancer," said the oncologists interviewed for the media report. Cross had revealed that her anal cancer was the result of HPV—most likely the same HPV type that caused her husband, Tom Mahoney, to develop throat cancer a decade ago, in 2009, the same year Fawcett died (SurvivorNet 2019). Women's bodies and their heterosexual lives seemed most able to desexualize anal cancer, drawing associations away from sex and toward a general health concern. When sex was clearly delineated as a source of transmission, it was in association with men or targeted to LGBTQ communities, and never as a "women's concern." At the same time, oropharyngeal cancer, the cancer affecting Cross's husband, was imbued with a gendered heterosexualization that would bring yet another HPV-associated cancer to the public's attention.

CHAPTER FIVE

A "Coming Epidemic" of HPV-Associated Oral Cancer

The first public (and notably intimate) link between sex and oral cancer appeared in June 2013. It had been well publicized that Michael Douglas, a winner of two Oscars and countless other accolades for acting and producing and a venerable member of Hollywood royalty, had been undergoing treatment for oropharyngeal cancer since 2010. Then fifty-two, and married to actress Catherine Zeta-Jones, Douglas is perhaps best known for his roles in the movies *Wall Street, Fatal Attraction,* and as Liberace in the biopic *Behind the Candelabra.* In an interview with the *Guardian* following a successful but brutal regime of chemotherapy and radiation and a thirty-pound weight loss, Douglas unequivocally said oral sex was responsible for his cancer when he told reporters, "this particular cancer is caused by HPV, which actually comes about from cunnilingus." The testimonial launched a media storm; Douglas's words in the "surprisingly frank" interview were widely re-reported. Douglas's declaration—rather than speculation—that the sexual act of cunnilingus was causally responsible for his cancer was unprecedented, as was the suggestion that others could be at similar risk of a disease caused by sex.

An expansion and diffusion of the sex-cancer link was traveling from cancer type to cancer type—cervical to anal and now oral—and from population risk group to risk group, taking on new gendered and sexual undercurrents along the way. Now the cancer in question was a subtype of throat cancer, oropharyngeal cancer (OPC), that affects areas deep in the back of the throat, tongue, and tonsils that share a common set of epithelial cell types.[1] While this cancer was designated "rare," just as anal cancer had been, it garnered more attention possibly due to its locus in a less stigmatized body part and because it had little in the way of a lingering stigma associated with sex. A warning of a *coming* epidemic, a designation based on rising rates of diagnoses, was delivered to a population group mostly unmarked by a harbinger of sexual risk. These cancers, largely outside of public awareness, were increasingly coming into a new form of public conversation around cause and concern. They had previously been widely attributable to smoking cigarettes, individuated into a health risk behavior and having gradually become an established component of preventive medicine. The known carcinogen of tobacco, whether smoked or chewed, had come to be closely associated with men and masculinity (Greaves 1996), and in particular (in the case of menthol cigarettes) with Black men. These "habits" are pushed through capital and marketing efforts to establish a hold in various bodies and communities.[2]

When the journalist Catherine Shoard (2013) reported in the *Guardian* that the "cause of Douglas's cancer had long been assumed to be related to his tobacco habit," she was implicating an already publicly and medically understood gendered contour of the throat cancer Douglas had gone public with. Yet now, with Douglas's assertion that cunnilingus—oral sex performed on women—was the behavior that had put him at risk, this cancer would reflect and produce a gendered sexuality that was potentially cause for concern *for anyone*. "HPV, the sexually transmitted virus . . . is thought to be responsible for an increasing proportion of oral cancers," Shoard wrote, echoing Douglas's remarks linking his cancer to a practice that, in mainstream understandings, is associated with heterosexual "foreplay." It is no surprise that given this sexual contour, the story went viral and was picked up by thousands of news and entertainment websites. The internet exploded with bold headlines, each proclaiming this specific sexual link to men's throat cancer. As Michael Douglas's story went viral, the symbolic associations between sex and this cancer type would differ significantly from those between sex and anal cancer.

The gendered sexual association for the HPV–oral cancer link contrasts starkly with that of HPV's association with anal and cervical cancer. With oral cancer, it was viral evidence itself that prompted research into transmission paths, rather than the other way around (that is, with suspected transmission motivating the search for a viral cause), as had been the case with cervical cancer. These at-risk subjects of oral cancer are adult heterosexually active men in their middle age. In contrast to the girls of Gardasil, these men were not identified (by themselves or others) with any particular social movement, and were largely unmarked as a risk category for diseases associated with sex. HPV has initially, and strategically, led many publics to become aware of the causal connection between HPV, cancer of the cervix, and "women's health."

Michael Douglas's declaration came at a decisive time for Merck, which had just expanded Gardasil's use to include adolescent boys based on a link between HPV and non-life-threatening genital warts. HPV-associated oropharyngeal cancers were on the rise not from these HPV strains, but from those associated with cancer. A narrative was beginning to circulate about this cancer and its risk categories as media picked up the story of Douglas's cancer and as the epidemiological evidence unfolded scientifically about HPV's role in the onset of cancer tumors in the back of the throat and tonsils.

White heterosexual men were rarely enrolled in narratives of cancer or of risk—that is, except as the abstract masculinist version of a risk-taker possessing strength and the capacity to protect deserving others from harm.[3] The cancers associated with HPV were no different. Cervical cancer was already inscribed as an unknown, silent killer of women, its prevention part of a long history of disease-testing and surveillance medicine: screening technologies and programs performed on individuals without symptoms or at no special risk. The media attention following Douglas's pronouncement of his cancer diagnosis, however, signaled that the gendered contours of HPV-associated cancers might be transforming to include middle-aged cis and heterosexual men. The media focused less on the cancer and its medical treatment or any personal story of triumphant survival, as often happens with a cancer narrative, and more on the sex that caused it. In the two months following the *Guardian* article, 2,840 unique stories appeared documenting Douglas's claim and the contribution of sex and HPV to cancer. His recovery from cancer is still regularly mentioned in profiles of the actor, though the source of the cancer has mainly dropped away from the story of Douglas's life.

Douglas's story captures the familiar symbolism of cancer as a gendered and sexualized category of disease, but in this case the disease is associated with men, masculinity, and (explicit) heterosexuality. Douglas's handlers, meanwhile, were eager to dial the sexual association back by identifying his cancer more specifically as tongue cancer, which in their description might conjure associations with disfiguring treatments, yet was also a cancer with a different behavioral association: tobacco use. Oropharyngeal cancer, in contrast, was gradually coming to be associated with HPV. Almost immediately following his initial disclosure, Douglas took pains to apologize publicly to his wife, Catherine Zeta-Jones, for the "embarrassment." The exact source of that embarrassment, however, was unclear. Was it from bringing Zeta-Jones's sexual practices and sexual self into public conversation, implying that it was her body that was the "vector" of his contagion? Was it perhaps the signaling of Douglas's or Zeta-Jones's previous sexual relationships and practices? Or was itr something else? Did this narrative thrust Zeta-Jones into a vulnerable subjectivity in need of protection from a cancer risk or from her husband's airing of his and their sexual history and practices?

Scientific, health, and other media began to report evidence of changes in oral and other sexual practices as they tried to make sense of increases in cases of oral cancer and the emerging narrative about a coming epidemic. In the US about 20,000 people will be diagnosed with this cancer annually ("How Many Cancers Are Linked With HPV Each Year?" 2020). Behind these numbers lies a medical search and a narrative explanation of whose bodies and lives are at risk of developing this cancer. Heterosexually active men who "go down" on sexual partners with vaginas were brought into a new "at-risk" identity. This identity and its indications of risk were gendered and sexualized as the proliferation of discourses on cunnilingual sexual practices attached to men's heterosexuality, rendering invisible women's and queer sexual practices more generally. HPV exists in epithelial skin zones found all along the "anogenital tract," so transmission would likely occur from tongues, lips, and mouths engaged in sexual pleasuring from the anus to the penile shaft or to vaginal lips and the clitoris—mouth to an epithelial zone. There was no mention of oral cancer risk to women—neither from performing fellatio, cunnilingus, or rimming nor from the other sexual practices with fingers or devices that also involve epithelial skin zones and one's mouth or vagina. This desexualizing of the domain of cancer risk was a parallel narrative and epidemiological research feature of HPV and oral cancer.

The *Guardian* article in which Douglas's assertion first appeared recognized that a causal shift at least partly "cultural" was underway, as they argued that these new cancer cases "might also be linked to the lack of safety of penetrative sex in the wake of the AIDS epidemic," referring to the ways oral sex came to be associated with safe sex (Shoard 2013). Like most of the others in my data search, the article desexualized queer sexualities in favor of a sexualization of hetero-masculinity. The social and cultural politics of sex, then, demonstrated the ways HPV and its associated cancers are part of an ongoing yet temporally specific politics of sexuality. Here, sex is neither tamed nor de-gendered; rather, it is the specter of the "other," better known (and more risky) gendered, sexualized actors associated with HIV/AIDS that were mobilized. The ghostly matters of gay, bisexual, and other men who have sex with men (MSM)'s sexual identities, with their presumably anal penetrative or receptive (and therefore "risky") sex practices, stood in contrast to the identities of heterosexuality, which were already seen as reducing their risk by engaging in other "less risky" heterosexual practices. Oral sex had already been mobilized, in other words, as a risk protection. Cunnilingus, at least in this context, was not only in the news and thus part of a proliferation of discourse about sex and disease; it was also associated with an awareness of "risk" for heterosexually active men, given their distinctive differentiation, it would seem, from not only "homosexual" riskiness, but also the risks for women.

This focus on masculine heterosexuality was largely uncontentious until 2013, when its association with containment of stigmatized sexual practices and identities was rendered visible in another attempt to suppress and govern sexual behavior. Regulating non-procreative sex for pleasure outside of heterosexual marriage emerged as a site of backlash. A corner of social conservatism in the US, the American Family Association (AFA), well known for opposing LGBTQ and other human rights in the name of "biblical principles" and morality, entered the discourse on HPV and oral cancer.[4] At the height of publicity around Douglas's Stage IV cancer diagnosis, the AFA appointed a spokesperson to call for a ban on oral sex among consenting adults, in explicit response to the developing news of rising HPV-associated throat cancers. Perhaps recognizing the lack of prior stigmatizing significations or corrupted or diminished identities associated with this practice of men providing oral sex to women, the proscription was bound to a ban on anal sex as well. Drawing on decades-old, legally hollow, and functionally fallow anti-sodomy laws outlawing sexual acts largely (though not exclusively) among same-sex people, and lumping anal and oral sex together as like practices of like people, the AFA was relying on familiar sexual politics used to target LGBTQ people, in particular non-heterosexual people and their sexual practices (through anti-sodomy laws, for example). Such laws against oral sex remain on the legislative books in eighteen states, despite the US Supreme Court's 2003 ruling in *Lawrence v. Texas* declaring that state's anti-sodomy laws unconstitutional, thereby invalidating such laws in all states.[5]

While the rhetorical attempt to ban oral sex was easily dismissed and was even met with some mockery, the AFA's broader intent was clear: to reignite sexual politics generally by bringing cunnilingus specifically into association with the stigmatized practice of anal sex. This message of abstaining from all non-procreative sex and sexuality outside of marriage repurposed these laws, which had been used against gay people to justify discrimination and raise public alarm in the later years of the twentieth century and especially as social movements for LGBTQ rights and then AIDS activism were underway. Sexual politics and HPV were co-constitutive and haunted by prior associations revealing the ways these sexual associations were hard to tame, even as they were protected by the cloak of masculine heterosexuality.

Douglas's public claim had brought blowback as well as attention to HPV, sexual transmission, and cancer risk. Some of that attention was plainly right-wing reaction to the threat of new cultural discourse around non-procreative sex and sexual pleasure, but much of it belied important cultural and public health shifts in thinking about risk and behavior and around bodies and health. Soon after Douglas's comments, research and media began to highlight heterosexuality and categorize oral sex as an "at-risk" behavior. It was heterosexual men who were found to be three times more likely to be diagnosed with HPV-related oropharyngeal cancer than the "general population," a production of a population risk that persisted in the public and epidemiological imagination.

Gathering Evidence and Making a Case for Straight Men's Oral Cancer Risk

Oropharyngeal cancers were initially classified in the scientific and medical literatures first as "upper aerodigestive tract cancers" (UATCs) and then as part of the smaller grouping of "head and neck squamous cell carcinomas" (HNCCs). What are now called oropharyngeal cancers (sometimes OPC) to indicate their specificity as cancers of the oropharynx and tongue were never thought to have any infectious cause, although some speculated that it might be linked to another large family of infectious viruses, herpes, rather than to HPV. This stood in contrast to cervical cancer, which historically had a material and symbolic association as "a woman's disease" (Löwy 2011).

The discovery in the 1980s of the molecular composition of HPV launched a scientific search for a viral-cancer association. Not only were rates for cancers in certain areas of the body where sexual pleasure and sex occur (specifically, oral and anal) going up, but the conjecture of an infectious cause was backed by reason: materially, the HPV virus is transferred across moist epithelial surfaces (squamous cells) covered by skin and/or mucosa. These "epithelial zones" exist in many areas of the body, including the cervix, vulva, anus, and penis, as well as the interior of the mouth, the throat, the tongue, and the tonsils. HPV transmission, or transfer, occurs between epithelial cells as the virus crosses the skin barrier, especially when that barrier is broken or otherwise rendered "vulnerable" by abrasion. Sexual contact between epithelial zones, where saliva and other bodily fluids are exchanged is understood to be the most likely transfer point for viral transmission. When scientists and clinicians use the term "oral" they are referring to the oropharynx, a part of the pharynx between the soft palate and the skin-flap at the upper end of the trachea referred to as the epiglottis ("Oropharynx" 2020).

There were other reasons to use the narrower term as well. No preventive approaches had been developed for oral cancer, and Merck did not conduct clinical trials to establish evidence of a correlation between an HPV genotype and oral cancer. In addition, no trials had ever been done showing that HPV in saliva or other fluids of the throat would be in any way significant for prevention. HPV would surely be present in these similar skin and moisture zones, since it is a common and ubiquitous STI. To establish knowledge of its presence, however, definitive proof that persistence of a high-risk HPV strain associated with the wider umbrella of head and neck cancers (HNCC), or specifically to a narrower subtype, would be necessary. Creating and validating such a diagnostic and/or preventive tool could be profitable for any company that could successfully develop, provide evidence for use, and ultimately market such an approach to cancer prevention.

Oropharyngeal cancer came with a set of puzzles that had not been seen previously in HPV-cancer research. Compared to other HPV-associated cancers, many of the oropharyngeal cancers seemed to be more responsive to standard radiation and surgical treatments, and their rates of diagnosis were increasing, especially among men. An established professional world of oncologists with specialization in the *treatment* of HNCCs already existed. Therefore, with general HPV scientific knowledge increasing throughout the 1990s and early 2000s, researchers began to gather evidence in support of an HPV-HNCC association.

The oncological specialists and clinical researchers who spoke at conferences and declared that we are seeing "rising rates" of a subset of oral cancers were not infectious disease specialists, nor were they part of the now established infrastructures of non-AIDS-defining cancers. I was able to speak with Maura Gillison, a leading head and neck oncologist and epidemiologist then based at Ohio State University, at the annual meeting of EUROGIN, the professional association of the European Research Organization on Genital Infection and Neoplasia, held in 2015 in southern Spain. A panel on oral HPV included expert presentations that began with concerns about a "coming epidemic." Gillison, indeed, confirmed the increase in rates she herself documented and treated over her twenty years as a clinician: "There was such a dramatic and rapid change in the patients that we saw in that very short period of time . . . it's one of the few cancers that we're documenting as actually going up right now." Gillison's interest in infectious disease and cancer had been sparked in 1994 following the publication in *Science* of research conducted by the University of Pittsburgh virologists Yuan Chang and Patrick Moore, who found an association between another oncogenic virus, Kaposi's sarcoma-associated herpesvirus (KSHV, also known as human herpesvirus 8 or HHV8[6]), and the human cancer Kaposi's sarcoma (KS). KS came to prominence with the onset of red skin blotches associated with AIDS (when HIV was not treated in ways that suppressed viral loads).[7] It was a sudden entrance into infectious disease: "This made me realize that if you study the infectious disease tumor associations, there'd be many more opportunities for intervention in terms of prevention, screening, therapy," she said. Gillison then turned to the stakes for care as the "patients" in her oncology practice came to the office with a new desire to know, "How did I get this?"

The "how" puzzle she raised was not one of sexual cause, given the study of infectious disease; rather, it was a question of "whether we are seeing similar rates among sexual partners . . . among these men's wives." Ultimately, there was a need to determine how the pathways and impacts of sexuality might be understood. Gillison described a relational and sexual risk that had emerged in the past decade concurrent with the cancer she and her colleagues specialized in. As her patients entered cancer care, she told me, many bore feelings of embarrassment along with the more expected fears of treatment effects and life expectancy.

Gillison was deeply involved in applying molecular biology to treatment studies for people with these cancers; as a molecular epidemiologist, she worked with population-based statistical studies to contextualize her research. Her research designs combined studies of biomaterial (e.g., tumor genomes) with behavioral and demographic survey data. These cancers had previously been linked mostly to smoking and, to a lesser degree, drinking alcohol. Using molecular epidemiology, Gillison was able to reveal not only the existence of a relatively unknown sub-cancer—in the far reaches of the throat and tonsils—but the surprising behavioral risk that seemed to be driving it: sex.

Researchers had begun to look closer at HPV to see whether there might be other cancers resulting from the infection since the 1980s. In 1995 the International Agency for Research on Cancer (IARC) of the World Health Organization issued a report on HPV that discussed in detail cervical, vulvar, vaginal, penile, and anal cancers, with a small, final section dedicated to "Other Cancers" that included a review of research into the presence of HPV at less-discussed biological sites. Cancers of the head and neck—mouth, pharynx, tonsils, and other sites—were included in these "other cancers" by evidence from case studies beginning as early as 1987, 1989, and 1985, respectively (International Agency for Research on Cancer 1995, 195). Acknowledging the relative dearth of attention given to these sites, along with the much smaller number of patients affected compared to cancers of the cervix and anogenital areas, the IARC deemed the evidence to date from research studies inconclusive: "the presence of HPV according to any technique does not constitute a proof of causality *per se . . .*" (International Agency for Research on Cancer 1995, 195).

In 1996 a scientific call came in the conclusion of an article published in a widely read medical journal from the American Association for Cancer Research (AARC), *Cancer Epidemiology Biomarkers and Prevention*. Researchers acknowledged the lack of evidence supporting HPV's role in head and neck cancer and called for the development of "a measurement tool to solve the uncertainty around the role of HPV in the development of UADT [upper aerodigestive tract] cancer" (Franceschi et al. 1996, 567).[8] Evidence came in 1998 through a population-based, case-control study examining cancer risk with HPV infection and the epidemiology of "sexual history." Its authors concluded that "oncogenic, sexually transmittable human papillomaviruses (HPVs) are etiologic factors in the development of oral squamous cell carcinoma (SCC)" (Schwartz et al. 1998, 1626). Sex behavior surveys (which included questions such as age at first regular sexual intercourse; lifetime number of opposite-sex partners; whether one had ever performed oral sex on an opposite-sex partner; lifetime number of opposite-sex oral sex partners; and prior diagnosis of genital warts),[9] along with HPV genotyping, showed that HPV-16 infection was associated with the development of a small proportion of oral cancers in the population studied, and confirmed that cancer risk increased in proportion to (declining) age of first intercourse, (increasing) number of sex partners, and a history of genital warts (Schwartz et al. 1998).

In 1999, Gillison and colleagues published a major review of the existing epidemiologic and virologic studies highlighting what they referred to as an "intriguing relationship: between HPV infection and HNCC." The authors noted the importance of sexually transmitted HPV as a possible and potentially important risk factor for head and neck cancer development, and sought to establish a causal relationship between them (Gillison, Koch, and Shah 1999). Then, in 2000, Gillison's team reported study results confirming that "HPV-positive oropharyngeal cancers comprise a distinct molecular, clinical, and pathologic disease entity that is likely causally associated; and demonstrating that cancer patients with HPV infection *had* [emphasis added] a markedly improved prognosis" (Gillison et al. 2000, 709). The improved prognosis indicated there was some difference between these molecular-based cancers and others of the same area. This led researchers to confirm that more than 50 percent of what were referred to as HNCCs in the oropharynx region, particularly in the tonsils and at the base of the tongue (where Douglas's cancer was diagnosed), contain oncogenic human papillomavirus (HPV) DNA, and specifically HPV-16 (Forastiere et al. 2001). This finding also importantly revealed an increase in the rates of certain head and neck cancers not associated with alcohol and tobacco use, as might be expected, but instead associated with HPV, leading to understandings of this cancer's rising rates.

Sexual transmission became the presumptive pathway and the causative role, and HPV the socially designated infection responsible for subsequent development of cancers of the oropharynx (Herrero et al. 2003, 1772). Scientific consensus converged around a need for more evidence to support this preposition, given an additional aspect of the puzzle: only about 20 percent of these malignancies are associated with viral infection; unlike cervical cancer, high-risk HPVs in head and neck cancer are neither a necessary nor a sufficient cause of cancer. As the lead researchers in the field indicated, it was not yet clear whether "tobacco and alcohol, the major risk factors for HNCC, are less frequent exposures among those detected with HPV in HNCC" and therefore not the causative driver of disease (Smith et al. 2004, 766). What was clear, however, was that from analyses of tissue specimens of oral cancers, US National Cancer Institute scientists had found that HPV DNA was present in almost a quarter (or 23.5 percent) of oropharyngeal cancer cases (Kreimer et al. 2005). This research supported that any biological explanation for a higher prevalence of HPV in tumors of the oropharynx compared with other sites in the head and neck remained unclear (Kreimer et al. 2005, 469; see also Saslow et al. 2007). In 2007, Gypsyamber D'Souza and colleagues at Johns Hopkins University in Maryland would provide the evidence: oral HPV infection is strongly associated with oropharyngeal cancer, with or without the established risk factors of tobacco and alcohol use. Consensus emerged around the data that at least one-quarter and probably a third of oropharyngeal cancers are caused by HPV infection (zur Hausen 2009, 262n10; see also 2007 IARC conclusions summarized by Muñoz et al. 2006), and specifically as *primarily caused* by HPV-16.

The IARC declared that there was sufficient evidence to support the viral cause of oral cancers in 2012 (IARC Working Group on the Evaluation of Carcinogenic Risks to Humans 2012).[10] Cancer epidemiologists at the American Cancer Society would include this HPV-associated cancer in the next report to the nation, due to be released in 2013. The report made the case to the public that the incidence of this cancer had more than doubled over the ten-year period from 2003 to 2013, that it did so among men, and that it was attributable to HPV (Jemal et al. 2013). This "men's cancer" was projected to surpass the number of cases of cervical cancer for women in the United States by 2020 (Chaturvedi et al. 2011), a projection often amplified with alarm by news outlets. Oral cancer causation's "viral infectious process" as HPV transmits through heterosexual contact

(Mundell 2008), presumably from women to men. Evidence was needed to understand whose bodies and practices were most at risk as well as most important to immunize.

Gillison and her colleagues proved a correlation between HPV and oral cancer and provided data confirming the sexual pathways of transmission. HPV data is regularly monitored by the National Health and Nutrition Examination Survey (NHANES), a unique data collection survey that combines interviews with physical examinations, including blood and other biological materials, and information on lifetime sexual partners and practices. Using 2009 and 2010 NHANES survey results, Gillison analyzed data from 5,579 men and women ages fourteen to sixty-nine in combination with results from oral rinse tests for HPV genotypes (Gillison et al. 2012). A narrative was beginning to unfold: the study found that 7 percent of this group had an oral HPV infection, and the infection rate was three times higher in men than women (10.1 percent vs. 3.6 percent, respectively). Polymerase chain reaction (PCR) analysis showed that of the 1 percent of the population with an HPV-16 infection, five times more men tested HPV-16 positive than women, correlating with their higher incidence of HPV-related cancer (Gillison et al. 2012).

The self-reported survey data on sexual activity included information on number of partners (lifetime and recent), type of sex (oral, vaginal, anal), sexual partners (same-sex or opposite-sex), and personal history of STIs. Taken together, these data provided a presumptive explanation for men's higher probability of HPV transmission through oral sex performed on women (in contrast to women's likelihood of having HPV through oral sex done on a man), as well as the statistical finding that HPV prevalence increased more sharply with increased number of sexual partners for men than for women. Men are three times as likely as women to develop HPV-related oral cancer; white men were at highest risk, almost nine times as likely as Black men to be diagnosed with HPV-related oral cancers (Gillison et al. 2012). In other words, it was either that performing oral sex on vaginas was more risky than doing so on a penis, or that performing more oral sex increased the risk of infection.

Gillison hoped to understand why the incidence rates were going up so dramatically for men and not for women. She explained, "When we looked at that relationship between sexual behavior, gender, and oral HPV infection, and we saw these dramatic differences, you know, I said, 'Oh my God, this explains exactly why we're seeing this increase. It's because this is completely consistent with sexual behavior changing, but women rapidly develop protection with their first three partners [while] men remain at risk to 30 partners.' So, that's why it's going up for men." For epidemiologists and oncologists, an understanding of men's continual risk was coming to light. Across the life course they are more likely to have HPV infections, and older men seem to be just as able as younger men to contract the virus. Women, in contrast, seem to be protected over time (although it is unclear why). In addition, the transmission pathway was gradually shown to be more efficient, and thus somewhat more likely, when it went from women's bodies to their sexual partners': "Vaginas may spread HPV into the mouth more readily than penises, since vaginas usually contain more fluids, in which HPV particles can reside, than the penile shaft or scrotum, the surfaces most involved in oral sex" (Harris 2012). While subsequent research would reveal that HPV resides in semen as well (Luttmer et al. 2015), a novel and significant concern was emerging: men, presumably cis and straight, not lesbian, queer or nonbinary people, were in need of protection from vaginas, as this body part was given a measure of responsibility for disease transmission. In turn, it was quickly suggested that sexual liberation and changes in sexual practices (including first sexual experience at an earlier age, higher numbers of sexual partners, and higher probability of oral sex) may be associated with the increasing prevalence of HPV infection (Heck et al. 2009). As research and a conceptualization of this cancer as a "men's cancer" predominated in scientific and popular imaginaries, women and their sexual practices with other women were curiously absent.

It was these scientific claims about men and men's practices through which oral cancers joined cervical and anal cancers in the uneven and gendered sexualization of HPV cancer prevention. Identities, groups, and practices were forming various narratives as well as affecting epidemiological facts linking some to risk (specifically sexual risk) and to a need for inclusion in cancer prevention. Adult men in their fifties or sixties, and in long-term monogamous heterosexual relationships, had likely not been concerned with their risk of oral cancer. These were the same men, however, who are part of a generation that had recently accrued other cancer risks, predominantly through the development of prostate-specific antigen (PSA) blood tests and establishment of routine guidelines for colonoscopies and stool-card samples for colon cancer screening. Former and current smokers were also part of a well-established risk group for lung cancer and other smoking-related diseases such as heart disease. None of these cancer risks, importantly, were known to be "contagious" or transmissible, or related to sexuality. They did not extend to sexual identities, practices, and cultures, nor to sexual partners. Today, these men find themselves assigned risk designations for a rare cancer of the tongue, throat, and neck, and a cancer with rates on the rise that brings their identities and intimate relationships into medical view.

But without a cancer screening tool like the PSA for prostate cancers (Faulkner 2012), these men had not yet been officially or strategically "made aware" of their cancer-risk designation. And this is a demographic group that had largely gone "unmarked," at least in terms of enjoying a normative place in the biomedical imaginary: heterosexual, middle-aged, and largely white men. Yet scientists, clinicians, and media were working to bring these men into "awareness" of both a sexual risk and a cancer risk with claims that their cancers could soon surpass the incidence of a vastly better-known cancer specific to women—cervical cancer. As diagnoses accumulated, oncologists found themselves at the center of a quiet sexual storm. Along with discussion of cancer diagnoses, prognoses, and treatment plans came a surprisingly new, and at times controversial, set of conversations among patients and their medical providers about sex and the risks it might pose. These patients were just as surprised as the doctors by the sexual conversations unfolding at the oncology office, as patient groups began sharing their experience either with their doctors or through emerging patient advocacy organizations.

Media Caution Men to Be(come) Aware of Cancer Caused by an STI

Media stories would gradually join a chorus of commentary about men's risk, amplifying the alarm over time and beseeching men to "know the link" between HPV and oral cancer. Not much time had passed since the public had been inundated with messages of the HPV-cancer link and Gardasil advertising that emphasized cervical cancer prevention. In 2007 and 2008 two leading newspapers ran stories by their prominent science reporters, bringing oral sex to the fore. Rob Stein's (2007) story in the *Washington Post* came with the headline "Virus Spread by Oral Sex Is Linked to Throat Cancer," and the headline of Nicholas Bakalar's (2008) piece in the *New York Times* read, "Oral Cancer in Men Associated with HPV." Reporting on the first study to firmly establish the link between HPV and oral cancer, Stein drew a line from the sexually transmitted virus that causes cervical cancer to the sharp increase in the risk of certain types of throat cancer among people infected through oral sex. He referred to research published in the *New England Journal of Medicine* finding that those infected with HPV were thirty-two times as likely to develop one form of

oral cancer than those free of the virus (D'Souza et al. 2007). Science journalists understood these findings as significant to public understandings of
STIs and cancer, as well as to sexualities and sexual cultures more generally. Stein included a quote from a medical researcher, Mark A. Schuster,
about changing sexual norms: "Many adolescents, and adults too, say they
engage in oral sex as a less risky type of sex," said Schuster, noting for the
readers that the strategy was ineffective, since herpes, syphilis, gonorrhea, HIV, and other STIs can spread through oral sex. In his *Times* article Bakalar stayed close to clinical trial evidence and the stakes for care.
He covered the newly published evidence that among people undergoing
OPC treatment, more than 40 percent of tumors in men were found, when
sampled and tested, to be infected with HPV. These cancers, shown to be
HPV-associated, responded positively to treatment (Worden et al. 2008).[11]
Cancer centers across the US would highlight the good news along with the
rise in rates: "HPV positive throat cancers" are now "surging" among men
(Memorial Sloan Kettering Cancer Center 2021), bringing newly identified
patient groups into cancer risk

Catchy headlines implicating men and their sexuality in cancer risk
would become more and more common, as health news raised the specter of a disease that was hidden, but on the rise. A media frenzy began in
Men's Journal, in which an article posed this question: "Can Oral Sex Cause
Cancer?" (Harris 2012). The answer to the rhetorical question was equally
blunt: "The cause is, shockingly, a common sexually transmitted disease."
And it came with a grave warning: "[A woman you go down on] is almost
certain to have been infected at some point with a virus that could, years
from now, give you throat cancer." The image accompanying the article
was a lower torso of a seemingly white woman. Her caution-tape–yellow
bikini underwear was printed with the word "WARNING" over the universal "No" sign—a red circle with a slash through it—superimposed over
a knife and fork. The text forewarned readers: "The next time you think
about going down on a woman think again."

Readers, likely intrigued and probably surprised, would be schooled in
the sexual trend of "the increasing popularity of oral sex—often seen as safer
than intercourse—among heterosexual couples." This safe sex approach,
readers were warned, "may soon lead to more male fatalities in industrialized nations from HPV-related infections than female ones—a surprising
turnaround after decades when women suffered higher death rates from
the virus, which also causes cervical cancer through vaginal sex" (Harris
2012). Another so-called surprise contained in the article was that women
had for years carried the burden of cancer diagnoses and death from HPV-
associated cervical cancer, a burden driven by their exposure from "vaginal

sex," *without* male alarm being conjured. It is only as the cancer concern and coming cancer burden is shown to shift from women to heterosexual men through men's practice of oral sex that alarm bells ring. In addition, unlike anal sex, which had long been silenced and stigmatized, heterosexual oral sex had largely escaped imputation. Yet, when associated with disease, these identities and practices could succumb to the same kinds of symbolic associations—the familiar shame and blame—as other STIs. There is little a heterosexual man can do to avoid HPV infection: "Virginity, monogamy, and [limiting oneself to] just plain old 'fooling around,' will not protect you," men were warned.[12]

When news broke that the legendary rock star Bruce Dickinson had been diagnosed with oral cancer, the public was primed to hear of the familiar viral-cancer association and sexual transmission pathway.[13] It was 2015, the same year that HPV-associated OPCs had surpassed cervical cancer rates in the US. Dickinson, the lead singer and songwriter of the heavy metal band Iron Maiden, was known not only for his strong stage presence, but also for his diverse offstage activities, including fencing, flying planes, and producing beer, as well as some of his conservative values. Echoing Douglas's earlier and much-publicized statements in an interview with Sirius XM radio, Dickinson asserted that he'd "contracted cancer from the virus transmitted via cunnilingus." As with Douglas, Dickinson's story was picked up by the media and carried similar headlines.

Billboard magazine's online headline announced: "Iron Maiden's Bruce Dickinson Blames Oral Sex for His Throat Cancer" (Brandle 2015). In contrast to Douglas's story, Dickinson did not backpedal or apologize for a sexual assertion, although he too asserted the direct causal connection between oral sex and his cancer. Instead, he declared that it was something unique in men and their sexuality that placed them at risk: men's "giving" nature, he speculated, was the likely path to his and other men's cancer diagnosis. He urged men to "stay vigilant" and to submit their bodies to the health care they warranted. He told the public, "guys should know if you get a lump here and you're over 40 don't just assume antibiotics will get rid of it" (Brandle 2015). In many ways, Dickinson and Douglas projected a common thread of masculine stereotypes: both seemingly unequivocally heterosexual, and each with a history of marriages and divorces. Developments in scientific and epidemiological research, coupled with the diagnoses of these two well-known men and the widespread and eye-catching media coverage of the topic in general, collectively brought this cancer into awareness. Socially and culturally, this cancer and its cancer risk took on a decidedly (hetero)sexual and masculine association.

Men's Health highlighted the concerning connection—not between HPV and cancer, but "how oral sex can give you cancer." Reporting provided the historical puzzle: this cancer had once been routinely attributed to smoking, but "from the early (19)80s to '90s, hospitals started seeing patients who had never smoked" (Hrustic 2017b). When clinicians found that these cancers in the tonsils were more treatable than the smokers' cancers were, scientists knew something was different. "The sexual revolution of the '60s," it was said, provided support for researchers' speculations about the likely culprit. "The STD can be passed by giving and receiving oral sex, and even by open mouth kissing alone," reporters advised (Hrustic 2017b). The public readership of *Men's Health*, presumably men, would learn that this STD could lay dormant for decades, an important clue as to why researchers were only now seeing a rise in what is being called an oral-sex-related cancer diagnosis. *Men's Health* reporting (Hrustic 2017a, Zickl 2017) would cite Gillison's research (2012) as they warned their readers that "1 in 9 men have this cancer-causing STD," adding that "some men" are at higher risk than others (Hrustic 2017a). They would also mention particular populations: racial identities as Black men were implicated alongside behavioral practices, such as men who smoke more than a pack of cigarettes a day or use marijuana, or report sixteen or more vaginal or oral partners in their lifetime, and each group was shown to be at a higher risk.[14] Yet media like *Men's Health* would pick up the story of a "coming epidemic," a "catastrophic rise [in]" and "surging" rates of a rare cancer. Media and popular culture figures, including Douglas and Dickinson, warned men about their (hetero)sexual practices, adding that "If your throat is infected with it, and you go down on your partner, you can transmit it to him or her, and vice versa."

While cunnilingus is not practiced only by heterosexual men, little news or risk-categorization ever appeared to make women "aware" of potential harm. Audiences would learn that condoms and the little-used dental dam were ineffective in "lowering your risk." These prevention tools (for other STIs and pregnancy alike), etched into the safe-sex organizing of AIDS activists and safe(r) sex campaigns, had little uptake in oral sex, among straight or queer gender and sexualities. Jerome Groopman, the well-known science reporter, had indeed warned, in his 1999 article for the *New Yorker*, of a coming sexual epidemic that "condoms cannot stop" (Groopman 1999). In doing so, he too was engaging in prevention biopolitics: the previously upheld prescription of barrier methods for prevention were of very little if any use in protecting against this viral concern.

Knowledge of an HPV–oropharyngeal cancer link worked backward from molecular certainty to evidence of sexual risk. The new molecular approach to gathering the evidence offered hope for a precision approach to prevention with a concomitant epidemiological narrative that brought heterosexuality and heterosexual men to the foreground of a cancer scare. Despite its very small numbers, the now established HPV-cancer risk would drive new questions about how precision medicine and preventive approaches might respond to this newly available information. While this cancer, like HPV-associated anal cancer, is uncommon in the general population, indeed holding the designation of a rare cancer, its incidence among some was emerging as a concern. It is a difference, however, not a disparity, and thus from a public health perspective it does not warrant critical attention. Yet in biomedical contexts, the newly emerging questions about treatment, care, and prevention would take on their own gendered sexual contours.

CHAPTER SIX

Sex at the Oncology Office

Oral Cancer Care and the Politics of Prevention

Oropharyngeal cancer in the US affects a relatively small number of people; yet of the almost 20,000 annual diagnoses each year, only 3,530 are women, and 16,245 are men ("How Many Cancers Are Linked with HPV Each Year?" 2020). Because of its status as a "rare cancer," it attracts little research funding and few dedicated professionals, and generates little in the way of medical approaches to its treatment and control as well as its prevention. HPV knowledge, however, accelerated a case for potential "innovation," in the language of science and medicine. In asserting a "coming epidemic," researchers and clinicians are not only making a case for attention; they are also forging a symbolic association between these newly produced "at risk" bodies and prior associations with sex, sexuality, and disease. The epidemiological story of a gendered cancer affecting heterosexual men sexualizes the meaning and practices surrounding this cancer in distinct ways. Viruses are social and interactional as well as material, and the ways they are understood and intervened upon sheds light on the social grid of power and its place in the shaping of health and disease.

(Hetero)Sex in the Oncology Office

As cancer specialists gathered evidence in support of HPV's role in oropharyngeal cancers, they were also gaining new expertise as sexual health educators. It was oncologists, not infectious disease experts—or even preventive medicine providers—who would integrate the domains of sexually infectious disease and cancer care into their clinical cancer practice. This commingling came first with disease diagnostics and then, as patients entered cancer treatment, with a new conceptualization of this disease. With evidence of an HPV link, health care interactions underwent a change of their own: sex entered the oncology office. Maura Gillison and other oncologists I interviewed described their clinical conversations as being no longer only about prognoses and treatment plans, but more frequently about "Who did I get this from," "Who gave this to me," and more particularly, "is this associated with (my or someone else's) infidelity or promiscuity?" These multi-surveillant conversations implicated past and present sexual partners and practices of the mostly middle-aged and heterosexually married people who found themselves in front of oncologists with a cancer they had very little knowledge of before. HPV ignited new questions not only about oneself, but about the others with whom one is—or had ever been—engaged in personal intimacy. A gendered sexualized dynamic accompanied conversations about treatment and care and came to occupy space and time in the oncologist's office. The non-patient wives of men diagnosed with cancer, it would seem, had questions of their own.

Interviews with leading clinical oncologists illustrated how these specialists would find themselves at the forefront of health education explaining to patients not only how viruses are causally implicated in cancer, but also how one's sex life and sexual partners play a role in what they are now finding to be a health concern. "We became sexual health educators," Ezra Cohen, a head and neck oncologist practicing in Chicago, exclaimed in our interview. It's not only that "men are at greater risk than women"; it also seems that the "number of lifetime sex partners that a person has correlates with the risk of developing an oropharynx cancer." Cohen felt unprepared and in need of some new ways to interact with the people who came to his office. Patient interactions were changing what he needed to do as an oncologist. Asked to describe a typical interaction, he begins: "We directly test all of our newly diagnosed OPC for the presence of HPV." Then, he explains how the conversation can be tricky: "We tell patients why testing on the tumor biopsies is indicated or thought to be otherwise useful." Cohen then often needs to do some education: "It's very helpful to know whether a patient's disease is related to HPV or not so we can talk to them about the psychosocial consequences of that viral presence and create a treatment plan." Once he begins the conversation, his patients find they "had no idea that there was a relationship between HPV and oropharynx cancers." And their surprise leads to questions about how and through whom the virus came to cause this cancer.

Lori Wirth, a Boston-based clinician and oncologist, described the cancer patients she sees: "They were completely floored . . . taken off guard." She too has found herself immersed in "a lot of very difficult discussions and peeling patients off of the ceiling," she said. Wirth told me of many examples of difficult discussions with patients that went beyond what she had been trained to deliver. "When people are coming into the medical oncologist to talk about their head and neck cancer, the last thing they are thinking about is a sexually transmitted disease." These conversations, she said, were "loaded" with sexual "baggage." She described these discussions and their dyadic nature as dominating clinical visits: "It was not what I had been used to as a provider . . . I needed to re-tool a bit. Over time, patients were less surprised. And so were their partners." In a short time, "more patients than not would understand that there's head and neck cancers associated with HPV," yet regardless of this information, office visits would inevitably include "'Who did I get this from?' or 'Who did I give this to?' . . . and for women, whether they are spouses of men diagnosed or people diagnosed themselves, they would often say, 'Who did my husband get this from? Certainly not from me!'"

Wirth also shared a typical clinical conversation, laying out the details of the encounter: A heterosexual married couple is in the office, and one of the spouses or members of that couple has an HPV-related oropharynx cancer. Wirth says, "We begin to talk about how they got it, what it means, and that it's a sexually transmitted virus." Immediately, "many begin to ask questions: 'What about my partner? Are they at risk? Do I need to inform anybody?'" Contact-informing practices are typical of sexual health and surveillance guidelines for STIs such as HIV, gonorrhea, and syphilis— STIs with transmissibility as high as that of HPV, but with very different materialities due to their more immediate health effects. Cancer is a distal and uncertain risk. As Wirth continued, "When we explain that first of all, this is contact they had a long time ago—probably decades ago rather than something recent," she says, "I think some of the stigma with respect to other partners is dissolved." There is a worry that drops away, and then, she says, especially their worry for their spouse lessens when she tells them "they are at very low risk for having an HPV related cancer, the risk is very low." "This is not gonorrhea or syphilis, that's acute and very highly transmissible. This is just the opposite. When we put it in that context, and I think rightly so, the patient and their partner begin to focus on the matter at hand and that is treating and managing their cancer."

Gillison too spoke of the ways sex and sexuality have become a salient part of her clinical work. "There were a lot of problems between couples. You know, when I treated patients, you could tell that this was causing stress in their relationship, and so I figured out ways to talk to people, to explain what we knew about HPV infection, and I addressed that right in the initial consultation, this issue of blame and guilt." She, like Wirth, describes a "normalizing of HPV" among her patients over time. For Gillison and other clinical oncologists the challenge of conducting sexual conversations led them to rethink their clinical encounters: "In the beginning, it was huge. Because, well, physicians weren't comfortable even talking about it [sex]." Research also drives physicians' reticence; they are encouraged to focus instead on treatment and to dismiss their patients' other, more emotional concerns. Gillison explained that her NIH-funded research into the connections between sexual history, HPV, and cancer hit roadblocks not from the usual recruitment of human subjects or data constraints, but from oncologists' inability to discuss sex. "Most people don't know [it] was a five-institution study. . . . We were never successful in enrolling cases from the other four institutions, because the physicians weren't comfortable with the questions we were asking their patients," she told me. "I think it was because the physicians weren't comfortable dealing with that issue at all, and no one had any clue what the answers were to the questions that the patients were asking." While oncologists were used to conversations about uncertain causality, at least those specialists known to her were not prepared to bring sex and sexuality to their clinical work. A social worker in her oncology practice told Gillison that "Patients from other oncologists were coming to them with 'marital stress.'" Gillison and the providers she worked with were retooling their approach to clinical interactions. She explained how she begins to reduce that stress: "The first thing I talk about is educating . . . you have no idea how long you had it. You have no idea who brought it into this relationship. You know, if you're human and you've had sex, you've had HPV. That whatever you swapped, you swapped when you first got together. You happen to be among the 99.9 percent who get it, never knew it, and you did not clear it. So, I specifically talk about you shouldn't change your sexual behaviors."

Oncologists, I soon found at scientific meetings, were most interested in talking with me—and their patients—about the relevance of sex and sexual transmission in these cancers and how a new conceptualization of cause, risk, and care was reshaping their clinical practice. It's not an epidemic, Gillison, told me, but "I can understand—I mean, for those of us who treat these patients every day, it feels that way because they're flooding our clinics." She says she is not in the "camp" that calls this an epidemic—that "it's not Ebola." "In the funding environment, you have to make what you're doing seem of critical importance. To say 'a 300 percent increase over a decade'—there are ways that you can say it that make it scarier than absolute numbers."

When I interviewed Ezra Cohen, a medical oncologist and currently the director of UC San Diego Health's Precision Immunotherapy Clinic, he brought women patients to the forefront. He described a clinical consult with an elderly woman, recently widowed, who had become infuriated, he told me, upon being diagnosed with cancer of the oropharynx or lower throat—infuriated not at her cancer diagnosis per se, he explained, but rather at her late husband. This example of marital stress caused by HPV held its own gendered dynamics. She was convinced she had contracted a sexually transmitted infection from his obvious and previously unknown "infidelity" and disloyalty, and Cohen described his clinical encounter with her as shifting from a discussion of how best to treat her cancer to one centered on education about distal risk, viral transmission, and the life course of viral infections. It was only after completing her treatment and delivering a good prognosis, Cohen reflected, that "I could just tell that something wasn't quite right and she wasn't ready to move forward as I would have expected." The widow had expressed her discomfort not to him, but to a nurse. "She was just as certain that [her husband] gave it to her and that he had not been faithful to her during the relationship. He was dead and she was having a hard time coming to terms with this." This was a sexual "finger-pointing," he said. "I think there are a lot of feelings related to the fact that HPV is a sexually transmitted virus that makes that association difficult for patients. . . . I think it raises a sense that patients have that this is associated with promiscuity." He then described his newly developed strategy of what he calls "normalizing" HPV. HPV is widespread, he tells them; "most people in our population who have had normal adult sex lives have come into contact with the HPV virus. And we don't understand why some people will end up with oropharynx cancer whereas [not] everybody who comes into contact with the virus [does]." Like others in my interviews, he brought up Michael Douglas and the media coverage of his diagnosis. Douglas's story helped stimulate the conversation, he told me. And helped Cohen move into a new role as a health educator.

As more people were diagnosed with OPC, it became clear that most had not previously, and especially recently, had their sexual matters entangled with health risk. Viagra, a little blue pill prescribed to help with erections and penetrative sex, was at the forefront of the ways their sexual health was pharmaceuticalized. A cancer diagnosis was the last place they expected to encounter sexual health education. Many of these men had at some point in their youth found themselves at the STI clinic seeking diagnosis or treatment for STIs, including genital warts, and many had likely been monitoring (or expected to monitor) noncommunicable and chronic diseases associated with cardiovascular health, occupational exposures, and smoking and alcohol reduction. These men, now cancer patients, were transformed by this reconceptualization of cancer as part of a risk group entangled with sex.

Risk without Pathology: Bringing Men into Surveillance Biomedicine

There is no technological tool (yet) that is tested and validated for specificity and sensitivity for the detection of high-risk HPVs in the body site of the (internal) head and neck on the market for use in screening and prevention. While cancer specialists detect HPV in tumor sites as part of clinical medicine and treatment protocols, the knowledge comes with a great deal of uncertainty. For definitive results, the presence of tumor tissue is required; in its absence the presence of HPV alone is inconclusive for disease. HPV can clear on its own, and without visible lesions to test for early signs of "precancer" or cancer, no screening test is available to offer these men who are newly aware of their risk.

The men in clinicians' oncology offices were largely not accustomed to designations of a masculine rather than a feminine sexual risk, nor were they presumed to be consumers of sexual risk prevention and surveillance. These men were otherwise unmarked as inhabiting "normative" sexual practices and identities. Bringing this concern to others already in place for aging men—routine colonoscopies; PSAs; cholesterol, blood pressure, and blood sugar levels, for example—was neither a clear nor an established route for preventive care. This was not part of the lifestyle turn in biomedicine offering medications to improve erections or reduce baldness.

Debates around HPV-anal cancer screening were well known among oncologists of the head and neck. Yet for OPCs the risk to health had not been sutured into medical care in the same way that HIV care and research was providing for other cancer risks. The risk of OPC was not previously designated as an AIDS-defining or a non-AIDS-defining cancer. Organizations advocating for these nascent risk populations were forming and had begun to demand inclusion in research and adequate (sexual) health education to prepare people who might find themselves in the offices of an oncologist. While Merck would continue to play an education and advocacy role to pharmaceuticalize HPV-linked risk, along with their partner cancer organizations, oncologists as well as patients and advocacy organizations were not prepared. There was, however, an ethos of triumphantly "taking on" cancer, with survivorship rather than victimhood (Sulik 2010) in place to draw on for messaging. There were none of the health movements around cancer that we see today, empowering patients to "Stand Up to Cancer" with a message reflective of another ethos, of neoliberalism and individual action as a moniker of self-control.

In 2013 I met with Pamela Tom, the founder of HPVANDME, a non-profit news and information website. Her husband's diagnosis in 2012 with stage 4 HPV squamous cell carcinoma, an OPC, had compelled Tom into near-immediate activism. Within the year, she had successfully fundraised, designed, and launched the organization HPVANDME (Tom 2012) with the goal of building public awareness about an HPV throat cancer pandemic and helping those who are and will be affected by this cancer. "Our Mission is to provide education about HPV infection, the HPV vaccine, and HPV-related cancers, specifically HPV-related oropharyngeal or head and neck cancers—now the #1 HPV cancer, surpassing cervical cancer. HPVANDME is about YOU. It's about everyone who wants to know more about HPV throat cancer—how to prevent it, how to fight it, how to live through it." Tom is an experienced journalist and communicator, and a formidable force in her own right, which partially explains HPVANDME's sophistication. But I wanted to understand the contours of Tom's decision to form an advocacy group, including the forces pressing her to do so in such an urgent and decisive fashion. I also had questions about whether the risk designation of heterosexual men and their sexuality would or could be part of established advocacy and activist cancer movements. Tom lived and worked near San Francisco, and generously agreed to schedule some time with me for an interview. It was a sunny afternoon when I drove north over the Golden Gate Bridge and largely along the Pacific coast from my home in San Francisco to Marin County. When I arrived at her home perched on the edge of a cliff and overlooking a beach on a gorgeous California afternoon, her dogs ran to greet me while she stood waving from an upper deck. She offered me something to drink, and then we sat in the sun and began to talk, with the dogs at our feet. I inquired about her husband's health, and she happily told me, "We count him among the survivors."

Before arriving for our scheduled interview, I had read through the website, which led me to place this newly established organization as closely aligned with the more general emergence of patient advocacy sites reflective of twenty-first-century biomedicalization. The site's direct address—to "YOU"—with information and expert guidance, yet with peer-to-peer content, was becoming fairly routine. These characteristics exemplify the "healthism" first referred to by the medical sociologist Robert Crawford (Crawford 1980, 2006), denoting the ways biomedicalization processes include a shift from treating disease to promoting and enhancing one's health. HPVANDME's enrollment of healthy actors to know their risk was reflective of social advocacy more generally—and, I thought, similar to previous HPV and pharmaceutical messaging to become "One Less."

Tom explained that HPVANDME was at least the third major cancer advocacy organization dedicated to research, awareness, and social support for patients and families with cancers of the head and neck—but the first to explicitly draw the connection to HPV and to lead with a goal of demystifying the science and communicating it to what she called "a new risk group." As a journalist, she told me, she started HPVANDME as a way to provide answers to the many questions she herself, as well as her husband, had about the disease.

When Tom's husband was diagnosed in March 2012, she told me, "It came as such a shock." First, "because he is an athletic, otherwise healthy non-smoking man." But then, "we never heard about it before . . . we were surprised to learn it was sexually transmitted."[1] Tom and her husband were not alone in their understandings: cancers were most often associated with nonsexual behaviors such as smoking, and otherwise mostly associated with either some form of "bad luck" or an occupational or environmental exposure to carcinogens such as coal dust.

After her husband's diagnosis, when she went online to find out, in her words, "What is it and how do you get it?" she said she had been unable to locate much information, and what was available was hard "for an ordinary person to really comprehend and digest." As a professional journalist, she was accustomed to going through a lot of information, so she anticipated that she would quickly become an expert. But in this case, she said, not only was there little information available; what she did find was difficult to parse. She was also surprised by what she learned: while many men were being diagnosed, she said, "People need[ed] to know that women can get it too."

Tom built and launched HPVANDME as an educational website just as news of Douglas's cancer was hitting the airwaves. Her initial goal was modest: she wanted to "find new ways to get the word out" and, using social media, "have more people share their story." From the outset, a surprising number of people wrote to Tom, telling her about their own husbands' HPV+ throat cancer and asking her the same questions she had previously asked. In response to emails, she says, "I try to tell them that this is like any other cancer. It's not as if you're wearing a big A—a scarlet letter A—on you; this is like any other cancer, and it can kill you!" The "Scarlet A" she was referring to was not the cancer itself, but its established sexual association. "That's why you have to get over any inhibitions you have about [talking about] oral sex because there are all kinds of ways to contract cancer, right. And different ways. And it's almost better if you know how you get it," she said. Tom increasingly advocates for what she calls the only known prevention against HPV: HPV vaccine awareness. "And here you can prevent this—because you know that this virus causes cancer, then you get the vaccine, and get it at a right age." While the HPV vaccine was not in-dicated or approved for the prevention of oral cancers, Tom shared what many researchers and clinicians quietly confirmed. Although Gardasil is recommended for boys based on genital warts and anal cancers, and not oral cancer, "behind closed doors, pediatrician to parent, are the pediatri-cians saying you should vaccinate your son to prevent oral cancer?" she asked. "Probably." In addition to promoting HPV vaccination, Tom was also focused on turning uncertainty into disease prevention. She instructs many: "if you know that if you start having a sore throat, it could be a sore throat, but if it's unusual and persists, it could be something else."

Tom also told me about her own reaction to learning of the STI link to her husband's cancer: "The HPV connection didn't bother me because it is a virus, like any other." She then turned attention to the then recent reports of Michael Douglas's cancer. "While I respect any individual's desire for privacy, I was surprised and disturbed that Catherine Zeta-Jones hushed up Michael Douglas's admission that his cancer was caused by HPV. Doug-las is popular and has a large audience. Had he been permitted to continue sharing his entire cancer story with the public, our movement to increase HPV vaccination and cancer prevention would have been propelled for-ward several years. Sadly, it was a lost opportunity."

Tom started HPVANDME in hopes of filling the silence and dispelling the misinformation around sex that accompanied oral cancer. We spoke of how Michael Douglas stated that his cancer was caused by the same vi-rus that causes cervical cancer, but never uttered the name HPV, relying instead on repeated mentions of his heterosexual marriage. Tom gained expertise in the sexual transmission of viruses, specifically of HPV and its role in oropharyngeal cancer, as the basis of her advocacy work: "Doc-tors whom I've interviewed say most of the time, these middle-aged men contracted the disease or the virus back in their twenties when they first became sexually active." She understands the ways the entanglements of sex and disease have historically stigmatized, shamed, and blamed certain groups. As a result, HPVANDME is designed to do the work of provid-ing information and raising awareness without invoking ghostly hauntings from prior sexual associations used to repress and discriminate. She told me, "most people will clear the virus and, of course, there's certain strains that cause cancer and certain ones that don't. But doctors say those who get an HPV-related cancer have a compromised immune system. Their bodies can't attack it sufficiently. And then HPV sits in their bodies for de-cades and emerges later as cancer." The awareness Tom aims to provide is a major part of her prevention goals: "We have an 'anti-cancer vaccine,'" she tells me. "Getting yourself or your children vaccinated is a no-brainer."

HPVANDME was formed at the same time as several other oral cancer advocacy groups that focused on patient support and medical research, including the Oral Cancer Foundation (OCF), founded by Brian R. Hill in 2007. Hill himself had been diagnosed with oropharyngeal cancer, and as a survivor he was deeply concerned with the ongoing health effects resulting from cancer treatments. OCF's mission has changed over the years, and the organization has joined forces with members of Hollywood's Paltrow family, including Blythe Danner and Gwyneth and Jake Paltrow, to form the Bruce Paltrow Oral Cancer Fund. I spoke with Brian Hill by phone from my office at San Francisco State University, offering my services as a researcher and asking if he would share his experience as an advocate for oral cancer. He explained—mostly paraphrasing what I learned on the organizational website—that OCF is a "public service charity designed for advocacy and service, created to promote change, through proactive means, in both the public and medical/dental professional sectors." But as we spoke further, Hill shared with deep conviction and animation about how patients, himself included, were suffering from side effects of the available OPC cancer treatments, and that people, mostly men, needed support, advice, and better treatment options that would not leave them disabled and stigmatized, many not able to eat and barely leaving their houses due to facial disfiguring. Change was needed, and he was dedicating his life to helping make this happen. Hill's organization would raise awareness of patient experience, and his message was driven by reducing the social and psychological impact of this cancer's treatment effects on patients and families while pushing researchers to find better treatment options. I was glad to be able to partner with Hill, the Johns Hopkins University oncologist and cancer epidemiologist Carole Fakhry, and an MPH student, Cameron Kephart, to conduct an assessment of the social experiences of patients seeking support through Hill's and the Oral Cancer Foundation's efforts. The UK's Throat Cancer Foundation (TCF), founded in 2012 by Jamie Rae, and the collaborative group HPV Action have missions similar to the OCF's: to provide a voice for patients "battling throat cancer."

These organizations, launched by people diagnosed with OPC or their partners, share a shift from advocating for treatment funding and research to advocating for screening and early detection. OCF stated on their website in 2019, "At the forefront of our agenda is the firm establishment in the minds of the American public for the need to undergo an annual oral cancer screening, combined with an outreach to the dental and medical communities to provide this service as a matter of routine practice." In the US and in other places with robust yet uneven health care infrastructures, cervical, skin, prostate, and other cancers that lend themselves to routine screenings and exams have seen lower death rates attributable to programs promoting early diagnosis, thus better long-term outcomes and lower severity of disease for those who undergo treatments.

Most oral cancers are not "hidden" within the body, in some inaccessible location where detection requires an invasive examination. The broader umbrella of oral cancers are not new cancers, and their diagnosis in other areas (especially toward the front of the mouth, where lesions are typically related to tobacco use) had already led to dental and other health care professional using visual inspection as a screening modality. Some cancers, especially those related to heavy smoking and alcohol consumption or (in a small number of cases) a genetic predisposition, often produce visible precancerous tissue changes that can be seen with the naked eye. In contrast, OPCs are found in the very back of the mouth and are now known to be more frequently related to persistent HPV-16 infection, the high-risk oncogenic viral strain that is commonly associated with cervical and anal cancer. These areas are hard to assess visually; surface changes are not visible to a screener in the same way throat cancers in other areas might be. HPVs often hide and go unnoticed, asymptomatic for years, when the immune system is unable to shed these infections. When the virus persists in the body it can cause cellular changes that lead to cancer. As a result, many advocates are working to produce and scientifically validate an effective screening and prevention tool that incorporates visual inspection with verbal questions about symptomology. The latter are already used, and guidelines to do so have been recommended by the American Dental Association.

When Bruce Dickinson told men to be "vigilant," he was using the media to do so (Britton 2015). The urgency intimated is part of the war against time, or more specifically, the "do not delay" assertions that helped support mass surveillance of otherwise healthy, symptom-free (i.e., no subjective experience reported by the patient) people and often sign-less (i.e., no objective observation reported by the provider) cancers (Aronowitz 2010, 210). Dickinson was saying: Precancers cannot be detected, but if you have signs of "early cancer," get checked. Tom concurred, telling me that she wants people to "talk about this like they talk about breast cancer," a reference I interpreted as a hope that this cancer would move from a quiet, undiscussed disease to one with a cadre of disease-awareness groups and organizations as well as a well-known preventive approach (like the mammogram). Tom's main goal in founding HPVANDME was crystal clear: "I want middle-aged men to know to go to the doctor early."

Preventive Biopolitics: Risk Assessments, Screening Tools, and Vaccine Guidelines

Cancer screening is an ongoing practice of body monitoring for status, change, and biomarkers of risk. People enter risk with preventive health guidelines as well as the product offerings of disease screening as commodities of care. I have been arguing that HPV vaccination is part of a prevention apparatus dominated by a pharmaceuticalized approach to public health that often erases the "we" in favor of the "me." Biomedicine, from prevention to care, includes multiple—often simultaneous—tendencies, from curing the ill to transforming the well. What my interviews attest is that knowledge of HPV is part of an HPV-associated knowledge-technology platform that includes cultural, social, and clinical formations—from diagnostics, risk-assessment, and vaccine interventions to cultural and social knowledge production about who comes to be at risk and how. Given HPV's sexual transmission, gender, sex, and sexuality have always been stitched into these multiple processes, always present yet differentially visible at each landing. People are brought into awareness, body monitoring, and disease prevention approaches for a risk of which some were already keenly aware, and others were not.

OPC is significantly more difficult to "find" hidden in regions located at the bottom of the valleys around the tonsils or deep within the tissues at the base of the tongue. Oncologists did not support the invasiveness of retracting tissue from these deep regions of the throat for biopsy as a prevention tool. Further uncertainty punctuates HPV's role in cancer formation, for instance about whether an HPV will persist or clear on its own. Without an easily available diagnostic test, what tool would emerge as the "right tool" to prevent HPV-associated oral cancers? Would screening plus vaccination be the recommended approach to prevent this cancer? "Vaccination does not replace screening," Merck has informed girls and women. Having HPV is not a cancer risk in and of itself; the virus may be necessary, but it is insufficient for the development of cancer. As is often stated, most HPVs (up to 90 percent) clear on their own. Yet some high-risk types, such as HPV-16, are strongly associated with the later development of precancer and cancers. While it is not known in whom and under what conditions this viral risk might clear, evidence indicates that it is the virus's presence and persistence that signals potential cancer risk. From its earliest product campaigns targeting girls, Merck variously—although infrequently—included a message about the importance of cervical cancer screening alongside vaccination.

Vaccination and screening were becoming entangled preventive processes not only for cervical cancer, but for the politics around anal and oral cancers as well. As Gillison stated, although many physicians were likely "confident that HPV vaccine will reduce HPV-related oropharynx cancers," studies had not yet provided evidence of this. Would some bodies undergo ongoing risk management, through screening tools, for the prevention of OPC?

The HPV vaccination expansion that came in December 2019 with the approval of Gardasil 9 for adults and for broader coverage of HPV strains was in part based on Merck's request that the FDA review the evidence for the vaccine's prevention of oropharyngeal and other cancers of the head and neck, specifically HPV-16 (declared in 2012 as oncoviral by the International Agency for Research on Cancer—IARC Working Group on the Evaluation of Carcinogenic Risks to Humans 2012). By June 12, 2020, accelerated approval for the expansion of Gardasil 9 had been granted based on a "surrogate endpoint"—not for OPC, but for prevention of HPV-related anogenital persistent infection and disease. An assumption and extension was drawn: Gardasil 9, it was argued, is "reasonably likely to predict its effectiveness in preventing HPV-related persistent oral infection and disease" (US Food & Drug Administration 2020, 1). The case included an epidemiological narrative based on the evidence: the epidemiology of HPV-related head and neck cancers showed that they "disproportionately affect [adult] white, male, non-smokers in North America and Europe." While studies have proven Gardasil safe and effective in "subjects from this population," FDA approval came with a caveat, requiring further clinical studies to address the "uncertainty of the surrogate endpoint to clinical benefit" (U.S. Food & Drug Administration 2020). Despite such demands, the official approval letter issued to Merck by the FDA requested and expanded the indication for Gardasil 9 to include these oral cancers, bringing newly vaccinated people up to forty-five years old into a cohort of oral cancer protection. In a press release, Merck asserted that while "both men and women can be at risk of HPV-attributable oropharyngeal cancer" based on CDC analysis, "this cancer affects men five times more than women . . . and has surpassed cervical cancer as the most prevalent type of HPV-related cancer in the US" (Merck & Co. 2020a). What of the men too old to receive Gardasil 9 and at a more proximate risk for diagnosis of this cancer?

Gillison had told me that she had long hoped Gardasil would include indication for the prevention of OPC from the start. "When you're an evidence-based scientist, you'd like there to be definite evidence for making public health recommendations," she told me. But, she said, "we don't have any data," signaling the ways of the current era of evidence-based medicine. She then added: "One thing I've noticed over the last decade is the field has become far more comfortable with extrapolation than it was 10 years ago." Extrapolation, in this case, may be another word for a clinical surrogate. Speaking of the various cancers she and others had previously studied, she wondered aloud, "We looked at vulvar and it was true, and we looked at vaginal and it was true, and we looked at cervical and it was true, and we looked at anal in a subset of men, and it was true. . . . So, it must be true. And so, the field almost feels like it's no longer necessary, we can just assume that it works. I don't think anyone who's a true scientist is going to be able to go around and say, vaccinate to prevent oral cancer." FDA approval, however, makes scientists more likely to support vaccination to prevent HPV-associated oral cancers.

The media reported on the new vaccination guidelines in much the same ways that they reported on the diagnoses of Douglas and Dickinson. Yet, instead of the good news Merck hoped for, these stories often presented the "bad news" for middle-aged men: there is no screening tool for the early detection of cellular changes or even for HPV itself in the mouths of those who are at risk. As men, largely cisgender, heterosexual, and in their fifties and sixties, were becoming "aware" that their sexual identities, practices, and cultures posed an oral cancer risk, there was little they could act upon. Yet, these older men, the likely clinical patients of Gillison, Fakhry, Wirth, Cohen, and other oncologists, were unaccustomed to bringing their sexual lives and practices from long ago—and their marriages and relationships in the present—into their thinking about their health and disease, nor into their medical care visits. If these men were aware of the recent health news about HPV, they likely understood the virus and its potential health effects as a gendered risk and a concern for their wives or daughters (if they had them), not for themselves.

Alongside those diagnosed with oral cancers—and their partners, spouses, and families—are those *not yet* patients, mostly younger adult men now included in a vaccine approach. Would these young men take on identities as patients-in-waiting and otherwise healthy actors in need of preventive tools? Would this cancer join vaccination plus other screening tools in prevention biopolitics? In the case of OPC, without an analogous screening tool like the Pap test for anal cancer screening, a first step was to understand and model potential risk. Researchers sought to develop risk-assessment technologies to gauge which bodies and lives might be at "high" and "highest" risk for OPC. As a researcher I interviewed stated: "Given age, gender, race, sexual behavior, smoking are the principal determinants of oral HPV infection, then take those five variables and factor in their variability, and try to figure out for any individual person, like a 50-year-old male who had 10 sexual partners, who also smokes 10 cigarettes a day and is white. What's the likelihood that a person with those characteristics has an infection?" In some oral cancers—for example, those occurring in tobacco smokers and smokeless tobacco users—HPV is superfluous to/as a cause; and even in oropharyngeal cancers, HPV is insufficient for cancer development. Because of these uncertainties, researchers are left asking what may seem like a very elemental question: Who *is* at risk? Accordingly, one approach in risk assessment has been the development of risk-assessment tools to help publics ask and answer the question "What is my risk for oral HPV?" Like many risk -assessment tools, this one was biopolitical in the ways it collected individual data, used the data to calculate and predict population-level risk, and then re-individualized that risk into a risk score for individuals who were keen to learn what their risk was (see Fosket 2004 for an analysis of the Gail model for breast cancer).[2]

Gypsyamber D'Souza and her research colleagues set out to ascertain and communicate risk levels to the worried public that was emerging as newly aware of HPV–oral cancer risk, asking who might benefit from a screening approach (D'Souza, McNeel, and Fakhry 2017, 3065). Researchers built a risk-model based on the incidence of oropharyngeal cancer cases collected by the Surveillance, Epidemiology, and End Results (SEER) registries (representing 28 percent of the US population) and oropharyngeal cancer mortality records from the National Center for Health Statistics (NCHS). Their goal was to ascertain whether the presence of the HPV-16 variant would warrant a screening approach. Concluding that it would not be useful, D'Souza and colleagues stated that "Most groups have low oncogenic oral HPV prevalence" (D'Souza, McNeel, and Fakhry 2017, 3065), and because of the large number of people who would have to be monitored, screening is not suggested. According to their study, the lifetime risk of developing oropharyngeal cancer, even among those with infection, remains low.

Asking and answering the question "Am I at risk?" was visually represented by a flow chart and risk score from "low" to "medium" to "high" accompanying their conclusion. Together these created gendered risk categories of "Very low risk" = women with 0–1 lifetime oral sexual partners, regardless of smoking behavior; "low risk" = women with 2+ lifetime oral sexual partners (and oncogenic oral HPV prevalence of 1.5 percent). In contrast, "low risk" for men was designated as including the presence of oncogenic oral HPV (1.7 percent among men with 0–1 lifetime oral sexual partners), and slightly higher risk was designated for men who did not smoke but had 2–4 lifetime oral sexual partners. "Medium risk" included men who smoke and had 2–4 partners (with oral HPV-16 prevalence of

7.1 percent) and non-smokers who had 5 or more sex partners (with 7.4 percent prevalence). However, prevalence as a biomarker is insufficient; HPV alone is not a cause, but had emerged as a risk factor for subsequent cancer (D'Souza, McNeel, and Fakhry 2017).[3] The tool normalized risk, refusing to configure a new surveillance market (at least for now).

The risk model tool begs the questions: What would happen if a similar tool was developed to screen for early signs and then risk of oral cancers? Would a new identity and risk group be solidified around heterosexual men and a "populationism" approach of risk, identity, and responsibility? In many ways cancers have long been established as the ultimate risky disease, putting patient and doctor in real and potential conflict with an enfolding, devastating narrative. With a generation of cancer survivors outliving the immediate threat of the disease, knowledge of the risks throughout one's lifetime—emanating from both the natural history of cancer and different (constantly changing) modalities of treatment—has exploded. The dimensions of this transformation are huge, in part because of the large numbers of people who constitute the growing group of cancer survivors, today's "remission society" (Frank 2013 [1995], Ries et al. 2008).

Combining risk reduction with symptomatic relief is a subset of the larger ways that risk reduction has permeated not just disease prevention for the healthy, but the management of existing disease for the "ill." Bundling risk reduction and symptom relief may be a good thing in itself, but it is part of a problematic, self-reinforcing cycle of fear promotion that is inevitably followed up with the marketing of tests and products that promise some means to reassert control—not necessarily over the disease itself, but over fear of the disease. These cycles of risk production and risk reduction in our primary and secondary prevention efforts have financial and psychological costs. Should we have a higher bar for accepting new practices and products whose primary goal is to reduce the risk of other practices and products? Recent debates about the cost-effectiveness of new HPV vaccines show that any substantial savings might ensue not so much from the reduction of morbidity and mortality from cervical cancer and other HPV-related diseases as from reductions in the expensive and intrusive workups triggered by HPV-related Pap test abnormalities. Further, such attention to risk and surveillance reproduces narratives about who "deserves" good medicine and good science.

As rising cases of oral cancers in men led to research support (and a narrative of alarm along the way), debates came to the fore about whether more and better medicine was needed to ensure their health. This included specific attention to the merit and availability of screening tools for this cancer type. *Men's Health* was once again part of the production of a cancer-risk imaginary. Ted Teknos, chair of the Department of Otolaryngology–Head and Neck Surgery at Ohio State University's Wexner Medical Center, asserted that cases of HPV-related throat cancers had risen 300 percent from the 1980s to the 2000s. Teknos provided a causal explanation: "We're just seeing the effects [of past sexual practices] now, but it's going to be much more common in the coming years and decades." "Much more common" signals medically that something unexpected is beginning to unfold, something of which publics might well take note. "Here's How Oral Sex Can Give You Cancer," the headline exclaimed, employing a distinctive and already well-established outbreak narrative entangling gender and sexuality. The subhead read, "The number of oral sex-related throat cancers are rising—here's why," and introduced oral sex as "one of the most common ways to spread sexually transmitted diseases, like chlamydia, gonorrhea, herpes, and human papillomavirus (HPV)."

VICE News concurred, reporting with a bold headline: "Oral Sex and the Alarming Rise of HPV-Related Throat Cancer in Men." The story line was alarming as well, stating that "by 2020, the rates of HPV related oropharyngeal cancer are expected to surpass those of cervical cancer." Conjoining outbreak and containment, the article asked, "Why aren't young men getting vaccinated?" (Lawson 2017). Given what media—using epidemiological data—were presenting as a "catastrophic rise" in oropharyngeal cancer and a form of HPV-related throat cancer affecting men, the news was implying that something about these men and their sexual practices and lives placed them firmly in a new risk categorization, specifically a cancer risk.

Beyond the rudimentary but cheap and relatively accessible visual exams that dentists may use to screen for OPCs, there are non-FDA approved screening tests appearing on the market that use saliva, or cells rinsed from the mouth, which are sent to a laboratory to be examined for genomic, proteomic, or molecular markers that might be characteristic of oropharyngeal cancer.[4]

The 2020 news that the FDA approved Gardasil 9 for a new and expanded indication to prevent oropharyngeal was a new push to protect men and their health. The evidence, based on the surrogate marker of anogenital diseases, and the new approval allowed Merck to expand its educational and product advertising efforts. "It's your time to act. HPV vaccination is a type of cancer prevention," was part of an update to the "Did You Know?" ad campaign launched in 2016. The 2020 "Not My Child" campaign relied on the familiar bright yellow tape to caution parents and adults alike in a web-based and video campaign with a clear message: "HPV Is About Cancer." The message was immediately followed by an adjoining caveat: "For most people, HPV clears on its own" (Merck & Co. 2021b). The uncertainty lingers over the phrase "for most people." The campaign urges parents to "get in the way" to protect their sons and daughters from cancer. There is "no way to know who will or won't clear the virus"—so act now! they are told (Merck & Co. 2020b).

"Not My Child," part of the larger "Know HPV" campaign, again features parents who speak into the camera. This time they aggressively tell HPV to "Back off!" exclaiming "You're not welcome here." The body language of these parents, pushing hands outward and directly toward the camera, suggests a strong stop. The ad was broadcast widely in June 2020, with an estimated 3,000 national airings on television and digital media, as well as with online banners, video ads, and in Facebook and Instagram ads. By August 5, 2020, a dedicated Merck campaign YouTube channel no longer had this content, Twitter had a single tweet, and Facebook had just a couple of posts. The yellow caution tape showed up yet again on a middle-aged man's running shorts in a commercial released in 2021—following the expanded FDA approval up the life course for Gardasil 9—when viewers of cable and streaming platforms, including YouTube and product websites, as well as print ads in medical offices, would meet a new Gardasil protagonist. This young (but seemingly on the cusp of middle age), masculine and white-presenting man with blue eyes, curly short brown hair, and a short beard and mustache looked directly into the camera. In the video version, the protagonist appears as he is about to begin a 5k race, his yellow athletic shorts in view as he sets out to join a collective. He stops to speak with a woman wearing a headscarf (a ready symbol of breast cancer) whose very presence invokes the thought of pink ribbons and cancer awareness fundraisers, and then heads off to join others for the race, in what references a collective health movement broadly associated with cancer "awareness." This man is "helping protect myself against some cancers, like certain cancers caused by HPV." As he heads off to the race, a voiceover provides information about the "certain cancers" from which he is "helping protect" himself. Was this the culmination of a material and symbolic association forged between HPV, cancer, and hetero-masculine men?

The presumption that knowledge compels action lacks any evidence of success. It is part of the well-worn if highly critiqued and disproved health belief model of public health and the marketing assumptions of industry; but that coupling is part of a symbolic trope that constructs "deserving" and vulnerably positioned good patients and strong people, and distinguishes them from those undeserving of good medicine and science. The enduring ideas are based in a racialized framing, positioning white women as needing protection, white men as serving good science and medicine, and racialized genders as (more) contagious, dangerous, and less deserving of and/or able to engage in (self)care practices. When epidemiology produces gendered, raced, and classed population groups, these "statistical trends create ideologies of race, gender, and difference" (Wailoo 2011, 4). While manifesting differently, the statistical associations support systemic power structures—Jim Crow politics, Chinese exclusions, and the pseudoscientific racism of eugenics and white supremacy, as well as the continued racism in medicine that addresses Black pain or Black skin or Black lung capacity as different from other people's pain, skin, and lungs. The logic of difference is sutured into our systems. The ways white mothers in particular were constructed as the modern, well-to-do protectors of family health had as much to do with protecting white norms as it did with defining nonwhite others (Wailoo 2011).

As knowledge and action was compelled from white active men, what happened to the gender diversity staged in the "Versed" campaign (Klahr Coey 2021)? And, I was left to wonder, what about the queer- and lesbian-identified adults who are rendered invisible by the oral cancer narrative and the new ad campaigns?

What about the Lesbians in a Cis-gendered, Masculine Health Concern?

I met Kate O'Hanlan, a gynecological oncologist, on a warm September afternoon near her office in the South Bay area of San Francisco. The interview was scheduled for lunch, and we sat outside at a café. O'Hanlan was very generous with her time. Her spirit was patient and welcoming. She was delighted to talk, and we shared our mutual sense of gratitude for the work we had each done in the field of lesbian health. The conversation led us to reflect on a question other than the one that had been posed for so long and had now been answered with a vaccine indication: "What's in it for the boys?" Where, we now wondered, are the lesbians and queers who sleep with people with vaginas? What does their invisibility in the face of a visible men's health and men's risk mean for the gendered production of sexuality and health risk of biomedicine? These groups have long been on the margins of medicine's objects of medicalization, at once subsumed into the leaky, unruly bodies of "women" and relegated to the margins of the sexual risk that came to congeal around the presumed sexual excesses of gay and bisexual men. "What's in it for the queer girls and women?" we mused. Would lesbian and queer women continue to be overlooked in conversations, research, and clinical care about the risk of HPV-associated oral cancer? Would a gendered sexualization allow the particularities of their lives and identities to be brought into the ways these infections are also omnipresent, yet with its own specific ecological and interactional risks for their sexual lives?

O'Hanlan told me of her professional work that included a clinical oncological practice, "mostly surgical care of women with uterine cancer, cervical, vagina, vulva and ovarian cancer," and a leadership and educational role as founder and medical director of the Laparoscopic Institute for Gynecologic Oncology. As we spoke, we shifted our conversation from these cancers to OPCs and whether she thought there was an over-emphasis on heterosexual men in oral cancer research, to the detriment of lesbian health. She told me that she too had not come across research on queer and lesbian women and/or nonbinary groups. "No one is working on it," she said. "No one is researching women who have sex with women." She was quick to add, though, that "lesbians do smoke more than heterosexual women. We know that from the Women's Health Initiative and the Nurse's Health Study." *This* small subset, she said, of lesbian smokers should perhaps be followed prospectively. Yet, as she stated, "It's hard when you're studying like 2% of the population. Let's say 30% of older lesbians smoke, 30% of 2% [is small]. It'd be interesting to see, but they're having sex with people who are pretty unlikely to have the virus." She paused and then modified this to say, "younger women are definitely more bisexual." She then stopped herself again, to say, well, "older women were too 'cause they came out with children from previous [heterosexual] marriages." "I wonder what the rate is and what the change in rate might be." It was only a matter of time, I speculated, until the rates of oropharyngeal cancers in lesbian, bisexual, and queer women would be on the rise. And until the media were reporting on a well-known lesbian public figure who would tell them she was diagnosed with this cancer.

O'Hanlan's response brought forward the risk profiles that had been generated by the small but visible field of Lesbian Health, which started in the 1980s and came of age in the late 1990s. Despite what may have been veiled signs for the use of dental dams and other latex products in the prevention of disease, perhaps even including HPV transmission via oral sex performed on women, very little disaggregation by gender and sexuality took place. A "minority-stress" theory of social discrimination, including histories of sexual assault and harassment, driving not only lower economic status, but also smoking and alcohol use and other risky behaviors, placed these "women" in a population group disproportionately at risk of some health concerns, including certain cancers.[5]

She and I wondered whether this population group—rendered invis-

ible—was more like heterosexual men in their risk, given their sexual practices. A logic of binary gender and heteronormativity means this question
has been largely overlooked outside of LGBTQ health and the broader
world of STI prevention. In this domain of LGBTQ health, I heard of new
research that was beginning to ask whether a percentage of the diagnosed
oropharyngeal cancers might be attributable to what the field is now
calling "women who have sex with women." We agreed that while some
studies have examined cervical cancer screening rates among lesbian or
women who have sex with women, non-heterosexual and nonbinary bodies who have sex with "women" were left out of the evidence base for HPV-
associated head and neck cancers. Instead, a cisgender and heterosexual
approach to oral cancer research reinforced the "reality" that heterosexual
men *are* at highest risk.

But despite the alarm among scientists and medical providers about this
rise in oral cancers, there had been no research (that I found) into LGBTQ
population groups based on sexual practices. As O'Hanlan and I spoke, we
wondered if and how one might identify the best "sample" to examine. We
noted that it was in the context of HIV/AIDS research that the designation
of MSM emerged for use in the study of behavioral risk, but a similar category of WSW is rarely used in medical research. Given low rates of throat
cancers, a large sample (likely in the thousands if not tens of thousands) of
WSW would be needed to prove anything epidemiologically, and qualita-
tive research with WSW and those who identify as lesbian, bi, or queer and
who have cancer or precancer has not been undertaken, to our knowledge.
Two exceptions can be found: The Gay and Lesbian Medical Association
included a session at their 2022 annual meeting, held in San Francisco, on
how best to demystify STIs and support safe sex practices that included
vaginal-vaginal, -digital, and -oral sex. And the American Cancer Society
(2020) published "Cancer Facts for Lesbian and Bisexual Women," which
lists risks for breast, colon, gynecological, lung, and skin cancers, but it does
not mention oropharyngeal cancers. There is hope for a particular sexualization to guide future research, as well as public health and medical care.

Nonetheless, there is little to no queering of oral cancer to date. The
face of oral cancer continues to be that of men like Michael Douglas, and
the sexual dynamics continue to be those that ossify around a notion of cisgender heterosexuality as these men and their female partners raise awareness of HPV-associated oral cancer. Douglas was diagnosed in 2010 and
has since been medically declared "cancer-free." He is now an outspoken
advocate for oral cancer awareness, emphasizing the links between oral
cancers and HPV and serving as an intermediary actor between pharma
and publics to advocate for Gardasil 9.

CHAPTER SEVEN

Cervical Cancer's Screening Politics

Dear Laura,
> *My daughter has just received an HPV diagnosis.*
> *What does it mean?*
> *What should she do?*
> *Any advice appreciated. Thank you*

A message like this would land in my inbox every few weeks, generally from a concerned friend or colleague whose young adult daughter had recently received "co-test" results from a combined Pap and HPV test given to them during a routine check by a primary care doctor or gynecologist. They were reaching out to me, someone they knew spent the bulk of their time thinking and talking about sex and health, for guidance. Unfailingly, there was concern worsened by uncertainty, and a request for information and help, each person hoping I could clarify and perhaps guide them in how to support their child as they made medical decisions and took the next steps in care together. Those contacting me were all already familiar with screening tests in general, especially the "annual pelvic exam" which includes a Pap test to screen for cervical abnormalities. They had been well-versed in the routine "no news is good news," and with the much later arrival of a report that indicates either normal cells or an atypical cellular finding and its associated expectation of "good health" or cause for concern. What they were less familiar with, however, were results reporting "HPV" status (the full name of the virus associated with some cancers and genital warts, "human papillomavirus," is sometimes not indicated). Many were certainly taken aback by an HPV+ result that arrives, now often in the "My Chart" electronic medical record and application on one's smart phone. The emails and texts put their shock and confusion into relief: "Should I be worried? Is this the same as the flu or more akin to Hep C or HIV?" (referring to other viruses, one common and the latter two also STIs best known to my colleagues and friends in the San Francisco Bay Area, most of whom were, like me, born in the late 1960s or 1970s). "Or is it something else altogether?" they asked. Some asked for direct advice: "What should I tell them?"

My response was rarely satisfying: "Don't worry," I would say, "the result is not cause for concern." What they all wanted to know was how to make sense of a new and underexplained screening guideline for cervical cancer known as "co-testing," in which testing of the presence of viral types of HPV is administered as a cancer screening tool and piggy-backed onto the Pap's laboratory test, depending on where one falls in the current guidelines in terms of age and medical history.

Co-testing brings together two knowledge-making systems: cytology, with its capacity to detect and define cellular abnormalities and lesions, and biomolecular technology, with its ability to isolate oncogenic and other viral presences within the plurality of HPVs. Decisions have already been made in the design of these investigative tools. HPV co-testing for cervical cancer screening includes testing for "high-risk" oncogenic types associated with cancer, and does not include the "low-risk" viral types associated with warts. Each of these outputs, which are technically different and come with their own ambiguities, offers a specific and contrasting rendition of what precisely is being identified. Yet, co-testing, to borrow from the feminist science studies scholar Annemarie Mol (2003), enacts a means for these two renditions to "hang together," even as translations of those renditions do not necessarily cohere. That is, cytological and molecular results do not provide the same information; they add to and supplement information from one another. Their "readings" arise out of two altogether distinct (and potentially discordant) knowledge systems. Yet, in each of these varying knowledge practices of medicine—and especially when they are read together, as Mol argues—realities about the body, disease, and the self are generated.

If you are over forty years old with a cervix, as I am, you can readily envision the routinized annual clinical visit complete with undressing, feet placed in stirrups, cold and concerned as a speculum is inserted into your vaginal canal and opened as a provider conducts a pelvic exam and Pap test that scrapes cells from your cervix. What is often referred to as "the annual exam" is encoded in many people's—providers' and patients'—psyches as the universal ideal of *good care for good patients*, despite these visits being, for many, fraught with tension or discomfort and, for some, judgment and biases. The Pap test guidelines changed in the 1980s, which changed annual exam expectations. For clinicians and patients, Pap tests were recommended at longer intervals, leading to a change in the nomenclature of this office visit from an annual exam to a less frequent wellness exam that now includes other health prevention and "risk" discussions.[1]

"The HPV detection test has been added to the Pap" was part of my typical brief initial response to the messages I received. I wanted to share what I knew to be true without going into a detailed explanation of the biomedical distinction between a screening tool and a diagnostic test; more than anything I wanted to hold back my own challenges with biomedical screening. I would quickly elaborate with the ambiguities of the knowledge-system in place: "A positive result can't predict if the viral type identified would clear or persist, or whether its presence is a cancer risk at all."

"What does that mean?" the person would shoot back.

My reply felt insufficient and awkward. "It's a risk of cervical cancer, but an uncertain one," I'd say, frustrated that I couldn't be more reassuring nor provide a fuller explanation. Then I'd usually add: "Keep an eye on it. Talk to the doctors." If I was loquacious in my response, I would tell them that co-testing is shorthand for the two knowledge systems that are now part of the current cervical cancer screening guidelines: Pap testing for cellular change, with an added molecular HPV test to detect the now known sexually transmitted virus and its risk types. I might add, depending on the person who wrote, that this was the near end of the molecular turn in medicine that began in the 1980s as biotech companies searched for new tools to commercialize. I might let them know I was coming to think of HPV tests as a new kind of test: one that measures a *risk* of developing a *risk* of cervical cancer.[2] Instead of being the kind of test that was unambiguous, like the risk of HIV and a need to treat and suppress the virus as a way of preventing AIDS, this information is causally uncertain, although it provides additional information (an HPV positive or negative result for certain HPV genotypes) that is considered helpful for monitoring risk and making decisions for next clinical steps.

"Don't worry," I would often sign off, pretty sure they still would.

Despite my attempt to reassure by writing, "It [the HPV detected on the cells] may clear on its own—wait and see," followed by "The doctor will likely do another test soon," I knew that ambiguity and uncertainty were baked into this screening approach. I also knew that like me, my colleagues were primed to worry about cancer, and more precisely, about pre-cellular changes hidden in our bodies. We also may have been part of a consumer base for HPV product offerings—from HPV vaccines to this new test—who are more decidedly pro-sex and feminist, thereby refuting any negative association between this virus and its health prevention and their daughters' sexual lives.

The Pap test, unaccompanied by HPV screening, was quite effective in decreasing invasive cervical cancer incidence and deaths here in the US, and also around much of the world. Yet this well-established tool had lost its decades-long distinction as what the sociologists Adele Clarke and Joan Fujimura refer to as the "right tool" for cervical cancer prevention (Clarke and Fujimura 1992a and 1992b; Casper and Clarke 1998).

My fieldwork was presenting me with a confounding puzzle: If cervical cancers have been reduced by almost 80 percent as a result of Pap test screening tools—a mantra heard at nearly every scientific conference presentation—then why was a molecular HPV screening tool necessary, even as a co-test? In what way, if any, was this tool becoming *more* right than the "right tool?" One thing was certain: cancer screening recommendations were changing as a result of new technoscientific tools in the diagnostic and molecular space, as well as the subsequent epidemiological and clinical proof used to push that change. The two-test or co-test approach was replacing the familiar and cellular-based classification of "normal," "abnormal," or "atypical" that came from a visual inspection of a Pap test. Instead, cancer screening approaches were now asking clinicians and their patients to parse what it means to be HPV+. My research found that given the uncertainties of meaning in these approaches, large-scale efforts to "optimize" and further refine, and thereby stratify, screening approaches for cervical cancer prevention were the object of "innovation" as well as justification for new clinical and public health guidelines. What test, for what purpose, and to be used when as well as for whom, had yet to be determined. I wanted to understand sociologically how a "better" tool and approach to cervical cancer screening was being constructed, what knowledge claims that construction was based on, and in what ways these interactions might reflect and be driven by larger organizational and technoscientific changes underway in medicine and public health more broadly, including how we, the public, understand ourselves, our risk, and our responsibility for health.

While in 2012 co-testing was not the standard and accepted approach to cervical cancer screening worldwide, HPV testing was increasingly part of clinical medicine and cancer control public health prevention in the highest-resourced settings with the infrastructure to support such testing (including laboratories and clinicians). My argument here is that the approach referred to technically as an in-vitro diagnostic device (IVD), specifically and expressly as a "co-test" in cancer screening and prevention, was evolving in a uniquely American form.[3]

The broad category of IVDs, of which HPV tests are a part, are used to collect and test biological samples to detect and map biological and especially genomic information (DNA and RNA) for use in diagnosing disease. (Think about how SARS-CoV-2 is identified by PCR or antigen tests to diagnose COVID-19). IVDs also are used to monitor conditions and states of biomarkers over time, such as the presence and levels of SARS-CoV-2, as well as hormones, blood sugar, or antibodies. IVDs' integration into medical practice is a principal part of biomedicalization, the technoscientific shifting inside biomedicine and technology driven by molecular and information technologies of the 1990s that alters not only the tools and approaches used, but also the infrastructures supporting everything from research to clinical decision making and services (Clarke et al. 2010, Clarke et al. 2003).

In the US, the Food and Drug Administration (FDA) regulates medical devices, like vaccines, sold commercially to assure their safety and effectiveness. Scientifically, effectiveness refers to the capacity of a diagnostic tool to identify true positives and true negatives.[4] To be considered "effective" a device must have a high rate of success at accurately finding the thing in the body being looked for (the "true positives"), also known as a test's level of "sensitivity"; *and* it must just as often show with equal certainty that when that which is being looked for is not found, "it" is indeed not there (the "true negatives"), which is known as its "specificity."[5] With the production of genomic information and the devices able to amplify and read this information, IVDs evolved into the essential tools of "precision medicine"—providing genomic-based information which is in turn used to identify a particular patient's condition or disease risk, and/or which individuals are likely to benefit from a therapeutic.

HPV IVDs were first used in the late 1980s as investigative tools, either for research or as on-site clinical decision-making tools to assist with triaging patients, in this case patients with abnormal Pap tests, to colposcopy or biopsy. The regulatory approval of HPV IVDs as an integrated tool in cancer screening was neither unidirectional nor preordained. This knowledge platform, in which the cervical sample (cells) collected during a Pap test undergoes molecular testing for a plurality of HPV genomic types classified along a spectrum of risk, is used along with the cytology information and classification of cellular composition also performed on the cells collected by the Pap. Taken individually, each result can indicate cancer risk—but with its own distinct ambiguities. When the two results are taken together, certainty is increased (but still not guaranteed). Each test holds different meanings for risk, disease, and identity.

Establishing Molecular Precursors: The Medicalization and Biomedicalization of Cancer Prevention

A new regime of cancer prevention, consisting of these shifting screening approaches plus a "cancer prevention vaccine," is now part of clinical biomedicine and population-level public health. How did this regime evolve, and specifically, how was the transformation of the use of screening tools in clinical and preventive care decided upon? In what ways were changes supported by clinical evidence and/or epidemiological narratives of population risk, and/or how were they justified by professional consensus guidelines?

I am arguing that this new regime is indicative of preventive medicine's crescendo into a technoscientific and biomedicalized approach to prevention. The shift began in the mid-twentieth century as cancer screening first looked for early signs of disease and increasingly brought aspects of people's lives under the medical gaze, with tools designed to search for early signs of pathology (Zola 1972; Conrad 1975 and 1992; Starr 1982). Then, especially in the 1980s, the approach integrated biological and molecular markers of disease risk and "pre-disease." That has moved us into a world "on alert," at times treating risk and at times monitoring early signs of disease—the presence of microscopic bacteria, viruses, and cellular or molecular changes—to ensure health and prevent death.[6] The talk of HPV as an omnipresent, uncertain, and somewhat mysterious STI that can, but is not likely to, lead to the development of cancer presses biomedicine to find ways to improve and expand with "innovation," "optimized" strategies, and new "precision" approaches to prevention.

Cervical cancer screening is part of the first "social transformation of American medicine," distinct in how it was shaped by a long history of suspicion that something was troubling about this cancer's formation, an unease that led scientists to look not just at the presumptively unruly bodies of women, but also at sex. Precision prevention of HPV, and the politics of that effort, are part of the new millennium prevention politics and the "molecular" tools to personalize and then target prevention to groups, places, and populations. Precision animates the approach with promises of specificity and capacity for eradication.

What are the stakes for people like my friends and colleagues and their daughters—and even more so for the ways cervical cancer is conceptualized and thus prevented and cared for in the US and around the world? What are the effects because this cancer is known to be caused by a sexually transmitted virus? Histories of cancer,[7] and "women's" cancer in particular, reveal the shape and consequences of a sexual cause. With external pathogens—bacteria or viruses, and likely sexually transmitted—as a causative factor in cancers of the womb (Javier and Butel 2008), researchers set out to explain the cause, determine its risk, and eventually develop prevention tools. "The father of epidemiology," the Italian surgeon Domenico Rigoni-Stern proposed in 1842 a causal link between sexual activity and "anogenital" cancers (Aviles 2015, Mammas and Spandidos 2015).[8] An external viral pathogen[9] and speculation about its sexual transmission led to studies of marriage and religion serving as epidemiological proxies—and narratives (Rotkin 1973, Proctor 1995, Prescott 2010, Löwy 2011). Lifestyle attributes, from diet to exercise, would include sexual roles and "morals." Levels of sexual activity, from celibacy to "unbridled sexuality" (later termed promiscuity), and their presumed virtues or excesses came into play. Each pattern of behaviors functioned alternately as safeguards of or risks to the so-called organs of maternity and reproduction, either maintaining a well-balanced maternal life or looming as potential causes of disease (Patterson 1987; Proctor 1995; Nolte 2008; Wailoo 2011, 15).

"Lifestyle" became a code word that masked sexual transmission and its many biological uncertainties (Braun and Phoun 2010, 47). Racist classifications and assumptions intertwined with gender and class in ways that increasingly stigmatized sexual activity as immorality and as a cause of cancer (Mei 2009). Examples include the associations of Jewish women's "sex hygiene" with low rates of cervical cancer; of working-class women's high birthrate with higher rates of cancer; and of the "broken marriages" or out-of-wedlock births experienced by adolescent and young adult girls with higher cancer rates (Prescott 2010). It was mostly women and their perceived "vulnerable biologies" and "aberrant behaviors" that figured in causal disease narratives in the twentieth century (Braun and Phoun 2010). By mid-century, studies of WWII war veterans suggested that sexual transmission of genital warts during sexual activity overseas was followed by transmission to the veterans' wives (Barrett, Silbar, and McGinley 1954), who later developed reproductive cancers. Vietnamese women's so-called wartime vulnerability—a euphemism for sexual coercion and rape—was also associated with high rates of cervical cancer (Mei 2009). By the 1960s and 1970s, sexual transmission was firmly established as a possible cause of various cancers, with the understanding of the mechanisms by which this occurred deeply intertwined with assumptions about sexual practices and their variation by class and race (Wailoo 2011).

Ilana Löwy's history of this "woman's disease" (2011) followed these shifting scientific claims through three eras and three patients—the computing pioneer Ada Lovelace in the 1800s, the Argentinian first lady Eva Perón in the mid-1900s, and the English television personality Jade Goody in the later 1900s—to demonstrate how cervical cancer had undergone radical change in its understanding, prevention, and treatment over a 150-year period, largely as a result of scientific claims. Löwy ends her book in the first years of the twenty-first century with a historical speculation about the restigmatization and sexualization of understandings and practices around this disease in the new millennium. Along with *Seizing the Means of Reproduction* (Murphy 2012), Löwy's book shows how the Pap test became part of the biomedical expansion, consolidating the fields of gynecology and clinical cytology and taking them beyond being what had in the early twentieth century been a strictly surgical field.[10] Specifically, the World Health Organization's (WHO) system for classifying results from Pap tests, launched in 1956, created a new technical entity, the "precancerous cell," that Murphy argued would gradually rearrange medical practice into a "risk-based, industrialized, laboratory-centered mode of diagnosis" (Murphy 2012, 112). Indeed, in the US the American Cancer Society hoped every doctor's office would become a cancer detection center (Aronowitz 2007) as they unleashed new recommendations for screening women's bodies. Women were encouraged to palpate their breasts for abnormalities, to see a doctor for "annual exams" including a Pap test, and ultimately to take responsibility for—and understand the reasons behind—submitting their bodies for a cervical "smear" test to detect early warning signs and prevent invasive cervical cancer. Over time, gynecologists and OB-GYNs (the combined specialty of obstetrics and gynecology) became the de facto "women's health care," with preventing cervical cancer via a cellular screening central to their approach. By the 1970s, mammography—another screening tool, used to visualize the tissue of the breast—joined the Pap test as preventive tools embedded not only in gynecological training and practice, but also in state legislation, insurance policy, and the commercial and nonprofit domains of various industries, professions, and organizations.[11] The seemingly healthy—and specifically "woman's"—body was transformed into a risky subject with ambiguous boundaries between the otherwise "well" and asymptomatic, and those primed for preventive actions, in need of biomedicine's interventions (as well as pharmaceutical therapies) to stave off potential illness. The intensification and so-called innovation of biomedicine would continue to transform preventive medicine and its infrastructural needs. In the case of cervical cancer prevention, in the 1990s HPV vaccines would be moving through the various stages of clinical study, with Merck anticipating its potential market. Along with pharma, biotechnology companies would launch and join a focus on developing new screening products intended to identify and treat risk in a growing prevention market and to identify and direct treatment plans for cancers.

With the establishment of HPV vaccines as a primary prevention approach to ignite an immune response and stop the virus from infecting and multiplying, a question emerged: what role would secondary prevention and screening tools—like the Pap test—play in the future? The risk that a virus, specifically one that is sexually transmitted, poses for the formation of a disease that might linger or persist, or for newer infections if immunity were to wane, was a potential target for preventive approaches. Further, screening technologies, like vaccines, are social and would likely be similar in entailing a need to manage sex and sexuality to support their uptake into biomedical and public health practice. Given the already established screening market, and the expectation of gynecologists and their configured patient populations, the field was wide open for—in the words of industry—innovation and growth.

In the thirty years following FDA approval of the first HPV test in 1988, a new regime in cancer prevention, including a distinct cervical cancer prevention trajectory, unfolded (see table 1). In the era of biomedicalization, individual responsibility, with risk largely conceptualized as a result of behavior (e.g., smoking), would incorporate biomarkers of bodily

TABLE 1. Stages of the socio-technical trajectory of HPV tests, 1988–2012

Development Stage	
1988	BLT becomes first company to gain FDA approval for HPV test (ViraPap kit)
1990	BLT sells its molecular diagnostics division to Digene
1992	Digene patents Hybrid Capture (HC) HPV detection technique
1995	Digene's first-generation HC HPV test gains FDA approval
Tinkering and Negotiation: Gathering the Evidence for HPV Detection	
1996	ALTS trial is launched
1999	Digene gains FDA approval for use of HC2 test in ASC-US triage
2000	ALTS trial is completed
2001	ASCCP guidelines state that HPV testing is better than repeat cytology or immediate colposcopy for triaging women with ASC-US, based on ALTS and Manos trial results **(HPV test enters as triage)**
Standardizing Co-Testing	
2002	ACS issues guidelines similar to ASCCP's 2001 guidelines. ACS also recommends HPV testing as additional form of screening (co-test) in women over age thirty
2003	FDA approves use of Digene HC2 HPV test as co-test (adjunct screening) in women over thirty. **First time co-testing FDA approved**
2008	ATHENA trial is launched
2011	FDA approves cobas* HPV Test for use with Pap or as Pap test follow-up (triage) **(First cobas HPV test approval)** [Based on ATHENA trial data]
2012	USPSTF new guidelines support co-testing every five years or cytology alone every three years ACS, ASCCP, and ASCP release concurrent new guidelines for the prevention and early detection of cervical cancer—preferred approach for women aged thirty to sixty-five is co-testing, but Pap alone every three years also acceptable. **(Co-testing becomes standard screening recommendation)**

Note: Bold indicates key turning points in negotiations.

conditions requiring ongoing screening (such as blood pressure or cholesterol), and would gradually include molecular risk (the presence of a specific gene or genotype). Sexual risk would be reframed as "sexual health,"
part of a change in biomedicine as well as in the nomenclature used in
other domains, from product sales to social activism (Epstein and Mamo
2017). In biomedicine, diagnostic tests (especially coupled with newly
available therapeutic treatments) were transforming the meaning and experience of the infections caused by intimate relations. No longer sources
of mystery, STIs from genital herpes (HSV-2) to HIV had a clear cause as
well as treatment. With the FDA approval of anti-retroviral medications to
treat herpes and other viruses in 1982 and then the availability of highly active anti-retroviral therapies (HAART) to suppress HIV infection in 1996,
these were no longer subject to the same degree of fear and worry, and
certainly no longer a source of moral shame or social stigma.

STIs, and in some cases their unique properties and effects, came to
constitute not only a risk of disease that could be diagnosed, monitored,
and treated alongside the symptoms of disease (think of treating HIV, for
example), but also the disease itself.[12] As scientific knowledge enabled the
molecular identification of pathogens such as HPV, the newly identified
plurality of HPV genotypes—and specifically the capacity to differentiate
its genotypes into "high-risk" or oncogenic types causally associated with
the later onset of cancers, "low-risk" associated with genital warts, and no-
risk HPVs not associated with any disease—were built into the machinery
and ways of doing STI prevention and disease control.

In the 1980s, companies began to compete to commercialize their HPV
testing capabilities as part of the diagnostic market of IVDs and to seek
product approval from the FDA to commercialize these tools. In subsequent decades, the numbers and types of IVDs multiplied to occupy a
seemingly important place in medicine and public health policy aimed
at combating and treating infectious diseases, a place that endures to this
day. From a medical device perspective, IVDs have relatively short cycles;
new products or indications for existing, already patented devices are introduced far more easily than other medical products like drugs and vaccines, which require more involved research and development, mostly in
the form of expensive and lengthy clinical trials. Device applications are reviewed by the FDA's Center for Devices and Radiological Health (CDRH)
committee, and the process is relatively quick from application to approval
and market—one or two years instead of the often ten or more for review
of drugs. IVD tests change particularly fast and often: every few months,
a new or slightly altered way of collecting biological specimens (such as a
blood test or nasal swab) is developed for use in diagnosing a previously

undetected virus, or strain thereof. Think of HIV, hepatitis, and most recently, SARS-CoV-2. Many of the tests available from retailers such as Walgreens and CVS for pregnancy or ovulation testing or to test blood sugar levels, for example, are also IVDs.

I sought to understand how and through what scientific claims HPV detection devices moved from clinical decision-making into cancer-screening guidelines, and from individual to mass-scale prevention tools—in this case as a co-test and then a primary (e.g., first and only) screening tool. How would this historically produced shift in prevention come to occupy (if it ever did) a new regime of risk and responsibility, and for whom? What would change mean for established cervical cancer prevention practice and the infrastructure of laboratories, clinicians, and patients already primed for cytological screening?

Further, I wanted to understand what I was coming to regard as a uniquely American approach of establishing co-testing in cervical cancer screening. This approach was first legitimized by the FDA's CDRH approval of an HPV IVD test, and then by its recommendation that the test be used as a companion or conjunction tool to be used along with cervical cytology. While many researchers and clinicians initially expressed concern about and opposition to this recommendation, others supported the decision, in part because of the assurance that the HPV test would join—not replace—the already established cervical cancer screening infrastructure of laboratories, pathologists, and cytologists, or the existing demand from an expectant user base of women already primed to screen their bodies to prevent cancer.

The introduction of co-testing would be the first step in the new millennium's transformation of cervical cancer prevention. The etiology and governance of this disease would morph from a distal and unknown risk to a sexual cause that could be managed and monitored, screened and prevented. No longer comfortably confined within the realm of "bad luck," this cancer would move into the realm of a scientifically proven association with an STI. Yet, uncertainty and ambiguity would remain, given that the viral presence, even if deemed risky, would be insufficient to cause cancer.

With co-testing, a promising possibility emerged to identify oncoviral risk (especially as the different genotypes gathered evidence of meaning) and to govern it on a mass scale through an infrastructure already in place. While it would take almost a decade to develop techniques with the capacity to differentiate HPV genomic types—into high-risk (HPV 16, 18, and about twelve other types); two low-risk types associated with genital warts (HPV 6 and 11); and over 200 types of HPV with a nuanced set of risk designations, including 100 no-risk HPVs (Meisal et al. 2017)—new information was reconfiguring cancer prevention as it unfolded.[13]

Materially speaking, it is worth remembering that HPV is extremely common, with most "contagion" or "infection" taking place early and often in most sexual activities. For the most part, HPV is also non-life-threatening; almost 90 percent of infections clear on their own in cases where the person's immune system is healthy. This clearance—known also as "regression"—and the question of whether and when it occurs is the basis of much uncertainty (and, I argue, effacement) in the medical and epidemiological worlds. The entire field of research is situated around the ways, not fully understood, in which some HPV infections persist over time, become chronic, and in some cases become cancerous. When types known to be oncogenic and high-risk (such as HPV 16 and 18) persist for two or more years, it is likely (but again, not certain) that at some point in the next ten to twenty years an invasive cancer will develop. This cancer, invasive cervical cancer, is, under the very best of circumstances (with optimal follow-up and treatment), life-altering, and at the worst, deadly. Medical screening identifies and monitors the presence, and processes, at different points in time and intervenes in ways that might help reduce or remove the potential adverse outcome of disease. It is part of a secondary cancer prevention model that seeks to identify or predict (and treat) precancers and cancer precursors that present a risk of developing invasive cancer, by diagnosing them early and stopping disease progression.

Sociologically speaking, uncertainty and ambiguity underscore knowledge about HPV and its role in cancer progression and incidence as scientists have amassed clinical and epidemiological research into HPV's role. The degrees of ambiguity have changed, but not its underlying presence. Uncertainty persists around which viral types are most high-risk, how to gauge viral persistence that matters most for disease, which outcome to measure (cancer or some surrogate marker),[14] and how to develop screening guidelines (inclusion and exclusion criteria by age and gender, molecular identifiers of importance, and for use in particular cancer types). Epidemiology, the scientific approach of collecting large quantities of data to predict incidence and ascertain cause as a means to help model and assess risk, was useful: through a feedback loop data could move from populations to individuals, to predict harm and shape prevention approaches.

Preventing Cancer: Diagnosing Cervical Cancer Risk

Health is "politics by other means," as the sociologist Alondra Nelson (2011) reminds us. The knowledge-making processes of who gets to decide what is "true" and what informs those decisions set the standards upon which life is governed. In health and illness, race and racism, gender and sexism, and sexuality and its heteronormativities entangle with beliefs and practices about "culture" and behavior. What we eat, do, and think; where and how we live; and what is conceived of as our risk are structured by the allocation of resources, power, and opportunity that define the inputs and outputs of medical knowledge. These, in turn, shape perceptions of health and illness, the structural opportunities and constraints that together bestow different degrees of care and neglect on bodies, lives, and populations (Epstein 2007b, Rosengarten and Michael 2009, Rosengarten 2009, Will 2009, Will and Moreira 2010). The concept of "risk" shapes the sociotechnical trajectory of cancer prevention—from the medicalization and biomedicalization of risk and its behaviors and social conditions to the ways precancerous cells and molecular precursors become the information upon which problems are identified and intervened upon. The variation—more specifically, stratification—of how to diagnose, monitor, and intervene upon risk makes up the biopolitical project.

When messages of "One Less" promoted Gardasil use, the narrative did the work of enrolling publics in the biopolitical project of managing risk and fear of cancer. Managing specific HPV types was framed as the best—if not only—way to manage this cancer risk. When my colleagues and friends emailed me to ask, "Is my daughter at risk for cancer?" the simplicity of their question belied another, far more complicated concern: How should they process their child's newly given embodiment as possessing a molecular risk with HPV's viral presence? Are they now "HPV positive," and part of a new identity category of individuals and groups thought to be risky, at risk, and/or potentially ill, patients-in-waiting? What they were really seeking was advice on how to manage this fear arising from uncertainty— fear of a potential harm lingering in the future.

Risk and governance conjoin—as strategies to control are bound with power (Bunton and Petersen 1997, Foucault 1979). With capacity to identify and screen external pathogens now inside the body, risk and responsibility are remade.[15] Screening tests imagine and anticipate subjects as good patients deserving good care. When HPV tests began to be adopted as a routine practice, claims for the importance of their use were often bolstered by assertions that the Pap test was an insufficient and also cost-ineffective approach. With HPV tests, savings were shown based not on the reduction of morbidity and mortality (the usual indicators of population health), but on estimates of cost savings driven by eliminating the expensive, intrusive, and often unnecessary medical workups that Pap tests often (and at times unnecessarily) trigger.[16] Such a claim seemed to ignore the clinical experience that co-testing sent more patients for follow-up care than Pap tests alone (as a result of the more sensitive yet less specific HPV test). Whether there are real and even important savings, there is also something futile and problematic about this kind of meta-efficacy, in which risk interventions reduce the costs and harms of other risk interventions, especially if such practices become dominant in our clinical and public health work (Aronowitz 2010). While diagnostic tests are a way to mitigate these secondary cost issues and refine and improve diagnoses, as these tests shift from the diagnosis of pathology (a lesion, for example) to the diagnosis of risk, thereby making risk itself into a disease, their use expands and multiplies—and so does treating that risk (Fosket 2010). In expanding diagnostic tests into screening modalities, companies were engaging part of biopolitics: producing the risk categories and risk identities for clinical intervention and population governance. With medicalization, and the proliferation of techniques to monitor bodies and lives, risk shifted from behaviors and identities (from badness to sickness) to clues already inside the body, including genomic profiles.

The commercial medical market for HPV tests now comprises a "high-risk HPV test," to detect but not differentiate between different types of HPV; an "HPV genotyping test" that detects and differentiates HPV types; and other tests that provide individual HPV genotyping results in addition to the results of pooled probes showing whether certain groups of HPVs are present. Taken with other processes such as clinical trial study design and implementation, interpretation of results, and regulatory decisions by the FDA and their associated professional guideline panels and advisory boards, these biomarkers of molecular risk combine to form the epistemic politics of HPV testing. Devices such as HPV screening tools bring people into different forms of awareness of a constructed risk with different "choices" to engage those risks to prevent disease (to monitor, to triage, to treat, etc.). These choices, along with emerging epidemiological evidence and statistical risk models, produce what Samerski (2018) calls "individuals on alert" and Weir and Mykhalovskiy (2012) call a "world on alert." People are expected to act accordingly (or at least to have an awareness of the expectation to do so) by performing or submitting to ongoing biomonitoring (by medicine, by public health, or through self-practices), and by submitting their bodies for treatment of any newly identified risk. From populations to individuals, predictions are individuated onto patients-in-waiting. Cancer has been an important part of population-level risk production and management: genetic screening for breast cancer gene mutations (BRCA1&2) or, in this case, detection of the presence of HPV, introduce potential, yet uncertain, risk (and fear) to be managed and controlled.

Cervical cancer prevention has changed in its scope, scale, and ontological effects, from centering around diagnoses of clear dysplasia—an alteration or abnormality of (potentially cancerous) cells—to diagnoses of precancers and early abnormalities, and then to the diagnoses of cellular, and later molecular, "precursors" (HPV viral types deemed oncogenic or tumor-causing). The shifts hinged on specific knowledge types, each with its own associated uncertainties, presumed *potentiality* (where presence was certain, but potential for persistence and sustained expression or regression over time was uncertain), and accumulative cancer risk: a risk of cancer risk. In its own way, each medical practice shapes perceptions, meanings, and ontological ways of being healthy, ill, and in between. Instead of being thought of strictly as a sudden and usually irreversible harm, disease has gradually been cleaved to the concept of chronicity: risks of illness and risks of *risks* of illness to be surveilled, managed, and controlled. Such "managed fear," as the historian of medicine Charles Rosenberg (2009) called it, is widely exemplified by common medical practices such as the diagnosis of hypertension and high cholesterol, as well as bone density and diabetes screening with risk classified into the well-known categories of osteopenia (a pre-osteoporosis) or pre-diabetes (resulting from the now common A1C test, which measures the percentage of hemoglobin proteins in your blood coated with sugars, and is thus useful for diagnosing diabetes).

HPV Molecular Risk Screening for Cervical Cancer Prevention: Tinkering & Negotiation

In 2012 "co-testing" (cytology Pap testing plus molecular HPV testing) would begin to compete with, if not supplant, the Pap test as the "right tool" in a mass-screening approach to cervical cancer control in the US. This capped almost two decades of technological development, with its accompanying debate and negotiation among leading professional societies and their members. The American transformation that gradually adopted a "primary HPV screening" approach exemplifies both a preventive health politics with diagnostic expansions and a privatized health care context in which companies negotiate the best approach for cancer prevention. Consensus, when reached, would be temporary.

As co-testing was becoming standardized as an approach to cervical cancer prevention, Roche[17] and other private (and public) medical and research organizations and actors were already conducting clinical trial research to make a case for regulatory approval of new indications for a primary screening tool. Pathologists and other professional leaders in cytology with jurisdiction over the clinical specialists, professional technicians, and laboratory infrastructures needed to interpret the millions of Pap tests performed each year would push back against a complete turn to molecular tests.

It was PCR—the polymerase chain reaction laboratory test, developed by Kary Mullis and colleagues at Cetus, a small San Francisco Bay area company, in 1983[18]—that provided researchers with the capacity to "amplify" or copy small particles of DNA for analysis, a necessary step in conducting research where significant amounts of the DNA particle are needed.[19] By "amplifying" small particles of DNA for analysis, HPV could be identified in the cells of cervical tumors and their precancers, confirming a causal role of HPV in cervical cancer.[20] Referred to by Paul Rabinow as "a machine to make a future" (Rabinow 1996, Rabinow and Dan-Cohen 2005), PCR technology had an immense influence on multiple areas of biomedical research and biomedicine more generally, perhaps most prominently in the field of genomics and the human genome mapping project. In cervical cancer, HPV identification produced the capacity to identify risk in the cells—an ambiguous potential, yet an identifiable risk. Cetus sold licenses for PCR use to multiple companies, moving the scientific knowledge of DNA sequencing into the technological practice of DNA identification and giving researchers and companies what they needed to identify and differentiate HPV into its genomic types. Not only did the genomic knowledge lead to the development of a new tool for cervical cancer prevention; it also ignited biomedical changes from the inside out. The "test, test, and test some more" mantra of the COVID-19 pandemic is in many ways a net result of molecularization and the competition to produce and market commercial products.

Molecular knowledge shifted professional training and clinical infrastructure needs. The cytology-based Pap test is read by laboratories employing cytology-pathologists trained to identify and scale cellular configurations on a microscope slide. As Pap testing grew over the twentieth century, the labor force needed to read the myriad smears collected—not just for the diagnostic or research purposes for which they had first been used, but also as part of the mass-screening cervical cancer prevention approach—increased proportionately. This in turn required a semiprofessional field of cytology-technicians to fill the workforce demand. PCR not only propelled a transformation in cervical cancer prevention, but would drive the technoscientific changes already underway in biomedicine as pharmaceutical and biotech companies joined academic and public researchers like those at the NIH to develop new tools for use "from bench to bedside," bringing "precision" approaches, which rely on genomic information, into medical care.

As venture capital and research funding accelerated in the 1980s, biotech companies hoped to develop, clinically test, and commercialize diagnostic tools. Bethesda Life Technologies (BLT), a merger of Bethesda Research Laboratories-Life Science (BRL) and Gibco Corp, was the first to gain FDA approval (in 1988) of an HPV molecular test, having launched research within eighteen months of zur Hausen's "proof" of the association between HPV 16 and cervical cancer.[21] The FDA approval it secured was for "ViraPap," a viral-type test kit that relied on hybridization processes to identify and type HPVs.[22] When Digene (also a Maryland company) acquired BLT's molecular diagnostics division in 1990, the small company obtained what it needed to ultimately develop, patent, and commercialize the "hybrid capture (HC) HPV detection technique."[23] This first HPV tool detected nine HPV types, the plurality of HPVs shown to be "high-risk" or oncoviral.[24] The FDA approval of HC launched clinical trial field tests, which would provide the evidence needed to gain the technique a place in clinical guidelines as a branded, commercialized product for cancer control and prevention.[25]

Cetus was patenting their own tool, another approach to amplification of HPV DNA led by M. Michele Manos. I was able to catch up formally with Manos in 2012 when she was a Senior Research Scientist at another Bay Area organization, Kaiser Permanente. Manos told me about the research on HPV she did while at Cetus. She and her team applied PCR to infectious disease diagnostics and developed what she referred to as "the gold standard for detecting and typing HPV," for which they secured a patent in 1989.[26] Cetus facilitated broad adoption of PCR as well as the new HPV detection technology, offering training courses and providing free reagents. In 1990 Cetus sold this tool and their molecular division to the biotech company Roche, which was hoping to grow its diagnostics unit.[27] As Manos told me, "I think the Roche test is a spin-off of the test developed in my, our lab at Cetus." Manos is an important scientist in the basic and epidemiological research into HPV. When we spoke, I wanted to understand from Manos the implications of the viral-cancer specificity, her role, and what she thought about the applications of vaccination and HPV testing in the changing landscape of cancer prevention.

Manos and I arranged to meet at a coffee shop in the North Bay of San Francisco. It was a warm afternoon, so we chose to sit outside. She told me that she began her career with doctoral training in the 1980s at the Cold Spring Harbor Laboratory in New York, where she worked alongside other researchers in molecular biology, including Yasha Gluzman, Barbara Mc-Clintock, Joseph Sambrook, and Steve Hughes, all regarded as pioneers in this emergent field. At the time, Manos was studying viral-cancer associations, specifically the Simian Virus 40 and the T-antigen protein that can modify cells to be oncogenic. She and others at Cold Spring Harbor were building on the work of Michael Bishop on sarcoma viruses and the RNA viruses, and as she states, "people were beginning to talk about HPV as maybe being linked to cervical cancer." As a virologist at Cetus, Manos was charged with thinking about PCR for infectious disease diagnosis. She put PCR to work to detect and type HPV: as she said, "I provided an accurate test." This was instrumental in the discoveries that would lead to the vaccine. As she told me, "If you think about infection, you think about immunology and the possibility of vaccines; that's what the drug companies were jumping up and down about." The commercialization of HPV testing was also of interest, particularly to molecular diagnostics companies. Then, she stated her conviction that HPV vaccination would "add pressure to make screening more efficient," confirming industry claims that molecular knowledge offered ways to improve on the Pap test.

Science studies scholars Stuart Hogarth and colleagues (Hogarth, Hopkins, and Rodriguez 2012; Hogarth, Hopkins, and Rotolo 2015) argued that molecularization had increased competition in ways that had reinvigorated the cytology of the time, but had not (yet) driven it out.[28] I followed their lead, asking for scientists' take on this potential improvement to the Pap test. To be clinically relevant, I learned, HPV tests would need to set their platforms apart from others. Researchers gathered the evidence base that medicine required to make change: launching randomized controlled or comparative effectiveness research, specifically by partnering with scientists in academia and at the National Institutes of Health (NIH) to design studies to evaluate HPV tests against other HPV tests, against "traditional" or "conventional" Pap testing, and for new indications given a (new) measured outcome.

Identifying HPVs and typing them by their high-risk genotypes exerted additional pressure on the search for alternatives to the Pap test, perhaps moving the needle toward what industry hoped to be more efficient and "optimized" screening modalities. From Digene's first HC tool (FDA approved in 1995) to its second-generation tool with the capacity to identify four additional HPV genotypes that were considered high-risk (in 1999), the capacity for "high-risk HPV DNA testing" would drive the Pap further afield from a screening approach.

Mahboobeh Safaeian, an epidemiologist and Director of Clinical Sciences for HPV at Roche, summarized the events: "Once the role of

HPV was established, between the virus itself, the carcinogenic types, and cervical cancer, you have to evolve with the times. Rather than looking at changes in the cells, you can look at what's causing the problem." The cause, I knew, was a molecular one—and more precisely, a genomic one established by mapping the virus, HPV, for its oncogenic types. The application of the current techniques of molecular biology was an example of how to keep up with the "times," and it was this expertise that would inform decisions around and establish the truth about the "right" and "best" approach to prevention. To do so, however, would require negotiation, evidence, and the support of a wide array of experts and organizational actors. After all, a molecular approach would need to not only compete with, but supplant the long-standing Pap test. This would include reconfiguring the Pap tests' interpretation by pathologists, trained cyto-professionals, and their professional organizations with molecular technologies and the machinery to identify and detect HPVs. It was companies already in the diagnostics business, such as Roche, Safaeian would tell me, that were poised to advance the field. To commercialize with broad use would require IVDs to move from diagnostics into screening tools. As Manos told me years earlier, "screening is important to get people into treatment." It was of no surprise to clinicians and researchers that the commercialization of oncogenic testing (HPV tests) could, and likely would, eventually upend the Pap test as the standard approach to cervical cancer prevention.

Parallel "innovations" in cytology were also playing a role in accelerating a new prevention regime. Two technosciences—each with its own epistemic politics—would apply pressure and drive change in cervical cancer prevention. One was the 2001 inclusion of "atypical squamous cells of undetermined significance," or ASCUS (now ASC-US) in the classification system for reporting test results. The classification system known as the Bethesda System reports Pap test results based on the shape and size of cells that fall in a gray area between normal and abnormal, "suggestive," it is now claimed, of a diagnosis of squamous intraepithelial lesion or SIL (Nayar and Wilbur 2015).[29] When Digene's second-generation tool was approved, it was as a niche triage test for any ambiguous cytology. ASCUS is applied to about 6 to 8 percent of Pap test interpretations—the equivalent of millions of test results each year. There was a lot at stake in understanding this ambiguous classification, both technologically and in terms of human health. Another development was the use of liquid in Pap test collection tubes. This approach, called LBC (for liquid-based cytology), was integrated as a prepping, storing, and testing approach for biomaterials collected by swab or brush.[30] LBC provided the basis and materials needed to run multiple tests using the same collected cellular biosample.

With LBC, Digene and the broader scientific community had the ability to design randomized control trials and other research tools needed to shift cancer prevention from a cellular to a molecular approach, and ultimately to transform it into a tool of precision prevention.

In 2001 and 2002, a clinical trial study design in which Digene provided the HPV testing research supplies free of charge, along with research conducted by Manos and other laboratory scientists, provided the "HPV world" what they needed to make a case for regulatory bodies to issue new cervical cancer screening guidelines. When we met on the Mission Bay campus of UCSF in 2020, George Sawaya, a UCSF obstetrician-gynecologist, said "HPV testing is better than repeat cytology or immediate colposcopy for triaging women . . . was the finding that made it into clinical practice for when pap-results return that are classified as ASC-US." He then added, "And just the name of that [ASC-US] tells you there's uncertainty, right?"

With evidence accumulating to show which viral types were most oncogenic and high-risk, under which circumstances and when an infection might clear on its own, and the length of viral persistence needed for cancer formation, substantive changes were underway. A set of molecular tools could be used to assess the *potential* risk of disease, and from the assessments those tools generated a new medical approach to cancer prevention would form. Given the capital investment needed from the public sector, I wondered, what processes of biomedicalization would be most easily controlled by power, and which would be funded and secured, even in the absence of (full) public interest and support? In what ways would some bodies and lives, and some places and populations, be subjects of health and screening, while others were by contrast objects of disease monitoring? And which others would simply be left out altogether?

Making the Pap Test the "Wrong Tool" for the Job of Cervical Cancer Prevention

Hogarth and colleagues (Hogarth, Hopkins, and Rodriguez 2012; Hogarth, Hopkins, and Rotolo 2015) showed that the evolution and growth of HPV testing included an accommodation to the Pap test: a reform, not a revolution. Baked into the evidence for molecular-based HPV testing as the "best tool" for cervical cancer risk prevention, they argued, were established "problems" with cytology and the Pap test that researchers and providers had known of all along. I followed their lead, and specifically the evidence and its trajectory into professional guidelines, to see if accommodation would continue or if screening approaches would develop around the complete replacement of the Pap test with an HPV test. The degree of "rightness" of HPV testing was cumulative, developing from the time it was first used as a research instrument to when it was used in follow-up, as a companion tool, and then gradually as it became part of a co-test in screening and then, in 2020, an (almost fully) accepted primary screening tool. Not only was the "rightness" of molecular tests baked into the "wrongness" of Pap testing; I also found through claims made by clinical experts and researchers that the "wrongness" of co-testing was baked in for some as well, as the "better" approach of primary HPV screening emerged.

The promise of the molecular tool was based on well-known scientific and clinical limitations of Pap screening. Somewhat new, however, was the assertion that the cancer prevention impact of fewer invasive cancer diagnoses and deaths were stuck at around 70–80 percent in the most well-resourced countries where Pap testing is most available (SEER 2021). The claim of a plateau in disease reduction, and one that is stubborn, persistent, and hard to break through, was joining another well-traveled assertion: that the Pap test, technically speaking, was a limited tool, and as the foundation of the mass-screening approach to cancer prevention had for decades been the object of reconsideration.

Safaeian declared, "You have to evolve with the times." She cleared her throat, and modulated her intonation; with palpable hesitation she confirmed the direction of her company's research. Safaeian worked first in HIV prevention, and is now in HPV research. At Roche she focuses on HPV screening and clinical research study design. "There are limitations of the Pap test," she argued, and these were what made the cytology-based test inherently the "wrong tool" for cervical cancer prevention—despite its also well-known effectiveness in reducing cervical cancers by 70 percent when performed with quality labs and professionals (Wingo et al. 2003), and its low cost, which allowed it to be fairly well established around the world.

Many have argued that the Pap test has "chronic ambiguities in classification, aetiology and diagnosis." Stabilization of this approach to prevention was accomplished through intense and active negotiation, messaging, and manipulation on the part of pathologists. Gendering of the division of labor took place with the formation of a profession of mostly female "cytotechnologists" to do the work previously performed almost exclusively by male pathologists. These semiprofessionals—not trained as MDs, but rather as specialized laboratory technicians who were paid less than pathologists—were justified and established as a needed workforce to make the Pap test the low-cost tool it is today. Yet, exploration into diagnostic alternatives as well as laboratory processes and regulatory enhancements were ongoing, two of the many negotiations Casper and Clarke described as "tinkering." The "rightness" and "wrongness" associated with Pap testing are constructs, "partial, situated, and contingent" (Casper and Clarke 1998, 257). Ultimately, the Pap test emerged and endured because it was "good enough" to do the important work of screening for early signs of cancer—at least until it was time for a better approach.

By 2012 many had become convinced that the focus on which test was right was a mistake. Eric Suba, a pathologist at Kaiser Permanente, was concerned that innovations such as HPV testing were being oversold with a "zombie argument" that Pap screening is not feasible in low- and middle-income countries (LMICs), where 90 percent of the world's cervical cancer deaths occur. A zombie argument is one that has been proven wrong again and again, but keeps shambling on because it serves political purposes. As Suba put it, "if you accept the zombie argument as being true, if Pap screening is really not feasible in LMICs, then research in LMICs on HPV screening, on VIA (visual inspection) screening, on HPV vaccines, those become fundamental humanitarian necessities for the parts of the world where 90% of the cervical cancer deaths occur." Suba's use of the zombie argument was strategic, highlighting his belief that the research underway to overcome the baked-in technical limitations of the Pap was driven by inadequate questions. The plateau of effectiveness, he argued, was not a technoscientific problem, but a moral concern: for Suba, it was well-financed and deliverable screening approaches that were "best" and "right." These other approaches would destabilize the Pap test, not because they are inherently better tools but because their developers are invested in making the Pap test the "wrong tool" for the job of cervical cancer prevention. Scientists, funders, and governance organizations from NIH's National Cancer Institute (NCI) to the American Cancer Society (ACS) have a stake, he argued, in shaping the standardized approaches to prevention, whether those include cellular pathology and Pap tests, visual inspection modalities, or molecular detection tools.

The Pap test's success as measured not by any one-time result, but by the test's regular and frequent use throughout a person's life—its repetition (enabled by the prevention guideline)—provided a cover for its limitation. "The [Pap test] became sensitive because it was repeated multiple times over a woman's life," Safaeian explained. This was the basis for "innovation"—not the unique promise and benefit of the HPV test, but the pitfalls and problems associated with the Pap. As evidence grew in support of just how "wrong" the Pap test was for the prevention of cervical cancer, and, by association, just how "right" the HPV test might be in light of problems associated with the Pap test (and less so for its potential to solve the problem of cervical cancer), so too did another assertion: HPV testing was not only the better tool, but also an important technology in the context of HPV vaccination. Researchers were building a case for HPV testing as a necessary and "right" tool for a new regime of cancer prevention in a context in which vaccine coverage was uneven. Personalized, precise, and predictive HPV tests, I would learn, would fill the gaps, and would do so without inherent problems like vulnerability to legal claims and legal payouts.[31]

HPV vaccination is far from universally available or accepted; it is also variable in its coverage of HPV types, making herd immunity out of reach and driving the ongoing necessity of cervical cancer screening. Evidence began to accumulate showing cancer reduction through vaccination in 2020. Screening is central to this measurement and declaration of success. Clinical research studies require an endpoint to measure "success"—in this case, cancer occurrence—and because the time from viral infection to cancer diagnosis is so drawn out (from ten to thirty years when persistence occurs), proving vaccine-attributable reduction in cancer has relied on the "clinical surrogate" of an "abnormal cytology" and "pre-cancers" from Pap tests, repeat testing, and/or colposcopy and biopsy, each a marker that appears in the interval between infection and invasive cancer. This is the same period on which screening guidelines overwhelmingly focus their attention to prevent (or, more accurately, treat) the risk that follows infection (specifically, the risk of viral persistence).

HPV tests indicate something qualitatively different in terms of potential risk from Pap test results. Pap test results classify cellular abnormalities on a range from lesions in need of removal to abnormalities that can be "wait and watched." HPV screening-based cancer prevention efforts do not really target the risk of cancer formation from abnormalities already underway—they target *the risk of the risk* of cancer. There is little certainty that the virus itself is a precursor, especially among young people, in whom the virus is especially prone to regressing. As one ages, persistence is more likely, as is a still uncertain likelihood of viral presence (the result of the same increase in persistence of infection) leading to cancer. In this way, the presence or detection of HPV types is a risk, but not a clear surrogate endpoint, nor an endpoint for invasive cancer; it is a risk of the risk of persistence by an identified viral type—one known to be oncoviral—that is the target of testing. How, when, and with what frequency to screen for HPV itself (as opposed to screening for a lesion or pre-cancerous abnormality detectable by Pap test) have been major, shifting questions for cervical cancer researchers, whether they are (also) using the less sensitive and specific cytology Pap test or the molecular HPV test. Evolving (albeit persistently uncertain) knowledge of the "natural pathway" of HPV to cancer only added urgency to the need for an alternative approach to the Pap test.

George Sawaya of UCSF confirmed the drivers of the Pap test—despite its inherent inadequacies—in clinical practice, adding that it was not only the Pap's lack of sensitivity when used only one time or infrequently that made the Pap test inadequate; it also had the capacity to do more harm than good. Harm occurred with the test's high rate of false positives and false negatives, netting an increase in erroneous as well as ambiguous results. It also occurred with the need to require subsequent clinical visits, the costs associated with repeat testing, the stress for patients when an ambiguous result was found, and the potentialities for legal claims when real cancers were missed.

HPV testing also came with its own set of challenges. These included high numbers of false positives—more than cytology. Significantly, the false positives returned by Pap tests, which justified "innovating" that tool, remain in place with the new approach. All of these challenges would create unnecessary anxiety, fear, and uncertainty, which, along with other potential harms of frequent Pap testing, were reliably shared with me along with the comparative promise—and not similar challenge—of molecular-based HPV tests.

These potential harms were technical by-products of the lack of "sensitivity" and "specificity" of the Pap test. The test lacks "sensitivity"—it misses actual positives (false negatives) and incorrectly identifies true positives and actual abnormalities (false positives), making it less than precise: "too many false negatives" leave too many people at increased risk of cancer despite screening. Low sensitivity meant results often incorrectly classified samples (and the people they came from) with cellular abnormalities as "normal."[32] The Pap test is unable to predict with accuracy the true rate of "positives," or people with (meaningful) cellular abnormalities. In reducing sensitivity, more false negative results were returned, and too many people with actual "pre-cancers" were going unnoticed (Löwy 2011, 157; Gaudillière and Löwy 1998). What made the Pap test work (and what specifically overcame this lack of sensitivity) was frequent repetition: abnormalities missed once or twice will eventually be identified. The Pap test also lacks "specificity"—readings do not have the precision to ensure certainty of results. This means that both false positives and false negatives are common enough to cause concern. This not only obscured the so-called true rate of negatives (normal people correctly identified as not having cancerous cells); it also led to unnecessary referral of people with false positives to further surveillance and/or cervical colposcopy. Colposcopy requires an additional clinical appointment and a somewhat invasive and uncomfortable exam, as well as additional cost. Given existing challenges to health care access, any additional clinical visit, especially an unnecessary one, was regarded as a reason to find a better screening test. Clinical providers of Pap testing would "adjust" for these potentials by either choosing to identify as potential pathology (or risk of pathology) only well-defined cellular white zones (signs of cancerous changes) that more clearly indicate something amiss, or to over-refer for colposcopy and biopsy.

Over time these cellular uncertainties, and the medical assertion of missed pre-cancers, would receive their own classification of ASC-US, a laboratory result that signals either a need for repeat testing and shorter intervals between tests and/or referral for colposcopy examination and cellular biopsy. Medical classifications like ASC-US shape people's identities and emotions, conveying both a potential self-image as at risk and a potentially unnecessary worry and fear. Would patients with ASC-US have a "pre-cancer" or a "precursor" and risk factor, or something else altogether? These uncertainties were not new; they were the objects of biomedical fixing with more stable categories of knowledge, and the basis for clinical decision making. With HPV testing and its increased sensitivity, however, greater numbers of people would subjectively experience *risky* chronic disease based on classification not of cellular changes (although they can coexist), but of viral status (if HPV positive is to be considered a pathological state, that is), as well as lowered thresholds for clinical diagnoses resulting in what could be called "pre-disease" conditions.[33] From a sociological standpoint, people's subjective experience and *identities* are shaped as they make sense of and integrate pre-disease and risk classifications as diagnostic categories into their lives.

While HPV testing provides a "objective" machine output, depending on the HPV viral type (and other factors such as medical history and previous pap and HPV test results), the HPV+ and ASC-US classifications inform triage decisions, and also impact subjectivity. Increased numbers of people experience risky chronic disease given the ways these classifications signal "earlier," and often, "pre-"disease. These tests produce affective states such as worry and fear, as well as what Howson (1999, 402) calls a set of normative expectations for compliance with power. "Even if you go annually for a Pap, about one-third of cervical cancers or high grade cervical precancers are diagnosed in women who have had normal Paps." A lot of cervical cancer is diagnoses, as Sawaya stated, "in women who thought they've gone for their screening and were ok."

This diminished benefit of the very low-cost, yet frequently repeated Pap test caused a bottom-line problem for providers and health care systems, and generated competition to commercialize a new approach. A key part of making the Pap "good enough" (but inherently wrong) was the purported inconsistency, and thereby "subjectivity," of readings by humans. Yet supplanting a professional world with a cadre of semiprofessional cytologists and medically trained pathologists would be needed if the field was to follow the Roche scientist who claimed: "[I]t was great when it [the Pap] worked, but now we have better technologies." As the HPV test transformed clinical medicine and public health practice, would this drive what the health writer Ray Moynihan (2006) calls diagnosis creep with its potentially expanded market, or what the bioethicist Jennifer Fishman (2004) refers to as the added reach of intermediary actors in configuring a whole new market?

CHAPTER EIGHT

The Precision Imaginary

Optimizing Cancer Prevention Tools

It has been said that oncology is a "natural choice" for applying the new tools of precision medicine to ensure a more "individualized approach with patients" (National Cancer Institute 2017). Precision is a charismatic as well as a biomedical name for a movement in medicine and public health that hopes to revolutionize its approaches to treatment and cure by bringing genomic knowledge and sequencing into clinical and public health efforts alike. The sequencing of the HPV virus was a needed first step in what is now a largely corporatized effort to produce and distribute a primary prevention vaccine coupled with new secondary screening tools applied to identify "residual risks" as well as prevention gaps in care.

When the US National Cancer Institute launched the "ALTS" trial (formally, the ASC-US-LSIL Triage Study) in 1998, it was scientifically designed with the hope of creating a clear approach for the millions of women and people with a cervix who received the Pap test result of "atypical squamous cells of undetermined significance" (ASC-US). The "mildly abnormal" Pap result was common, occurring in about 6–10 percent of all Pap tests. The clinical trial assessed how best to evaluate and manage ASC-US and what was understood as its equivocal classification result of LSIL, "low-grade squamous intraepithelial lesion." Mark Schiffman, who also developed HPV vaccination and research into Hybrid Capture HPV tests, led the ALTS study at the NCI (Schiffman and Solomon 2009).[1] The trial was also designed with the hope of including the additional information of a sequenced result of HPV's oncoviral or high-risk genotypes into that calculation.

ALTS compared screening approaches following ASC-US classified cytology results into one of three options: (1) to refer the person for colposcopy and biopsy, (2) to call for a repeat Pap test to confirm or disprove the prior reading, or (3) to conduct a "co-test" with HPV testing to ascertain the presence of HPV (Schiffman and Adrianza 2000). Trial results found that HPV testing is not shown to be useful (given the prevalence of HPV

TABLE 2. Stages of the socio-technical trajectory of HPV tests, 2013–2020

Destabilizing the Co-Test	
2013	Roche submits FDA Premarket Approval supplement for cervical cancer primary screening indication
2014	(March) FDA Microbiology Medical Devices Panel of the Medical Devices Advisory Committee meets to consider application from Roche (April 11) Coalition letter to FDA Commission in opposition to approving cobas* HPV Test for primary testing (April 24) FDA approves Roche cobas* HPV Test for primary screening in women twenty-five and older (**First FDA approval of HPV primary test**; based on ATHENA trial data)
2015	ATHENA primary HPV testing results are published
2017	Finalized guidance change for primary testing by the FDA (US Food & Drug Administration 2017)

The Pathway to Primary HPV Screening	
2018	(February) BD Onclarity HPV Assay gains FDA approval for use as primary test (**Second HPV test to gain primary approval**; also approved for co-testing and triage use) (August) USPSTF guidelines include HPV primary testing every five years as a screening option in those age thirty to sixty-five years
2020	2020 ACS cervical cancer screening guidelines are the **first to endorse primary HPV testing** as the preferred screening strategy

Note: Bold indicates key turning points in negotiations.

positivity, over 80 percent) and that HPV information is somewhat useless for decision making (Schiffman and Adrianza 2000, Schiffman and Solomon 2003). Nonetheless, HPV testing was found to be useful in detecting "underlying lesions" in ASC-US diagnosed cervices, supporting the conclusion that HPV testing was "better than repeat cytology or immediate colposcopy for triaging women with ASCUS" (Schiffman and Adrianza 2000). This would drive what was considered an "optimized" approach to cancer risk assessment, yet it left uncertainty in place (see table 2 for the trajectory of professional guidelines).

With two divergent knowledge systems—ASC-US Pap classification and HPV molecular results—came a new development: the production of a *risk* of cancer risk. ASC-US with an HPV positive molecular result transformed this risk from something "common and normal" and "undetermined" that affected up to 10 percent of Pap tests to a new "high risk of cancer" risk designation. That is, normal Pap results plus HPV+ "high risk" (hr) types indicated risk "equivalent" to that of someone with the singular HPV negative test; a moderate risk for ASC-US results accompanied by HPV negative indicated a designation as low risk. It is the now understood higher risk that attaches to ASC-US when accompanied with an HPV positive test for a high-risk genotype that opened questions about *which* next steps are best for prevention and care. Yet, even with a new question, the finding of additional HPV information was just that: additional.

The ALTS trial provided the evidence needed to "get HPV testing through to screening," as Sawaya indicated—first as part of clinical decision-making and a triage tool, and gradually as a means to shift the risk paradigm altogether. A patent race was on as HPV test developers (Digene, Hologic, Roche,[2] and BD[3] among them) hoped to dominate the coming market by positioning themselves and their HPV detection tools for consideration of integration into new clinical practices and prevention guidelines (Division of Cancer Prevention 2021). Roche's HPV division acquired the intellectual property rights to PCR testing from Cetus (along with many staff members from the PCR group, but not M. Michele Manos, who had led the HPV PCR development at Cetus) and was well positioned to command the market. Acquiring the rights to PCR (and giving others free PCR reagents) in the 1990s allowed Roche to develop "fast, sensitive and specific" diagnostic tests and to move into a leadership position in HPV diagnostics (Hogarth, Hopkins, and Rotolo 2015, 96–97).

The turn to HPV detection as a screening approach would take time; it would need more evidence to infer population-level effectiveness and then different infrastructures to run the lab tests and convey the information to "patients." Knowing the best way to translate two knowledge systems said to be "equivalent" risk measures into a single replacement approach would take time. It was Roche who would submit the first request to the FDA, in 2013, to use a molecular test as a primary screening tool, rather than as part of co-testing. Mahboobeh Safaeian, a Roche scientist, confirmed the steps taken to supplant a co-test and triage approach to screening altogether. During our interview she began by affirming Roche's dominance: "[we] now have a better technology," she said, that had been confirmed in the ALTS trial and other clinical trials that followed.

ALTS provided "predictive" yet uncertain information; triaging to colposcopy helped reduce what oncologists refer to as "cervical intra-epithelial neoplasia," the most severe form of cervical dysplasia, or abnormal cellular changes.[4] Because this severe form of cervical dysplasia (CIN3) is deemed a "pre-cancer," it is treated, which in turn, adds to the tools included in a clinical care regime. Along with FDA approvals of HPV diagnostic tools and now this new evidence, multiple professional worlds—corporate, governmental, and clinical—were feeling the pressure to "innovate."

ALTS study results led the American Society for Colposcopy and Cervical Pathology (ASCCP), the American Cancer Society (ACS), and the US Preventive Services Task Force (USPSTF) to convene their advisory groups to consider new screening guidelines. Guidelines are technologies of governance, shaping the incorporation of certain bodies, lives, and population groups into classifications of risk and disease, and what lies between. They also drive identity formation, be it "patient" with disease, or (now stratified) risk designation as low, medium, or high with "pre-cancers" and "patients-in-waiting" (Timmermans and Buchbinder 2010). As a technology of governance, these guidelines impose assumptions about good patients, good science, and good care. Each regulatory body would propose a new formula for screening that would consider age, intervals, frequency, and which tools to deploy as the final steps were underway to overcome what were accepted imperfections of the Pap. Once in place, the USPSTF guidelines would be followed by the US government, which sets reimbursements for Medicare, Medicaid, and the insurance plans mandated by the Affordable Care Act. Other insurers would likely follow.

The ASCCP chose to include HPV detection as a triage tool in 2001; the ACS followed in 2002. The ACS went a step further and recommended that clinicians use the HPV detection test as a "supplemental test" or companion tool, to be used simultaneously in triage decision-making for women over thirty. The ACS decision would especially affirm co-testing and would be the basis for approving Digene's second-generation HPV test (HC2) as a triage test *and* as a "co-test" for screening women over thirty. The FDA agreed with the evidence pointing to the finding that HPV testing is better than repeat cytology or immediate colposcopy for triaging women with ASC-US. FDA approved the test and its use in 2003, moving the co-test approach closer to a standardization.

Digene invested in sales and marketing, and approached physicians and laboratories that perform reference measurements (usually private entities that provide calibration, quality measures, cost-effectiveness, and other kinds of support testing for devices). They did this, rather than choosing against the more common route of approaching clinical laboratories, to expedite the adoption of the HPV test and to secure what was "62 percent of the ASC-US triage market" and profitability (Hogarth, Hopkins, and Rodriguez 2012, 241). In 2003, regulation approvals expanded to include a co-test at a later interval when following an HPV negative test and a normal Pap result. In these cases, a patient does not need to be retested for three years—a longer interval than was previously designated. The FDA's 2003 approval of the use of Digene's HC2 as a co-testing tool with the Pap test for women over thirty was said to be a significant cancer reduction step for this age group only; anyone younger would likely have HPVs that would still be amenable to clearance. The approach confers confidence of minimal cancer risk and would reduce unnecessary testing, costs, and patient visits.

The FDA was now recommending "adjunct" screening only for those in whom the virus may have persisted over time, increasing cancer risk.

With a recommendation from the USPSTF that clinicians offer a co-test to women over thirty, a pathway was established to eventually standardize the HPV test in primary preventive politics. Roche and others hoped this approach might overcome other persistent problems associated with cancer screening—specifically, low screening rates and clinic-based and laboratory infrastructure limitations. Digene partnered with Olympic gold medalists and MVPs from the Women's National Basketball Association to promote the importance of obtaining a human papillomavirus (HPV) test for women thirty years of age and older. The campaign bore an uncanny resemblance to the "Know HPV" campaign launched the same year by Merck for their coming vaccine. As Nikki McCray, Lisa Leslie, and Becky Hammon shot hoops and signed autographs for fans, cervical cancer prevention materials were distributed among the crowd encouraging women to "choose to know," with the familiar tagline, "Ask your doctor." The direction to "ask your doctor" was said to compensate for the relative newness of the tool for routine screening (WNBA 2005). The campaign to "spread the word" allowed viewers to send e-cards to friends, thus enrolling them in a new generation of cancer prevention actors.

Another tool, liquid-based cytology (LBC), first used in cytology and Pap testing, was built into the design of the molecular HPV tests, and it helped to smooth the pathway for the inclusion of HPV tests in a new cancer prevention regime. Instead of the dry biomaterials sample smeared on a slide for visual inspection under a microscope, LBC uses a vial filled with a liquid solution to store the sample. The ability to use the single vial to run multiple tests was significant for a shift to a new cancer screening paradigm. There were other "advantages" aside from a co-test, Sawaya told me: it also introduced a "second billing point" and the opportunity to replace human interpretation with automated technologies. As he put it, "In thinking about mandated re-screening of a certain number of normal cytology tests," finding "a way to have a machine read these negative Paps again" would be ideal. "And [then] we can only have human eyes focus on these that appear abnormal." LBC was more costly than traditional Pap, providing a higher reimbursement rate. "With that being a new system, it allowed it to have a new price-point of $35 above and beyond the $8 pap smear" (two to four times the usual cost of a Pap test). Sawaya continued, "maybe we are paying for more efficiency, and maybe we're paying for a little more of something else?" LBC was said by the FDA to be more effective than a dry sample, opening the gates to displace the Pap test altogether. Yet, as Sawaya indicated, "there were [no] comparative trials at the time . . . one study in Europe showed no benefit of liquid-based versus conventional cytology in terms of disease detection." However, it also did not "show that there is any particular harm . . . no increase in false positives." The USPSTF commissioned a large review of the literature on LBC to decide for themselves, finding "really no difference between the two." Sawaya continued, with a shrug, "So, you're then kind of left with, 'Oh, wow; we just now paid four times more for a Pap smear. But what is the benefit to the population or society—or to women?' I mean, that's a reasonable question to ask."

The other benefit—a second billing point, driven by automation rather than human labor—was instrumental in the shift to molecular testing standardization. Complete system approaches would come to dominate diagnostic company offerings. Hologic's ThinPrep™, for example, is a platform around which automation, algorithms, and multiple tests (assays, molecular, cytology review, etc.) can be performed. For each output, a unique version of what the test is looking for materializes; yet the versions of the "it" found are different. As Annemarie Mol (2003, 66) states, "reality multiplies"—medicine is an enactment in practice that might "hang together" but "not quite as a whole" (p. 84). Translations between disparate versions are sufficient for medical work to cohere, as is the case with information output. In an LBC platform like ThinPrep, the medium used to preserve cells and the collection device in which they are stored multiply and diversify the forms of information to be generated by the machine. In this case, an alcohol-based fluid preserves cells upon collection; at the laboratory, the vial itself is what allows for "out-of-vial" human papillomavirus testing and automated slide processing. The cells are distributed (e.g., smeared) on a slide in a thin, even layer for analysis. Where cytological testing is concerned, this automation is considered a better approach: subjectivity is eliminated (replaced with an objective approach), as are unnecessary repeat cytology tests (and the pathologists needed for interpretation); sensitivity has "increased accuracy"; and the quality of the sample is improved. Most of all, the technoscientific platform allows for multiple testing options beyond cytology, despite the samples' coming from a single LBC vial. With ThinPrep, a single sample vial can be used to run a molecular HPV test and also a test for chlamydia and gonorrhea (*Trichomonas vaginalis* and *Mycoplasma genitalium*).[5]

To ask "What is the benefit?" of LBC and of complete system technological approaches to screening and diagnostics is to ask an important sociological question: How do technosciences participate in constructing and overcoming problems of prior cancer prevention approaches? What problems, what people, and what organizations are poised to benefit most from a given solution? As various knowledge systems come together—cytology and molecular—each can give meaningful outputs even as the distinct "it" found by each is very different. Translational work allows medicine's work: "We are paying for more efficiency," Sawaya states, and "maybe we're paying a little more for something else."

QIAGEN's promotion message for the Digene test was not about cancer screening, but about STDs.[6] In 2002 QIAGEN provided guidance on talking with your partner about STDs, indicating cancer was significantly shaped by sex.[7] Over time, a redirected website would de-sexualize the domain and promote a "continuing legacy" in cancer prevention, with QIAGEN's three tests (QIAscreen™, QIAsure™, and the *care*HPV Test™) able to "objectively detect the presence of biomarkers associated with cervical precancer and cancer." Biomarkers were found "in the PCR lab, using the same sample from an HPV or liquid-based cytology test" (QIAGEN 2019).

LBC continues to drive change. Xavier Bosch, a cancer epidemiologist and oncologist in Spain, spoke in an interview of preliminary evidence that Pap samples could be used to test for molecular biomarkers for other cancers, such as endometrial and ovarian cancer, as well. The "objectivity" provided by automation contrasted with the "subjectivity" of Pap cytology readings, even though most of these had been automated as well. Whether HPV testing would supplant the established cytology technology was still unknown, but it was deemed likely, and pressure was mounting. At the time, it seemed, HPV tests had reinvigorated, but had not (yet) replaced, cytology. Like Sawaya, I was eager to find out whether the new approaches would ultimately reduce cervical cancers, and whether they would remain in place as a companion screening tool. The anticipation of an HPV primary tool led many to voice concern.[8] It was feared that HPV detection as a co-test and future primary screening tool would create new problems of its own, such as higher costs to providers and different infrastructure needs for clinics and laboratories, as well as training demands for those who would oversee their results and interpretations.

Primary HPV tests, in particular tests that returned positive results for HPV 16 or 18, for example, would lead to increased colposcopy as a result of the genotyping. This could, as many researchers in gynecology and oncology anticipate, lead to increased detection of what is called CIN-3 and thus drive decreases in cancers (Melnikow et al. 2018).[9] What is innovative technologically might also reproduce the multiple tendencies of biomedicine that drive individual choice and better health for some who are seen as "good" and "righteous" health-seekers, while producing mandatory mass-screening tools to prevent death for others, and leaving still others outside of care altogether (Murphy 2012). Certainly, screening could not address the relatively unspoken problems of social determinants of health and of cancer risk: from affordability and accessibility of health care to the social and structural upstream determinants of equity, rights, and justice. Yet the charisma of precision just might be able to shift into a new public health paradigm to enfold these settings in its preventive reach.

Over the next five years industry competed for market dominance with mergers, acquisitions, and new investment in R&D.[10] Roche was one of the clear front-runners (with Hologic and QIAGEN) by the time the FDA approved their cobas® HPV Test, an automated test run on their cobas 4800 system, on April 20, 2011. Cobas is a laboratory "total system" that allows for loading multiple sample vials at one time (in the same run) and selecting multiple options from a consolidated menu for testing, in this case in virology, sexual health, and microbiology.[11] The cobas® HPV test was FDA approved specifically as a tool for "Identifying Women at Highest Risk for Cervical Cancer," with high risk classified as showing the presence of high-risk HPV genotypes. The test specifically identifies HPV 16 and HPV 18, while concurrently detecting the other (now twelve) oncogenic types.[12] If test results are positive, the infection is presumably more than a cursory exposure, neither so recent nor so brief that it might shed on its own and regress so much that it could give a false positive result.

This use approval was granted within the bounds of then-current guidelines for cervical cancer screening, allowing for either cytology or co-testing to determine the risk of cervical cancer. HPV testing—and 16 and . 18 genotyping in particular—it was claimed, could identify more women at risk earlier than Pap alone. The "additive" information for the two "highest risk" genotypes of HPV for cancer, as the professor and pathologist Mark Stoler stated, "can provide predictive information about a woman's risk for having cervical pre-cancer or cancer" (Roche 2011). Predicting future risk was the new business model, yet whether more information, even of these high-risk HPV genotypes, would lead to lower rates of cancer deaths was unknown.

In fall 2011, three professional organizations—the ACS, ASCCP, and the American Society for Clinical Pathology, ASCP—endorsed the FDA decision and proposed new guidelines for the prevention and early detection of cervical cancer. At a symposium held in November 2011, a working group with delegates from twenty-five different organizations reached consensus. These associations worked together, but independently of the USPSTF, to review the existing evidence and develop draft recommendations; they coordinated their press release with the USPSTF to ensure minimal confusion for providers and the public. Recommendations were adapted into a final guideline (from the ACS) recommending a testing reduction—fewer tests performed over one's lifetime—to minimize any risks and optimize any benefits. The preference, these groups agreed, was for co-testing using the cytology platform of the Pap test combined with a molecular platform for HPV testing, and doing so for "women age 30 and over." The ACS-ASCCP-ASCP guidelines recommended that all women start screening at age twenty-one, making age, rather than sexual activity or onset of sexual activity, the entrée to cancer screening. This replaced the recommendation for women under twenty-one to begin screening three years after starting vaginal intercourse and shifted standards from sexual risk, with its subsumed assumptions of (hetero)sexuality and heterosex, to an age-based risk. Younger people, between twenty-one and twenty-nine, should receive Pap tests (conventional or liquid-based) every three years. For women thirty and over Pap tests are recommended every three years.

The move was significant for its extension of what had for decades been considered the optimum interval for Pap tests—one year—as well as for another key change: Pap testing plus an HPV test every three to five years for women aged thirty and older. It was also recommended that providers not screen with any test or combination of tests more often than every three years.[13] These guidelines, however, would undergo another shift from 2011 (when Roche submitted an application to the FDA for their cobas® HPV test) to 2020 (with new ACS guidelines) when replacement as a screening approach began to make inroads. The decisions were tightly entangled with the regulatory speed at which devices move through FDA approval processes.

(De)Stabilizing the "Co-Test" to Make Way for a Primary Screening Approach

In January 2014 the US FDA announced an upcoming review by the Microbiology Devices Panel of the Medical Devices Advisory Committee.[14] The meeting would review the fifth and latest "indication for the use" of the cobas® HPV Test "as a first-line primary cervical cancer screening test to detect high risk HPV, including genotyping for 16 and 18" (FDA 2014).[15] The co-test was about to hit shaky regulatory ground, and the language used in the description of the meeting was the first clue of what was to come; by questioning its role as a "screening test" and thus signaling the beginning of a possible shift from HPV tests as detection tools (in follow-up Pap decision making) to HPV tests as screening tools. In March 2014, the FDA announced that it would consider the application submitted by Roche Molecular Inc. for this "new indication" for the cobas® HPV Test.

The evidence presented to the committee was from Roche's ATHENA trial, which had been launched six years earlier in 2008 and ran for four years, to 2012.[16] It was this clinical trial that would provide the evidence needed "to get testing through to screening," as Sawaya had phrased the transition. Roche designed and implemented the ATHENA trial, "Addressing the Need for Advanced HPV Testing," to clinically validate Roche's own HPV test: the cobas® HPV Test (first approved on the basis of ALTS data) for triaging people with ASC-US Pap results. Cobas was approved for triage based on the concurrent presence of hr HPV 16 and 18 in those with ASC-US Pap, and thus as a co-test for people thirty years and older (it was also FDA approved to detect HPV 16 and 18). The ATHENA trial would drive approval by FDA in 2011 for four additional uses beyond a triage tool. The evidence presented would answer the lingering clinical question of "What do you do with these millions of women" (with ASC-US classification)? Safaeian answered: if a Pap test was ASC-US and the patient is also HPV positive, we know "the risk is high" and we would manage the people as being at high risk of cancer. For Roche, this led to the FDA approval of the second-generation Hybrid Capture HPV test, "HC2," with its capacity to differentiate four additional hr HPVs, and approval as a triage tool. It also continued to establish the pathway for a new screening approach, and for Roche to lead the way.

As interpreted by Roche scientists, the findings went beyond answering the question of comparative test performance, showing that HPV primary screening for women twenty-five or older was "as effective" as the prevailing cytological screening strategy for twenty-five- to twenty-nine-year-olds, and the co-testing strategy for those thirty and over. Additionally, Roche reported, it was good news that HPV primary screening of this type would require "less" screening overall (Wright et al. 2015, 189). The possibility of less screening was appealing, the authors claimed: it could reduce cost, it would reduce barriers of access, and it could reduce discomfort. No comment was made as to whether it would reduce cancer.

In the documents submitted to the FDA, Roche stated that "1 in 10 women, age 30 and older, who tested positive for HPV 16 and/or 18 by the cobas® HPV Test actually had cervical precancer *even though they showed normal results with the Pap test* [emphasis added]." This classification emerged as highly significant to the screening approach. This finding meant that an HPV "screening tool" would be able to provide the information needed to engage precisely in the clinical decision making to prevent infections, specifically those designated as pre-cancers, from causing invasive cancers. The claim by Roche was not that the cobas® HPV Test was better per se, but that it had the "equivalent effectiveness" of a combined approach (a co-test).[17] The hope was that the FDA would agree, making

Roche and their cobas® platform the leading company in a potential new market, and at the same time creating a pathway for professional organizations to consider recommending primary HPV screening.

Roche was amplifying the pathway they hoped for, buying exposure through their conference industry booths as they distributed materials and spoke with clinicians and researchers about their trial results. At EUROGIN, the European Research Organisation on Genital Infection and Neoplasia, in Seville, the exhibition hall on the ground floor required attendees to pass through a corridor lined with industry booths. At the center of these displays were the big players in HPV vaccination and HPV testing: Merck's Gardasil booth was the largest and most centrally located; another for Cervarix, the HPV vaccine approved in Europe, was close by. Then diagnostic companies like Hologic, Roche, and QIAGEN highlighted their sequencing, assay, and DNA tests. Attendees would take note as they walked by, returning for more information and conversation, as well as for the conference coffee, snacks, and other drinks offered next to these booths.

Roche got what they hoped for when the Medical Devices Advisory Committee Microbiology Panel—comprising academic pathologists, microbiologists, and gynecologists—voted unanimously in 2014 to approve the new indication for cobas® HPV testing. The vote affirmed that Roche's cobas® platform HPV test *could be* used as a primary screening approach for "women 25 and older" (although they did not immediately do so). The committee held a panel review the following month to gather experts to consider harms and benefits before announcing the new indication's approval. Supporters readily affirmed the inclusion of the primary test in the cervical cancer prevention field, asking rhetorically, as Dorothy Rosenthal, a professor at Johns Hopkins Medical Center, did, "Has our Pap, as we know it, outlived its time?" Rosenthal's question underscored a position that the Pap had hit a wall in its capacity to prevent deaths, at least in the United States, and a suggestion that another, better approach was available. Given the elusiveness of further reductions in cancer rates, Rosenthal claimed, "a tremendous gain" would result if the FDA approved moving more fully to HPV primary screening as a cervical cancer screening approach.

FDA Approvals Come with Opposition and Dissent

Others, however, voiced concern and some opposition as a distinctly American approach to standardizing co-testing became entrenched, at least for a time. In a statement made to the FDA, the American College of Obstetricians and Gynecologists (ACOG) objected to the possibility of a new indication for the cobas® HPV Test platform, citing a lack of evidence that a transition from a co-test to a primary tool would add any benefit. "There is little comparative effectiveness data comparing primary HPV screening with co-testing," they argued, and since co-testing was the preferred method agreed to by ACS, ASCCP and ASCP, ACOG stated that if the cobas® HPV Test was approved, "providers will not be able to adequately counsel patients regarding the relative benefits and potential harms of primary HPV screening compared with currently accepted methods, particularly co-testing." Evidence was still needed, they argued, to adequately understand the potential risks and benefits (Cancer Prevention & Treatment Fund et al. 2014).

In a letter sent to FDA commissioner Margaret A. Hamburg, and copied to Jeffrey Shuren, then director of the Center for Devices and Radiological Health, a coalition of organizations also voiced concern and opposition to this new approval. The letter was authored by the Cancer Prevention and Treatment Fund and cosigned by professional associations including the American Medical Student Association, the American Medical Women's Association, and the American Public Health Association, as well as cancer advocacy and health activist organizations such as the National Organization for Women and Our Bodies Ourselves.[18] Collectively, these experts expressed "grave concerns" about the potential new indication for the cobas® HPV Test as a primary screening tool for women over twenty-five. While the substance of the opposition was detailed, the net claim by these groups was that this would be a "radical change" to current USPSTF guidelines. The guideline in place at the time was considered a "hybrid" approach based on age and was determined to be the best and right tool for cancer prevention by these co-authors. Pap testing for young women in their twenties was preferable, given the frequency of HPV clearance; "co-testing" ought to begin at age thirty. The letter and its signatories meticulously laid out the ways in which the potential change to primary HPV testing would be both "radical" and unwanted, effectively replacing what was an otherwise "safe and effective" and "well-established screening tool and regimen." This regimen, the authors asserted, was successfully preventing cervical cancer in the US. The proposed new primary screening approach, they argued, was neither proven to work in a large US population nor supported by any evidence-based US guidelines. Like the authors of the ACOG statement, this coalition saw the new approach as an interference with the practice of medicine.

Many opposed to the change also warned that HPV testing would create unnecessary harm to patients: a positive result would identify viral infection, not abnormal cells. This information would lead to unnecessary colposcopy, they argued—an expensive and invasive procedure, and one that might deter people from clinical follow-up visits. Instead, they argued, the logical next step for screening is Pap testing to determine whether cellular abnormalities are present as well. It would be better, the letter argued, if the Pap test remained in place as a co-test. If there were no abnormalities found, then a colposcopy would not be needed: "The Pap smear is effective in detecting cellular signs of pre-malignancy that can be caused by HPV or other causes." HPV screening, they asserted, would not only be insufficient to provide the information needed for triage, but would also miss other causes of cervical cancer beyond HPV (Cancer Prevention & Treatment Fund et al. 2014).

To understand the opposition requires a closer look at the evidence provided by Roche to support their request to the FDA. The ATHENA trial consisted of a baseline measure, as well as a three-year follow-up phase of data. The baseline consisted of two cervical samples collected for HPV testing (using cobas® HPV Test, an investigational use only [IUO] hr HPV test, and an IUO HPV genotyping test) and Hologic ThinPrep LBC. HPV testing was performed at five different laboratories; LBC testing was conducted at four of these five laboratories. Cytology samples were classified according to the Bethesda System (2001 criteria) of low- or high-grade or ASCUS findings. The trial included an algorithm for triage decisions for both the proposed primary screening with HPV test and the traditional cytology screening (see the trial design algorithm in figure 1).

For primary HPV testing the algorithm began with three possible results (HPV negative; HPV positive for 16 or 18; and HPV positive for the 12 other "pooled" HPV oncoviral types). Low-risk was deemed certain for HPV negative results, and patients would continue routine follow-up. However, when HPV 16+ or 18+ results were returned, patients would be designated high-risk and referred to colposcopy immediately; if positive for any of the 12 other pooled HPV oncoviral types, the patient would be referred for cytology evaluation to determine need for colposcopy. Cytology results of ASC-US or greater abnormality would be referred to colposcopy; if cytology was normal (Negative for Intraepithelial Lesion or Malignancy—NILM), the patient would be returned to the standard interval of a follow-up screening protocol. The cytology alone algorithm—the comparison arm of the study—was for ASC-US or greater cytology abnormalities, with the step of referring for colposcopy (a normal result in the routine screening protocol).

ATHENA study findings, and the conclusions presented by Roche, were that the cobas® HPV Test was effective "for use in women 25 years and older

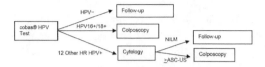

Figure 1a. Primary Screening algorithm (16/18 genotyping
with 12 other hr HPV positive to cytology)

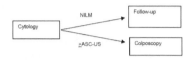

Figure 1b. Cytology algorithm (cytology alone)

as a first-line primary cervical cancer screening test to detect high risk HPV, including genotyping for 16 and 18," with potential for clinical practice to put the primary screening algorithm into the regime (FDA 2014).

Those opposed to primary screening asked the FDA to look critically at and to look beyond the data highlighted by considering what was left out of the study design in the first place. Roche had not included information on cellular pathology (only normal and ASC-US readings, not abnormal results), thereby—as opponents asserted—misconstruing their findings and subsequently misreporting the case to the FDA. When Roche went to the FDA for their original application in 2011, they specified that the "same sample vial as the Pap test" would be used as a "streamlined co-testing platform." In evaluating the cytology plus HPV detection co-testing platform, the FDA concluded in 2013 when reviewing the supplement for a new indication that this new platform "includes other diagnostic categories such as infectious organisms (candida sp., Trichomonas, Herpes viral changes, atypical repair, abnormal endometrial cells, etc.)," but would result in overlooking "non-HPV cancers of the cervix, such as choriocarcinoma, melanoma, metastatic carcinoma, and some adenocarcinomas from other primary sites, which the HPV test also cannot identify." It was in light of this information that a co-test was recommended. As Roche asked the FDA to approve the use of cobas as a primary screening tool, those in opposition asked: "How can loss of this information be justified when it can be acquired from the same sample at little added expense?" This would be an "unprecedent and significant shift," and one that would affect millions of women for the majority of their adult lives, they argued; therefore they "strongly urge[d]" the FDA to reject the application.

The groups' objections were detailed. Harms and adverse events could, and will, occur if more people, and younger people, are unnecessarily referred for invasive follow-up procedures (e.g., colposcopy and cervical biopsy). Young people especially could be over-treated. There is consensus that it is in young people "where it [HPV] is most likely to regress." No other governance body—not the CDC, the USPSTF, ACS, ACOG, or the American Association of Family Practitioners—had recommended HPV testing as a first-line primary screening tool in any patient population, citing professional and evidence-based reasons to maintain the co-test approach.[19] For these organizations, choosing a course of action that would increase both the chance of unnecessary health risks *and* costs raised questions about the very nature of the practice of medicine. What's at stake, some—like the National Women's Health Network—argued, is the "corporate pitch of innovation" over the jurisdiction of medical providers to decide on care. Even when a device is acknowledged as having "flawed" design, when professional organizations make their decisions they are considering potential gains—and in this case whether increased detection is worth the potential jeopardizing of patient compliance, increasing of patient harm, and devaluing of professional judgment. Opponents of HPV as a primary screening tool made appeals to health equity and justice: "Most cervical cancers occur in women who have never been screened, were not screened in the last five years, or did not have appropriate follow-up treatment." In other words, the problem here is one of health care access, not of a subpar tool of prevention in need of a replacement. "It is underserved populations who already suffer from disparities in cervical cancer survival" due to lack of access to screening who are most at risk of disease. This new indication "threatens to accomplish the very opposite of its intended purpose, which should be to reduce barriers to screening and to save lives" (National Women's Health Network 2015).

After only a few weeks of deliberation, the FDA panel largely disregarded these concerns, publicly announcing their decision to approve the tool's new indication as a primary screening tool on April 24, 2014.[20] With FDA approval, the cobas® HPV Test became the first and *only* test approved by the FDA to be used for primary screening. Yet despite statements affirming safety and effectiveness as reviewed by the FDA, even supporters hoped for better guidance over which tool was the "right" tool for prevention: in their decision, the advisory group recommended primary HPV screening as an "option," not a replacement for the standard US screening co-test approach. The co-test, then, was still in place, but it remained on shaky ground, and while a primary screening approach was possible, it was not yet the "right tool" for the job of cervical cancer prevention.

The committee refrained from offering a clear and powerful next step for cervical cancer prevention. Were they taken by the opposition's concerns? Had they succumbed to industry pressure (tacit or otherwise)? Or did they disagree in some way with the evidence? Perhaps it was the total system of contracts in place among diagnostic companies, laboratories, and health systems that worked to apply pressure against choosing one approach over another. It could also have been that the clinical option recommended was a nod from the committee that they agreed with health advocates that any clear decision for HPV screening alone would interfere with professional judgment. They also may have succumbed to professional pressure by pathologists and techno-cytologists, as well as gynecologists and other well-entrenched (and -reimbursed) providers who perform Pap tests as part of their laboratory and routine office work. Laboratory companies such as QIAGEN and Hologic, as well as office-based and lab-testing facilities that employed cytologists and received reimbursements, were sure to take a financial hit. The US context of insurance-based billing and the long-standing business model of cytology (despite being subject to low reimbursement when performed on its own) was a well-established profit base. The primary screening approach would ensure unfair advantage to Roche's cobas® HPV Test, given that other molecular HPV tests were not (yet) FDA approved for the "use" of primary prevention.

Diana Zuckerman, president of the Cancer Prevention and Treatment Fund, expressed disbelief not that the panel came to this decision but that they were "passing the buck to experts." In her statement she accused the FDA of "not taking responsibility" for their own influential decision to approve the test as a replacement first-line approach for the Pap test (for women over twenty-five). Andrew Pollack, a biotechnology journalist for the *New York Times*, published his take under the headline "Alternative to Pap Test Is Approved by F.D.A." (Pollack 2014), reporting that the test would not erode the Pap, which, according to him, would "not go away quickly, if at all." The reason, Pollack speculated, is that many doctors would not adopt the primary use until professional societies like the ACS recommended it in guidelines, decisions that would likely take several years.

Business interests aside, many asked what precisely the detection of HPV would indicate, even when oncoviral types are found. They wondered, as I did, how one would know if these HPV infections might regress or clear on their own. Roche had built into the clinical trial study a response to this question of indication and potential evidence for its benefit: the detection would indicate presence of the two high-risk (hr) HPV genotypes 16 and 18, with good specificity, and given the evidence that these hr types account for 70 percent of HPV-associated cancer cases, the potential benefit was clear. In other words, by using their oncotype specification tool, Roche had already built in the answer to their comparison: a benefit already existed to type HPV 16 and 18. The HPV test was shown to outperform Pap testing in specificity—a widely acknowledged limitation of the Pap. What Roche ensured in its design was not only to detect the presence of oncogenic types, but also to detect and predict the development of precancerous lesions. A negative result on the HPV test was found to be a better predictor than a negative Pap test in the measured outcome: that the cervix would remain free of precancerous or cancerous lesions for the next three years.

The switch to HPV tests as a screening approach would require professional and patient expectations to shift as well. Since 2001, when the leading professional guideline boards recommended that women, beginning at age twenty-one, undergo Pap test screening every three years, and that most women should not be screened annually, much of the public was already primed for changes to the timing and contours of cervical cancer screening. Many providers worked hard to find ways to be responsive to changing preventive guidelines that dropped the "annual exam" in favor of a new concept, the "well woman visit" or "wellness exam," with goals to bring new expectations to patient-publics. Patient advocate groups had raised concern, as they do now, that fewer preventive visits could negatively impact the health-seeking behaviors, medical care, and ultimately the health outcomes of patients. Others supported the change to reduce unnecessary harms (e.g., over-referral, unnecessary treatment, stress, discomfort, etc.) as well as over-medicalization of women's bodies.

In an unusual editorial, the New York Times covered the new medical guideline on May 14, 2014, asking its Sunday readers in a bold headline, "Are Pap Smears on the Way Out?" (2014). The question emphasized the editors' puzzlement, and in their commentary they reported that in announcing their approval of a "rival" to the Pap test in a "genetic test that looks for the viruses implicated in causing cervical cancer," the FDA had not indicated "which test is better." The committee chose instead to withhold judgment on what platform and specific tool was the right tool for the job of preventing cervical cancer in asymptomatic people. "The F.D.A.

made no comparative judgment," the editors wrote. "It simply said that a well-designed study by Roche provided reasonable assurance that the test was safe and effective when used as a primary screening tool" ("Are Pap Smears on the Way Out?" 2014).

As the FDA was approving the HPV test but leaving the choice of whether and exactly when to use it up to clinicians, a similar advisory committee in Australia was also saying that an HPV test would be more effective, save more lives, and be just as safe as a Pap test. In Germany, women's health advocates were fighting to ensure that HPV screening as a primary test would enter their guidelines (Lindén 2021). Was the decision to maintain a co-test uniquely American? After all, research indicates that HPV testing has some advantages over Pap tests: it was and still is a better predictor of whether a woman who tested negative would remain free of lesions for the next three years. The HPV test is also more objective than Pap tests, which rely on the judgment of health professionals viewing slides under a microscope.

In July 2020 the American Cancer Society endorsed primary HPV testing as a screening strategy.[21] This deviated somewhat from the USPSTF guidance in 2018 that included the option of HPV tests every five years for women over thirty (US Food & Drug Administration 2017). Yet what had unfolded was a complete "accommodation" to the HPV tests in cervical cancer prevention and a near supplanting of the Pap. Whether this was a better tool, and for whom, continues to be asked and considered in local contexts. Was it the case, as some argued, that women who were HPV negative would justifiably feel that they are safe from the disease, at least until their next screening? What about those who don't test negative, I wondered? Further, as the opposition letter made clear, many people will test HPV positive who may not have had an abnormal Pap. What impact will positive results have on them, on their clinical experience? Would less frequent testing leave some, especially those where HPV vaccines rates are low, in the gaps, perpetually concerned about their protection? Would less frequent primary tests lead the worried well into direct-to-consumer purchasing of HPV self-sampling tests (now available) to alleviate worry? Whether the changes were "optimizations," as was scientifically suggested, whether these were "better" tools, or whether they merely yielded small differences remained points of concern. "Pap smears aren't going away. . . . We still need the Pap smears to work up the women with the positive HPV tests, and we still need the Pap smears for primary screening of women who are too young for primary HPV screening," as a pathologist in San Francisco explained.

A Uniquely American Decision: HPV Primary Testing Deferred as Precision Approaches Escalate

When Roche expectedly, and in some ways finally, submitted materials to the FDA requesting a new use for the cobas® HPV Test as a primary preventive tool, they stated that a primary cervical cancer screening approach was already in use in a host of other countries, including Australia, Brazil, China, Indonesia, Japan, Mexico, Russia, Singapore, Taiwan, Venezuela, and some countries within the European Union (e.g., Denmark in 2015), including Serbia. It wasn't corporate greed or competition, but health advocates who pushed for primary tests in many other countries. As Lisa Lindén showed, women's health activists in the European Union demanded the HPV primary test be implemented as part of routine screening in national health programs. Activists called for guideline changes, and for them to happen fast. In the Swedish case, patient advocates brought evidence forward to support their position and demand health care policy change. Lindén described this as translating "credentialized knowledge" (from medical journals, for example) into evidential claims to advocate for the adoption of primary HPV tests as a screening tool (Lindén 2021).

In the US the evidential claims were underway, supported by FDA approved tools, clinical trial evidence, and professional organization committee consensus. Yet the US seemed to be different: not only with a slower paradigm change that included a seemingly long period of co-testing as the "best" approach, but also with a context in which women's health and patient groups more often advocated for co-testing as the best approach because it left in place the well-established Pap test tool. It is not the tool per se, they argued, but affordable access, participation, and quality of health care that matter most to reducing disease and mortality. The US approach to health care as a commodity and not a right is part of the failure in preventing cancer.

Michele Manos's prediction was playing out: the one thing HPV vaccination seemed to be doing was making "cervical cancer screening more efficient." In August 2018 the USPSTF released new prevention guidelines with a primary HPV testing approach. The guidelines included HPV primary testing every five years as a screening option for people aged thirty to sixty-five. In doing so, they capped a decade-long trajectory of destabilizing the Pap and endorsed a molecular approach to prevention. Many opposed the full-stop shift to primary HPV screening on grounds that the new use had not been adequately tested, would create confusion, and might lead to expensive, invasive, and potentially harmful follow-up procedures. Nonetheless, with the full weight of a cancer advocacy group, in July 2020 the American Cancer Society recommended primary HPV testing in those aged twenty-five to sixty-five. The new guidelines significantly expanded the age range, allowing a younger group to begin their screening lives and demonstrating that a major shift in cancer screening was underway. An option of co-testing every five years or cytology every three years remained in place, deemed "acceptable" only when availability is limited: eventually, the ACS asserted, co-test screening with Pap and HPV tests would be eliminated in favor of primary HPV testing.

The opposition to the political, commercial, and governmental support of HPV primary testing that had formed years earlier remained in place. There were assertions of imperfect science and evidence; concerns over more expensive testing; and arguments that fewer tests would lead to less, not better care for those already in most need of adequate and effective health care. In the US worries that screening "participation" was the real driver of cancer risk left many to wonder if people would seek care less often. "The Pap is not something that we should look at as replaceable," many asserted, fearing people would go to a medical provider less often (Hauck 2020). A less frequent HPV screen would result in less medical care, with those more likely to receive less care placed at greater risk. "This would be bad for health disparities; bad for women of color," said Gwinnett Ladson, an OB-GYN who spoke to the US newspaper the *Tennessean* in 2021, adding, "We know how to do better, and these tests are better together" (Ladson 2021).

The decision to allow primary screening may be less about patient-provider relations, though, than about laboratory-medical organization contracts and capacity. As the ACS stated in their guidelines, "Although the FDA approved the first test for primary HPV screening in 2014, as of 2017, only 40.6 percent of laboratories reported that they offered primary HPV screening, and, among those that did, primary HPV screening was a very small fraction of all HPV-associated testing" (Fontham et al. 2020, 16). Most clinicians have little if any control over laboratory contracts or the testing platforms used. My claim is supported by industry opposition from Hologic, who opposed primary HPV testing in 2020;[22] Hologic has an HPV test approved for co-testing, and none for primary testing. The standardization of primary HPV testing would likely drive them out of the market unless they seek additional regulatory approval for primary HPV testing. The ASCP (whose publication *ePolicy News* is sponsored by Hologic) has expressed commitment not to the Pap test per se, but to the use of co-testing as a combination that offers optimal screening especially for pre-cancer detection. ASCP positioned its interest in maintaining not only appropriate use, but also appropriate reimbursement, for co-testing.[23]

Through its work with the Cytopathology Education and Technology Consortium, the ASCP argued that the move to primary testing was not reflective of the capacity of the US health system (most US laboratories do not offer primary HPV screening on FDA-approved testing platforms), and on the evidence that a sizable portion of cervical cancer patients test negative for HPV and would not be flagged for further testing or treatment ("ASCP Articulates Serious Concerns with ACS Cervical Cancer Guidelines" 2020). For ASCP the now highly destabilized co-testing approach would remain in place.

A Precision Regime: Optimized Risk Stratification

Epidemiologists affirm that the large decline in this cancer is attributable to regular screening (National Institutes of Health 1996, "Cervical Cancer Statistics" 2021) regardless of the tool with which people are screened. Further, studies have shown a 1 percent decline in cervical cancer in the US, and a larger 4.6 percent decline among women aged twenty to twenty-four, over the decade since co-testing began (American Society of Clinical Oncology 2021). Such a seemingly small percentage has not slowed the "revolution" to optimize screening tools. It is not surprising, given the concurrent evidence, that in the US and around the world "Most cervical cancer cases occur among those who are not being screened for cervical cancer" at all, as the epidemiologist Rachel Winer told me. Winer echoed a common sentiment that health care disparities are driven by medical infrastructure, especially when infrastructure is unavailable or inadequate. The overwhelming cancer rates and deaths in low- and middle-income countries with such structures make this clear. In terms of screening in the US, there is a persistent gap in Pap testing that functions as a cause for the 20 percent of cervical cancers not reduced with this screening. Even if primary screening were the standardized approach, structural, socioeconomic, and other barriers to screening uptake would need to be overcome to get to zero. For Winer and others, education is needed for patients, "many of whom are unaware that HPV causes cervical cancer," and for "providers who are likely to fear litigation and thus more likely to use [the] HPV test as a co-test to help prevent missing people at risk." What is most important, as Winer explained, is to "engage more individuals in screening and increase HPV vaccine coverage."

In the US, screening "participation," and the health care gaps it reveals, are seen as the real driver of cervical cancer risk, rather than the inefficiency of any screening tools. The US CDC issued a press release in 2014 reporting that despite evidence that cervical cancer screening saves lives, about eight million women aged twenty-one to sixty-five had not been screened in the past five years, adding that more than half of the new cervical cancer cases in the US were diagnosed in those who have never or rarely been screened (Benard et al. 2014). Regional differences told the full story of the disparities that underlie the differences in screening participation: the US South had the highest rate of cervical cancers (8.5 per 100,000), the highest death rate from them (2.7 per 100,000), and the largest percentage of women who had not been screened in the past five years (12.3 percent)—numbers likely attributable to racial inequities, the US fee-for-service health care system, and other social forces.

Addressing the pervasive gaps is presumptively built in to what is emerging as a new precision approach of public health vaccine guidelines plus screening tools punctuated by speed and molecular stratifications. Others seek to (also) address the social determinants or root causes of health disparities, like poverty and discrimination, that coexist with and shape medical care and its access. Among the leading cancer prevention advocates, many call for not only HPV tests in cervical cancer, but also the development of screening approaches for the "other" HPV-associated cancers (American Society of Clinical Oncology 2021). For the marginalized in the US, the situation is not much different from that in the most poorly resourced countries around the world. Evidence-based research on which tool is right, or "right enough," cannot address these determinants.

This chapter has shown that the problems facing full-stop acceptance of HPV screening were problems of knowledge and data (e.g., do we have enough data on HPV regression/clearance or know the best intervals of screening regimes?); of professional jurisdiction (e.g., what about the workforce of pathologists and cytologists?); and of infrastructure (e.g., the number of laboratories and their technical capacity). Harder to hear were the voices of those scientists, clinical experts, and advocates who regarded the scientific norms, actors, and organizations as part of an enterprise exerting pressure and influence to ask the wrong questions, to tinker in the wrong places. For Rina Nissum, a women's health activist and gynecologist in Switzerland, "The best thing to do for health is to improve general social conditions. There is no shortcut." Nissum repeated this as we sat in a café in Geneva. Human rights, degrees of social equity, and social conditions are where questions, research, and funding should be focused. It is through expansions in rights that we might understand scientifically *why* certain viral strains have sustaining tendencies and how to interrupt this persistence and ensure viral shed or regression, Nissum explained. "This is research worth funding . . . and I suspect the answer will be found in general social conditions; for women, for rights and equity, and around housing and food and living conditions." What we need is "to encourage strong immunity." Nissum's interview emphasized her opinion that "if people are malnourished," if the "social conditions are poor," the vaccine won't work either, "the vaccine will be a disaster . . . it will only work in otherwise healthy environments, with food, housing, water controls, human rights." So, while screening can and might fill the gaps, this, she and others argued, should come after every effort has been made for equity in social opportunity as well as in health and health care provision and infrastructure.

Nissum's weak support for vaccination did not reflect an anti-science or anti-vaccination position, but rather an appeal to shift prevention "upstream" from technological to social solutions. In this view she differed from most of the scientists and clinicians I was interviewing, yet her argument resonated with my perspective as a sociologist of science and medicine. And, importantly, it resonated with M. Michele Manos, who told me during our interview back in 2012 that she had started her work in HPV because of the global burden of cervical cancer. "To be frank," she said, "I think we would get farther by assuring the rights of women and girls." "Health is politics by another name," as Alondra Nelson, a sociologist at Princeton University and the US Deputy Director for Science and Society, said so well (Nelson 2011). Ensuring that women have bodily autonomy and positions from which they can shape the policies and practices of their lives would be extremely useful in ensuring opportunities for a good life, however measured. Science and biomedicine require critical attention to who is establishing the truth of what is needed, who is part of imagining the future. These voices are seeking to hold science and society accountable to ensure a future that asks not only how to develop newer and more technically advanced biomedical products, but in whose interests and with what implications those products are developed.

An imaginary of precision cancer prevention is underway with fantasies of targeting screening and cancer eradication. Technologically, the imaginary prescribes vaccination plus routine screening at set intervals with follow-up as needed, plus other risk measures that make up complex risk score algorithms. While precision public health seeks to capture geo-markers of ZIP codes and population areas, precision medicine is working to capture biomarkers and risk scores. The public health "we" will take place side by side with a precision clinical approach to the "me." A cervical cancer risk-based management guideline was released in 2019 by ASCCP. The guidelines include a cancer management tool, an app that can be downloaded to a handheld device, that directs health care providers on how best to evaluate risk using vaccination status along with HPV and Pap test results and one's screening history (Schiffman et al. 2017). The app is used in office decision-making as these are considered along with variables such as "age, hormonal contraception use, history of sexually transmitted infection, parity, cigarette smoking, obesity, and sexual behaviors including age of first intercourse and multiple partners" (Perkins et al. 2020, 125–26).

To provide more nuanced information about an individual's cervical cancer risk, the ability to stratify and assess risk and management depend on the amount of information available from collective data on screening programs and patient records (Baltzer et al. 2017). A toggling back and forth from individuals to populations is needed for us to understand risk and its clinical management.[24] With HPV vaccination increasing, it is believed that prevalence of pre-cancer, as well as cytology and pooled HPV tests, will perform less effectively (e.g., will be less predictive of cervical pre-cancer) in vaccinated populations than in unvaccinated populations. The aggregated data, therefore, are likely to become even more critical, as Mark Schiffman states, "to push simultaneously toward greater precision and simplicity, supported by a computer-based decision tool" (Schiffman et al. 2017, 87).

The ASCCP guidelines—and the corresponding cancer management tool—are used to identify those most at risk of cervical cancer and to optimize population-level impact (Baltzer et al. 2017). They are intended to help navigate clinical decision making for patients with abnormal cervical screening results based on the Clinical Action Thresholds (risk categories corresponding to various clinical actions) determined by ASCCP. An algorithm is used to assign each patient a risk score, which is then mapped onto thresholds for clinical action to determine appropriate follow-up for the patient. Assignment to a risk group is, therefore, based on risk score rather than on specific risk factors, behaviors, or identities.

Alongside the acknowledged understanding that cancer risk lies in the social-structural topography, at least in the US it is precision innovations that are deemed to be the best drivers to move cervical cancer from its onetime status as a leading cause of cancer death to designation as a "rare cancer," with hopes of getting to zero altogether. What drives the epidemiological decline will continue to be negotiated along with the production of risk—the risk of *cervical cancer risk*, and how best to decrease its effects. While a precision stratification approach to cancer prevention renders sex and sexuality largely invisible as the complexity of cervical cancer risk intensifies, the crucial questions will be which vaccine (e.g., 4-valent, 9-valent) did the person/population group receive? How many doses were given? At what age? Will screening recommendations vary by HPV vaccination status? Can predictive models account for whether people or their partners have been vaccinated, and when? How might this impact the age at which cervical cancer screening should begin, at what interval, and when it should cease? Governance of these social categories is in development: ACS included a category for "HPV vaccinated," predicting that vaccination status will eventually be integrated into screening guidelines (Fontham et al. 2020, 17), while ASCCP opted to wait to do so (Perkins et al. 2020, 125–26).

A new prevention regime with molecular tests and stratified risk prediction models is almost complete, with inclusion of HPV vaccine status as a category of molecular risk and protection. Type-specific genotype persistence is now dominating understandings of cervical cancer risk, which is said to be much greater than the risk associated with "new" genotype infection of any "high-risk" (hr) type. The scientific claim is that it is not merely knowing *whether* someone has an hr HPV infection, but rather what *type* of HPV infection, and whether this has persisted and for how long, that is now emerging as a dominant precision approach, and one poised to supplant the now standard practice of immediate colposcopy for hr HPV 16 and 18 (Mello and Sundstrom 2021).[25] Clinical practice is moving in the direction of this risk-based assessment model.

For a public health approach, HPV researchers are hoping to reach zero through what they refer to as "faster" and "even faster" approaches to eliminating cervical cancers: one consists of offering screening and vaccination concurrently to "maximize" impact (Bosch et al. 2016; Dillner, Elfström, and Baussano 2021). If screening confers a negative HPV result, with vaccination people will need less frequent screening visits, and intervention can thus be made in the "participation" gaps. "Even faster" modifies this with population data on HPV reproductivity rates, the reproductive number (or R01) used to assess when and if herd immunity is realized, and importantly, with the end goal of diminishing the HPV reproductive rate to zero and thereby conferring herd immunity. Here, this measure can inform screening campaigns rather than the more distal effort to ensure infrastructure. Determining "optimal" age for screening and vaccination, and especially contribution to the reproductivity rate of HPV, is information that might get us to zero.

In all, the tension among "we" and "me" is converging with population vaccination strategies and the automation and algorithmic processing of precision prediction, with applications for easy use. These technocentric tools may also reducing workload, variability, and bias, introducing a cost-effective way of reading results (Menezes et al. 2019) and the capacity to process and determine outputs with speed. The goals of "optimization" and "precision," while not homogeneous across geographic contexts, emphasize technical problems and solutions for greater objectivity in decision making. Other problems—of infrastructure, equity, and justice, for example—are absent from these automated algorithms but no less present in the processes and outcomes in cervical cancer research, care, and prevention. It may be those who are most likely to seek cervical cancer screening who are also most likely to have received the HPV vaccine (Silver and Kobrin 2020). Those most likely to develop cervical cancer, given how they map to lack of opportunities and resources for health more generally (rights, education, jobs, etc.), may remain in the gaps. This is true of subgroups in high-resource countries like the US as well as in low- and middle-resource locales.

The narrative and dreams of precision cancer prevention—increased surveillance and data gathering, customized biomedical interventions, and targeted risk-reduction strategies—are almost fully put in place. Whether these exacerbate the very inequalities they seek to address—by reducing pressure to build infrastructure, for example, thus further stigmatizing already marginalized individuals and populations without changing their social and economic circumstances; or by shifting funding and attention away from strategies for addressing health disparities that are not framed explicitly in the terms of biomedicine or bioinformatics—has yet to be known (Kenney and Mamo 2020). Simple and low-cost tools should not always be driven out by more complex and higher-cost ones. While such an approach is good for biotech and pharma, as Sawaya pondered with a shrug, "So, you're then kind of left with, 'Oh, wow; we just now paid four times more for a Pap smear [given the co-test standard]." He asked rhetorically, "What is the benefit to the population or society—or to women? I mean, that's a reasonable question to ask." I agree—the US approach to health care as a commodity and not a right is part of the reason the gaps and disparities in preventing cancer persist.

CHAPTER NINE

Commodities of Sexual Health Care

When I went to San Francisco's Kaiser Permanente with a colleague to interview Eric Suba, a senior pathologist, I hoped to take stock of the global shape of cervical cancer screening. We phoned Suba from outside the main entrance of a non-clinical building after working hours; Suba immediately came to the front door to guide us through what felt like the bowels of a medical building to a rear suite of lab spaces and then into a small office, where he sat at a large desk, motioning us to sit in two chairs across from him, and almost immediately began speaking about the role of pathology in cancer prevention.

Suba told us about the ways public health began to frame the problem of cervical cancer as one of technological innovation rather than what he regards as the core issue: saving as many lives as quickly as possible. He told a story of change that began in the late 1980s, when it became clear that the Pap test had not eradicated cervical cancer in the United States. He affirmed the sociotechnical politics around the prevention approaches that are described in this book. Pathology laboratory failures in Pap test analysis (around sensitivity and specificity) led to an explosion of academic and commercial interest in finding alternatives to the Pap test. He added that, with a baby boom ending in low- and middle-income countries (LMIC) in the 1990s, overall disease burden shifted from diseases of childhood toward cancer and other diseases of adulthood. "These converged to create an environment in which the research community and the biotechnology industry sought to retire the Pap test just as low- and middle-income countries were beginning to realize how much they needed cervical screening," he told me in our interview. He added that "the primary challenge of global health is one of distribution" and "in most cases, basic tools suffice; technological innovation is not necessary." Innovation, he argued, should have no role as an ethical driver of medicine and public health. Instead he asserted "The Golden Rule"—a phrase he would repeat often during the two-hour interview and then again in a follow-up interview a few months later. The rule, as he passionately described it, was simple: the public health version of the medical doctor's Hippocratic Oath to "do no harm." For Suba, it was "to save as many lives as quickly as possible." The question Suba's Golden Rule pushed him to ask himself, and which he posed to us during the interview, is whether the world's leading scientists and researchers in cancer prevention, and groups like the Gates Foundation that support them, are driven by a similar ethical edict, or perhaps by one more aligned with capital than with equity.

Suba's quick and loquacious start indicated that he was eager to share his perspective. He spoke passionately about his experience, and frustration, as he pushed back against the cervical cancer establishment and what he regarded as unethical research conduct in a clinical trial on screening tools in India. That trial was financed and supported by the National Cancer Institute of the US National Institutes of Health. Although we arrived at the interview prepared to deepen our understanding of how changing tools in cervical cancer detection and screening affected clinical care, instead we were introduced to a clinical trial study said to be guided by claims of equity and justice for the Indian women enrolled as participants, but opposed by Suba when he came to see the study's design as guided by a racist and incorrect assumption: the "zombie argument" that Pap screening is not feasible in LMICs.

In 2005, researchers at the International Agency for Research on Cancer of the World Health Organization emphasized that "Our results clearly show that good-quality Pap screening can be implemented even in a rural setting of a developing country with reasonable investment, while HPV screening does not give any better detection of high-risk cervical lesions, despite the higher investments" (Sankaranarayanan et al. 2005). Yet the study aimed to validate what was known to be a less accurate screening tool, enrolling poor women as the human subjects of research. The trial, initiated in 1997 and conducted in Mumbai, reportedly had the goal of investigating whether visual inspection with acetic acid (VIA), a screening tool first introduced to clinical practice during the 1930s, could reduce incidence and mortality of invasive cervical cancers in a place without a cervical cancer screening program (that is, without Pap). However, documents obtained through the US Freedom of Information Act established that the Mumbai trial actually investigated the effectiveness of unaided visual inspection (UVI), a cervical cancer screening test that cannot detect precancerous cervical lesions and had been scientifically discredited before the Mumbai trial began (Suba, Ortega, and Mutch 2018). As Suba spoke, his emotion and frustration were palpable. The trial violated the golden rule, and therefore should not have been funded nor conducted; instead, based on the evidence of cervical cancer declines with Pap testing, what was most needed was funding for a Pap screening program. The problem with the study design and implementation was, as Suba and colleagues pointed out in 2022 in the *New England Journal of Medicine*, that the trial delayed Pap screening throughout India for more than fifteen years, and therefore contributed to the preventable cervical cancer deaths of at least 500,000 Indian women (Suba, Ortega, and Mutch 2022).

This almost sixteen-year study was designed to compare the effectiveness of a discredited cervical screening test to the effectiveness of no screening at all, leaving the exposure and control groups of women unprotected from cervical cancer risk, disease, and ultimately death. This design was ethically problematic, and an injustice to Indian women. Millions were spent to look for an even cheaper alternative to an already cheap tool, the Pap test, when what was needed was funding for adequate screening programs to reduce cancers and deaths—and to follow Suba's Golden Rule.

Suba anticipated my focus on how HPV testing might supplant the long-used Pap test, and the implications of that change for pathologists like himself. Yet he steered the conversation to what and who is rendered less visible in the shifts underway as the inadequacies of Pap tests are displaced with a new cancer prevention paradigm. The ethics of the drivers of change, for Suba, were no longer things to be concealed, given the ways they legitimize research findings and randomized clinical trial designs that lead to some tools becoming the presumed best tools for the job of cervical cancer prevention. He asserted that large investments made by NIH and other funders to answer technical questions on the minds and in the labs of well-funded scientists were not designed to address systemic social and structural determinants of health and illness. His view is that cervical cancer rates and deaths are shaped by discrimination and gender inequality, and in this case, the assumption that an adequate screening program would not be feasible for poor women in India. People are dying more from discrimination and neglect than from lack of technical specificity and sensitivity in prevention tools. The Golden Rule, he explained, is a lens through which to direct and invest in reversing the root (e.g., social) causes of disease.

In 2017 Suba and his colleagues, Robert Ortega and David Mutch, published their opposition to the trial. Based on documents collected using the US Freedom of Information Act, they showed that "the US National Cancer Institute leaders avoided accountability by making false and misleading statements to Congressional oversight staff" (Suba, Ortega, and Mutch 2017). The article was published in *BMJ Global Health*, which had planned a press release to publicize the findings, but *BMJ* canceled that release and retracted the article because their attorneys feared a potential defamation litigation in plaintiff-friendly British courts (McCook 2017). *BMJ* editors had no concerns about the scholarship of the retracted article, an updated version of which was published in 2018 by the National Center for Bioethics in Research and Health Care at Tuskegee University (Suba, Ortega, and Mutch 2018). Prior to these events, a piece was published in the *Indian Journal of Medical Ethics* that garnered responses from two of the leading researchers in India and the US (Suba 2014) refuting Suba's claims on the grounds that his assertions about the trial design and its effects on its human subjects were misleading and potentially biased (Sankaranarayanan et al. 2016).

Suba's interview confirmed for me that technical questions concerning sensitivity and specificity and which screening tools were best can also be the wrong questions to ask. Saving as many lives as quickly as possible with already proven tools is the reason for his emphasis on a need to provide care to those who don't have (enough of) it. The research questions and methodological approach of many randomized controlled trials (RCTs)—the gold standard of evidence-based medicine and clinical trial research, and the type of study that receives millions of dollars in funding from places like the US National Cancer Institute—are increasingly driven by technical questions found in precision medicine. This is an example of the "me" medicine approach superseding the goal of helping as many of the "we" as quickly as possible.

Like me, Suba was concerned with the consequences science and medicine, and the disease narratives of risk and harm they construct, hold for whose bodies and lives are protected over others. He rendered visible the ghostly matters of women who have died or are currently at risk in India, and by extension in all settings and regions (including some in the US) where adequate care is neither available nor equitable. When I assert sociologically that there are stakes involved as HPV genomic sequencing "innovates" vaccination and HPV testing tools, I am asking whose bodies and lives would be most protected and whose would be rendered less protected and seen as less in need of protection. The answers are driven by the particularities: the multiple tendencies and topographies of the biomedicalization and "economization of life" (Murphy 2012 and 2017) and the ways settings/places are socialized for precarity and/or abundance (Benton 2015). While sex had for almost a century been suspected as a causal factor in cervical cancers, poverty and place are significant co-drivers of whose bodies would become the objects of research for a mass-surveillance tool and/or the subjects of "consumer choice" to ensure health.

When disease-awareness advertisements for everything from Viagra for erectile dysfunction to cholesterol-lowering drugs for the prevention of heart disease began to saturate US media in the late 1990s, publics and the markets they made up were already primed to consider their presumptive "choice" to protect their health. Yet many were also primed to be skeptical of the scientific advances claiming to "guard" women's bodies against deadly disease, especially in the domain of gynecology and "women's health" where ghostly matters linger. Health and critical activists and scholars have extensively documented the long and varied forms of exploitation and use of women's bodies, and especially the bodies of Black women and other people of color, to preserve the social order—including the social control of reproductive and sexual matters. Many of the diagnostic categories and assumptions used throughout the twentieth century, some of which remain in place today, about women, race, and sexuality are residuals at best and continued ideologies at worst, formed in the logics of racial, gender, and sexual difference.[1] Critical race scholars are more recently asking "us" to consider "what lies in the wake" and in the afterlives of slavery and other racial injustice (Sharpe 2016).[2] What are the effects, from diagnoses to death from cancer, if we also consider biomedicine's infrastructural failures and the political economies of public health that render prevention of infectious disease more visible than the need for preventing chronic disease in some settings or among certain populations and not in others (Banerjee 2020, Livingston 2012)? What are the omissions that linger after humanity is refused or when settings are socialized for scarcity and without financing, treatment, and prevention? What community-based and other forms of collective organizing formed in response to and as a result of systemic exclusion and harms?

My intention in focusing on the ghostly haunting of HPV-cancer connections is to confront and engage these from a different and discomforting vantage point, to see how they might be what Donna Haraway referred to as "the blood that shaped the eyes from which she sees" (Haraway 1991). Studying the scientists and scientific claims around cancers has, in many ways, obscured researchers' view of the lives and actual cancers they study. In her book, *Improvising Medicine: An African Oncology Ward in an Emerging Cancer Epidemic*, Julie Livingston documents the birth of an oncology ward from 2001–2009, as a cancer epidemic rapidly emerged—or, more precisely, was made visible, as the global south experienced a surge in cancers. The sociality of cancer care is made visible on the ward and in the bodies of mostly women with later-stage cancers. Livingston's ethnography carefully details what it looks and feels like for those with oncology, as well as for those without it. Biomedicine is shown to be at once necessary and vital—a means to exacerbate inequities in an already unjust world. For Livingston, the cancer ward in Gaborone, Botswana was also a metaphor for the ways bureaucracy, vulnerability, power, biomedical science, mortality, and hope intertwine and shape early twenty-first-century experience in southern Africa (Livingston 2012, 8). Bringing oncology to health care reflects the widely accepted "epidemiological transition," first proposed in 1971, which holds that as a society "modernizes," making gains in various economic and social indicators, the "distribution" of disease and death will shift from epidemics of infectious disease toward problems of chronic, degenerative conditions. Cancers represent diseases of chronicity; their visibility, however, is far more complicated than the anticipated epidemiologic transition. As Livingston argues, the separation of diseases into the distinct stages and types that the "epidemiological progress narrative" depended on—infectious disease vs. chronic disease, STI vs. cancer, "diseases of poverty" vs. "diseases of affluence"—was fuzzy rather than neat, and precarious rather than inevitable.

In Botswana public health efforts had long focused on "pre-transition" issues like infectious disease, malnutrition, and childbirth, even as a cancer epidemic was silently taking hold. Livingston shows that the cancers on the oncology ward were facilitated by and synergistic with endemic infectious diseases, most especially HIV/AIDS (and, curiously, its treatment), that rendered bodies susceptible to cancers, a fact that also escaped notice because of the "conceptual impossibility" of cancer in Africa. In Livingston's analysis, when cervical cancer is rewritten as an STD, this fits the epidemiological narrative of African public health as an infectious disease. This, therefore, allows for HPV technologies to fit seamlessly into the infectious disease logics embedded in the public-private partnerships that were restructuring global public health at the time of Livingston's research.

While it is valuable that Merck, in partnership with public health entities including NGOs, has donated mass quantities of Gardasil vaccines, their efforts have not only *not* produced vaccine equity; more importantly, their actions—as well as those of powerful actors like WHO and the GAVI alliance, among others—have reduced the complex pathology of cancer to a vaccine-preventable STD. Doing so may be necessary to maintain the attention and funding in a way that fits within the logic of many public health systems, such as Botswana, where an infectious disease rather than a chronic disease model dominates conceptualization and practice. There are also risks associated with this rewriting of cancer as infectious disease. Preventive vaccines, as she argues, obscure the complexity, synergistic realities, and sociality of cancer as a disease. Cancer rates are as much about the lack of comprehensive health services as they are about the sexual networks that the STD logic and HIV co-infection imply. The STD model, then, allows for and is productive of a "pharmaceuticalized" (as well as behavioral) approach instead of a more broadly conceptualized form of care (Livingston 2012, 46). Many carcinogenic invisibilities follow—of toxic waste and tobacco industry markets, among others—that many anthropologists and public health activists argue reflect the environmental and economic disorders rooted in material practices, practices that vary among nations arrayed along a continuum from resource rich to resource poor (Burke and Mathews 2017). Approaching cancer as an STI obscures the lack of knowledge and commitment to understanding other linkages, such as chemical exposure and cancer causation (Jain 2013).

The expensive and inaccessible "pharmaceutical" technologies and drugs are needed for equity; they also must not be allowed to render invisible the complex and multifaceted drivers of (global) cancer burdens and disparities (Burke and Mathews 2017, Farmer et al. 2010). Attention must be paid not only to vaccine and screening approaches, but more broadly to strengthening existing health systems, particularly primary health care, as well as to community-based knowledge and research. Further upstream are the social conditions shaped by historical structures of power such as poverty and its connection to economic opportunities that shape exposures to toxins, stress, and harm, as well as to resources to protect and provide care.

I conclude *Sexualizing Cancer* by joining others in conversation about what lies "in the wake" of scientific "fact-making" and uneven biomedicalization, and specifically about the ways we protect and guard some bodies and lives over others. It has been my hope to also illuminate the resistance and reconfiguration of binary models of risk and inclusion, as many seek inclusion and create counternarratives and pressures to ensure health and equity. This fact-making is performed in the context of increased attention to the precision approaches of "me" biomedicine with an accompanying investment in not only surveillance biomedicine, but self-surveillance practices more generally designed by entertainment, health, and social companies to produce ever more ways to enhance the health of the already well.

The mid-twentieth-century introduction of a Pap test to continuously monitor cellular changes and a new type of technical entity—the "precancerous" cell—that once dominated "women's health" has shifted for many into a responsibility to monitor risk of a cancer precursor, an oncoviral type that might persist and go unnoticed. The Pap test would continue to shape others' preventive possibilities, having at first merged two of medicine's preventive subjects—the figure of women *not-yet-ill* (and in need of protection) and the figure of *at-risk* women (in need of treatment of early-stage disease). With the additional information provided by the HPV test, these two figures of risk diverge again in how they are made into the objects of preventive care. A "me" medicine of precision clinical care has transformed cellular abnormality into a molecular presence, a specter of risk from an oncovirus in need of monitoring for persistence. Gendered bodies and gendered health care practices, subjects, and disciplines deemed responsible, and in need of being made more responsible, continue. Cervical cancer screening practices, and all screening practices, are part of surveillance medicine's expectation that we all should "participate" in and for our own health.

At the same time, this shift integrates the "we" approach to mass surveillance and disease prevention and the "me" approach to clinical medicine. The pharmaceutical and biotech industries play an outsized role as a source of information, disease prevention, and promotion of health care activities (Wailoo et al. 2010; Williams, Martin, and Gabe 2011). In the US, cancer disparities litter the wake of massive biotechnology investments in precision biomedicine and the newly configured hope for a precision version of public health.

Cancer disparities follow racial and socioeconomic lines—affecting screening, incidence, and death rates. People living in rural, mostly poor counties have higher cancer incidence rates, and Hispanic and non-Hispanic Black women bear a disproportionate share of the burden of incidence of disease and rates of mortality. It is pervasive economic disempowerment and inequity that reproduces the social effect: Black people, especially women, are sicker and die quicker. These "facts cannot save" us, as Ruha Benjamin (2016, 3) has argued about the ways we continue to measure racial disparities. The inequities that continue along the intersectional dimensions of race and racism, place, and economics are forged over topographies (Murphy 2012). They map onto national as well as global patterns of wealth, power, and inequality (Busfield 2006). The formula is well known; as risk markets are produced and treated, it is first and most often those regions and groups with the greatest consumer demand (and ability to pay) that will reap benefits in terms of the alleviation of suffering. While these efforts may alleviate suffering and promote expanded notions of a right to access health via biomedicine, they may also occlude attention to a broader right to health that would be secured through improved health care infrastructures and improved living conditions.

In 2021, when the WHO livestreamed its global strategy to eliminate cervical cancer by 2030,[3] they chose to simultaneously honor Henrietta Lacks and the family-led foundation[4] set up in her name. The story of Henrietta Lacks, and the history and origin of the HeLa cell line, are at this point well known. Lacks died of cervical cancer in October 1951 in Baltimore, Maryland. Her story, her cells, and the work of her family to ensure that her name and the cancer that took her life are addressed equitably continues. The HeLa cell line was used in the research that led to discovery of HPV's role in the development of cancer, and thus Henrietta Lacks and the HeLa cell line are ghostly matters in the story of the transformation in cancer prevention. Lacks's body and cells from the cervical cancer tumor that ultimately took her life are now known to have been linked to the presence of HPV 18, an oncoviral type with a high rate of infectivity. The story of the HeLa cell line—a name taken from the first two letters of Henrietta Lacks's first and last names—was in part the focus of Hannah Landecker's (2007) book, *Culturing Life: How Cells Became Technologies*, which maps a genealogy of the technical processes of culturing cells as central to the development of immunology, virology, and ultimately the infrastructures in place today around cell biology.[5]

The understanding that HPV is common in sexually active people is now also medically unremarkable, well documented and understood. The suspicion of a linkage between sex and disease, however, including the possibility that cervical cancer was linked to sexual activity, shaped the various ways this disease was understood and addressed over time. These and the ways people were treated and cared for linger today. Henrietta Lacks's tumor cells were extracted as researchers were searching for the cause of cervical cancer. The field of tumor virology was entering heady days, with a viral-cancer program soon to be established at the US National Cancer Institute in 1958. It is worth noting that Lacks had been a patient at the Johns Hopkins Hospital in Baltimore. She was admitted to "Department L," a hospital area named for "lues venerea"—an abbreviation likely chosen because it would be legible to "experts" but not to publics. It is surmised that this ward was the syphilis clinic, and that shortening its name might prevent patients embarrassment and social stigma (Reverby 2009, 136; Jones 1993, 16–29).[6] While Rebecca Skloot's book *The Immortal Life of Henrietta Lacks* makes only a brief mention of Lacks's diagnosis with syphilis, it is in a book review of Skloot's book where the historian Susan M. Reverby writes: "The fact that Lacks also had syphilis . . . provides insight into broader health policy issues" (Reverby 2010, 739). For me, that fact also reveals a ghostly haunting of the ways sex and STDs were stigmatized in ways that follow established lines of power. Stigma reveals already present inequities and their effects, which in this case included how cancers and STDs varied across the color line. Skloot had written that Lacks was not treated for her syphilis but gave scant attention to why, mentioning only that she may have opted out of treatment—it may have been her choice. Cancer had yet to cross the color line—a line of segregation with Blacks assigned to the world of STDs and whites to cancer, demonstrating the ways racism and sexism intersected with science, medicine, and patient expectations (Wailoo 2011). When Reverby reviewed Skloot's book, she asked: Why, in the mid-twentieth century in the United States, wasn't Lacks treated for syphilis; and what were the effects, if any, on her and her children's health of the progression of this STD?[7] For me, it is the ways gendered expectations and racist stereotypes converge around sex and hold consequences for care that makes this aspect of Henrietta's cancer and her care important as a ghostly matter. As I listened to the WHO convening and thought of Ilana Löwy's worry about stigmatized cancer, I hoped that in showing how these often interconnect and linger in disease and prevention, I might contribute to a wider refusal to allow sex to be managed and tamed.

Almost fifteen years prior to the ceremony honoring Lacks's contribution, HPV vaccination was introduced amid great hopes of establishing cervical cancer as a preventable disease, even as cervical cancer's incidence was highly uneven. The Lacks Foundation and the community efforts of this organization and the family that directs its efforts are part of community response to educate and agitate for social justice. Cervical cancers are now approximately the thirteenth-ranked cause of death in high-resource countries like the US. In low-resource countries, cervical cancer continues as a top cause. Solidarities formed in struggles for economic, racial, and sexual empowerment emerge through the hauntings of past systemic exclusions.

The American Cancer Society reported significant reduction in cervical cancers in the US (65 percent) among young women ages 20–24 from 2012 to 2019. These young women are the first generation to have received the HPV vaccine as young people. I too expect and hope that reductions in cervical cancers will continue as people age, and that there will be new reductions in other HPV-associated cancers. It is also my hope that vaccination strategies for this and other STIs will demystify the particular ways gender, sex, and sexualities affect how microbes pass from body to body. Further, I hope to render visible how HPV exposure and its effects follow lines of social and structural inequity. These can be geographic, such as US state policies that rejected Medicaid expansion; or they can be raced, gendered, and sexualized. As the molecular knowledge of HPVs produced a vaccine (almost twenty years later), other technologies began to "innovate." I hope to reveal the social nature of these innovations, and to examine whether and how they shape health and disease. Access to a direct-to-consumer product is needed in contexts of denied care, as conservative efforts to limit reproductive, sexual health, and gender-affirming care escalate, for example. Yet this approach to medicine and health is likely to follow similar patterns concerning who is protected and who remains outside of "good care."

Fifteen years in, HPV vaccines in the US and elsewhere have not been fully implemented in places where poverty is prevalent and health care and other infrastructures are fragmented or absent. The WHO was calling for a cancer prevention strategy: for 90 percent of girls to be vaccinated with HPV vaccines by 2030, as one of three preventive tools (also including 70 percent screening with Pap or HPV tests, and 90 percent treatment of people with pre-cancers or cancers). The WHO strategy was to put HPV vaccines where they were needed most, and to join these with other tools for prevention, detection, and early treatment. Merck was already reporting Gardasil sales of US$1.2 billion in 2021—a surge that the company claimed was also responsible for an overall increase in previously slumping vaccine sales globally during the early years of COVID-19, yet was also far short of the multiple billions in revenue they expect from this vaccine.

The WHO meeting called for increased attention, funding, and health care resources for cancer prevention and care, yet by honoring Henrietta Lacks it also called for social justice to address the ways poverty and precarity continue to shape people's lives in places where cervical cancer burdens are highest and access to the vaccines is lowest. When Groesbeck Parham, a professor and clinical researcher at the University of North Carolina-Chapel Hill spoke, he showed without pause and with great clarity the synergistic ways in which social injustice continues in the science and practice of cancer prevention and in the organization of society more generally. The injustices Parham called out were not around sex and stigma, but rather around structural inequities of poverty and the profits of pharmaceutical companies and the high-resourced countries from which they operate.

Parham shared his own professional trajectory, recounting his memory of opening a copy of *Ebony* magazine in 1976 to a story titled "Miracle of HeLa" that profiled "an obscure Black woman, who [had] ironically become a pivotal figure in the fight against cancer."[8] Parham went on to develop one of the largest cervical cancer screening programs in the world in Lusaka, Zambia, where he is now based. To successfully fight cervical cancer, he said, a five-tool "arsenal" is needed: the HPV vaccine; screening tests for curable pre-cancer; early surgical intervention for early-stage cancer; chemotherapy and radiation for late-stage cancer; and an infrastructure of pathology labs.

Yet, as he explained, when one looks at a map of the world, the places with the most meager arsenals are also the places with the most misery, pain, and death from cancer. He named some of the places where tools, technologies, and human resources to prevent and treat cervical cancers are least available: sub-Saharan Africa, India, Brazil. This is "racial injustice," "human injustice," and "an international tragedy," he exclaimed.[9] (It is also the "tropical scourge" in Brazil referred to in Löwy 2011.) Parham then invoked Henrietta Lacks's spirit to call for justice. "She would be asking us, 'Why does this situation exist in the first place? Why does it continue?'" He challenged organizational and scientific actors: "When will pharma make the vaccines against HPV available at an affordable price? When will we produce more doctors and nurses to screen and treat women with affordable tests they need?"

Parham brought these ghostly matters (Gordon 2008) forward, asking us to see the people rendered invisible by contemporary structural inequalities who are at risk of or dying from cervical cancer. He wanted to understand where the world stood on science justice, and the ethical aspects of technology design, use, and accessibility—specifically, where they stood on reaching toward health equity. He asked rhetorically, "When will corporations lower prices of treatments and technologies needed in low-resourced settings, and when will tech from high-income countries be transferred to low-income countries so 'we' can develop schools and institutes of science and develop the intelligence of kids to be the workforce needed?" Parham noted that without the political, social, and corporate will among high-income countries to deploy existing solutions, we could only "admit that we are no better than a photographer looking through a camera lens at a vulture as it devours a child weakened in an open field."

The metaphor of a child being devoured conjures the ghostly matters of this cancer and its prevention, and of the racial and social disparities in health and medicine produced through systemic injustices. It includes a haunting figure—echoing too closely Parham's "child weakened in an open field"—in the ways processes of gendered sexualization and racism persist in health and medicine, especially as these are part of the infrastructural "natureculture" (Haraway 1991) of biomedicine, and specifically of cancer prevention and care.

Inequality and discrimination are rampant—whether from gender, sex, and STIs, or the ways place, race, and other dimensions converge and intersect with disease, prevention, and care. These linger and haunt the ways HPV sequencing has "innovated" the field of HPV-associated cancer prevention. Sexuality is always already inscribed into the sociality and preventive apparatus of disease. These continue to matter for understandings of health and disease, for the distribution of care, and for practices of ensuring health equity. To see the sociality of viral exposure and its stakes is to see the inequality that characterizes the most precarious lives due to discrimination, poverty, and other already sutured lines of power.

While too much has already been said about the workings of biopower, by me and by others, the term remains helpful in understanding the management of life through systems—of thought, government, organizations—that exert control in ways that not only administer death, but also support life (Foucault 1980). What social problems are addressed as greater degrees of precision and prediction not previously available become available to some? As molecular epidemiology directs biomedical intervention to where it is needed most, it also supplies the categories upon which disease narratives take hold; real and symbolic associations with gendered, racialized, and sexualized categories; and, at times, how policies are linked with behaviors and identities (including those deemed "deviant," "immoral," and "contagious").[10] Who and what is rendered invisible in the risks of living in precarity and poverty and by the "injuries of inequality" brought on by sexism, racism, and other forms of power (Watkins-Hayes 2019)?

The "cancer vaccine," admittedly remarkable, would first enhance the opportunity for health already in place for those well-provided with health screening, human rights, and the structural social justice protections needed to live free from exposure to the many causes of ill health. Stopping a virus is a social, economic, and structural project as well as a medical one. Screening technologies were imagined as able to fill some of the gaps that existed due to age, health care access, or transnational migration. Cancer screening would always be necessary, whether for prevention of cancer among those who fall through the gaps or live in places where health care is unaffordable, inaccessible, or nonexistent, or in the context of health care decision making. The girls of whom Parham spoke are at risk as a result of the continued injuries of inequity, which include (albeit less so depending on your approach) the ways development and health care financing are locked into a pharmaceuticalized approach that simultaneously, yet unevenly, offers commodities of care and strategies to increase "participation." Such injuries are not exclusive to low-resource countries in the global south; they exist in the folds and valleys of the topographies of privilege and inequity. They are often found as human rights and bodily autonomy are pushed down and in places where resources are limited.

A Twenty-First-Century Precision Cancer Prevention Regime

Sociotechnical imaginaries are the visions of desirable futures that are animated by shared understandings of forms of social life and social order attainable through, and supportive of, advances in science and technology (Jasanoff and Kim 2015). These imaginaries comprise specific practices of storytelling and visualization that organize space and time and structure pleasure and anxiety. They inform what kinds of futures are possible and desirable, how problems and solutions are framed, how we respond to threats and contain uncertainty, and ultimately what we hope for, expect, and fear from science, technology, and medicine.

Pap tests were imagined as the best tool to prevent cervical cancer death, yet over time the test's effectiveness plateaued at 80 percent reduction of potential deaths, leaving 20 percent still exposed. What kind of future was imagined, desirable, and possible that would not only address this remaining 20 percent, but also reduce the much higher rates of unmet reduction challenge (about 40–60 percent) in low-resource countries around the world? The challenge of understanding and addressing that problem most often led in my research to the precision imaginary that emerged with genomic sequencing, and eventually to the newest hope of bringing scientific and technological efforts from high-resource areas into low-resource areas.

HPV testing, and a liquid-based collection tool, might be the easier and more effective approach that was needed, when performed with "self-sampling." This practical solution to increasing participation and reaching the "hard to reach" could also provide a more convenient approach for those already protected. And it might be welcome news in contexts where health care is either largely unavailable or a site of discrimination, or in countries like the US where conservative politics have restricted sexual and reproductive health care. Cervical cancer prevention continues to rely on the discourse and objectives of "women's health" and its newly formed relative, "reproductive and sexual health." As the historian Michelle Murphy argued, for feminist health it was the Pap test that emerged as a "lifesaving and instrumental [tool for] the arrangement of professional gynecology" and was simultaneously "proximate to sometimes coercive, racist, and unequal medical practices" (Murphy 2012, 114). The ontological organization of "reproductive health," to use Murphy's conceptualization, included cancer prevention and care in the category of "reproductive tract cancers," a category that included cervical cancer. Feminist NGOs would come to emphasize biomedical and social goods—needed quality of care, equal rights for women, family planning services beyond demographic targets, and issues of sexual and reproductive health and cancer screening—with associated recommendations for redirecting vast streams of resources toward a new formulation of the "problem" of women's health. The field is now widely referred to as "Sexual and Reproductive Health," sometimes with a second "R" included for sexual and reproductive health and rights (SRHR), and at other times as the shorthand version "sexual health," a strategic modification that may seem at first like an elision of rights and social justice calls but is on closer examination more strategic and political (Epstein and Mamo 2017).

Self-sampling for cervical cancer prevention in this framework is simultaneously a strategy to right the many imbalances of power and institutional control described by Murphy, and an effort to address a problem of women's lack of power and therefore vulnerability to health threat. HPV testing used for screening, more recently referred to simply as HPV self-sampling,[11] is emerging as a commodity of care (Fan 2021), and one that entails complex agencies as people negotiate biomedical power to take these into their own hands. In cervical self-sampling, a collection device is inserted into the vaginal canal, rotated to collect cells, and placed into a small tube (these can be incorporated into clinical appointments for privacy and autonomy), then screened for HPV genotypes using either cytology or molecular testing.

In contrast to many other types of self-tests (e.g., blood-based sugar tests or COVID-19 antigen tests) where samples are self-collected, HPV test results cannot be "read" by the patient. Instead they are mailed to laboratories, shifting some (but not all) control from patients/consumers to providers. Which test is deemed "better" and then made into the "right tool" for the job is a social production—both of which tool, and for what job. While HPV test kits for cervical cancer are available, tests for oral or anal or penile HPV-associated cancers are not yet part of medical monitoring and preventive guidelines.

The technical approach to self-sampling for an HPV test is similar to the colon cancer fecal test now routinely sent to people at home as a prevention screen in place of inpatient colonoscopy. As Roche clinical scientists said:

> where [patients] don't have access to buses to take them anywhere, where some of them can't even go because the husband will not allow them to go, can you give them a swab and say "look and see if you detect HPV?" . . . The uptake of self-sampling compared to going to a clinician to do a cervical exam was 84%. This was in their home. So, women are more likely to screen, and then we can do a test and you can look for the virus that's causing it.

Literature confirms that self-collection is a way for individuals to take a more active role in managing their health (Marshall, Vahabi, and Lofters 2019), a more convenient and private approach, with less discomfort than having a Pap test (Madzima, Vahabi, and Lofters 2017; Reisner et al. 2018), and an approach able to provide care without inefficiencies. This approach is now consistently referred to as "an innovative extension of in-office screening" (Aninye et al. 2021, 1; Tranberg et al. 2018). Appealing to areas where health care and health care systems alike are limited, the approach is said to be advantageous for women who have limited access to a provider, or have access but feel some hesitancy about the internal exam needed for screening (Arbyn, de Sanjose, and Weiderpass 2019).

Marc Steben, a family physician with expertise in sexual health, described self-sampling as the future "disruptor" of the standard of care: "When you look at the studies, very few are showing that women are worse [at taking a self bio-sample] than doctors and nurses. Most are equal. And there are some that show that women are *better* than doctors and nurses and midwives."[12] Putting the test in the hands of women and people with a cervix was "scientifically shown to be as good as (or better than) leaving it in clinicians' hands" is an important evidence-based claim for expanding access to preventive tools, and it is also part of the production of a commodity of care in the form of self-surveillance for HPV and cancer risk. That is, it provides a rationale for bringing the technoscientific capacity of the HPV test to identify and differentiate HPV genotypes into public health expansion along with consumer-driven health care.

Rachel Winer, an epidemiologist at the University of Washington who conducts research within a large health care system, and Julie Graves, a family medicine and public health doctor in the US, agree. For them "disparity gaps" defined groups of concern and how to direct health care efforts. These disparities hold for those outside as well as within health care systems, and often among those with lower income and wealth, among Black or Latina communities, and among the unhoused. Graves, also associate director of clinical services at Nurx, described self-sampling as a strategy to "shrink some of our disparity gaps," adding that the approach would also be a means to fix discriminatory care: "They're not going to go get their Pap because they're . . . sexual assault victims. They're trans. They've had a doctor be rough and difficult and they're scared. Overweight women who will not go because they won't step on a scale and you can't get to the doctor's office until you step on the scale."

Graves describes self-sampling as also a needed good to ameliorate the failures of biomedicine. "Our health system doesn't treat women right," she told me. "You're always at risk for having a bad experience when you go in for GYN care." Self-sampling is a solution to a set of failures: not only of biomedicine, but also of a cis-centric, heteronormative, and patriarchal culture. For health systems, self-sampling could be used to ensure that "you can get your screening done in a more efficient manner, and free up resources and time for other things—whether at the individual level or for the greater population," Winer stated. Xavier Bosch, a clinical researcher, described the evolution of self-sampling: "initially, it was considered as a resource for women that were not participating voluntarily into the screening programs. They send it to the non-attenders, right? But now we are transitioning very rapidly into everybody, so if the person prefers to take the specimen at home and send it via post or through the pharmacy network or whatever system, the country will adopt. They [all participants] have the choice."

Self-Sampling Tools as Commodities of Care

The self-sampling test for HPV is at times used opportunistically and at times to fill disparity gaps; it allows for complex agencies in settings where access is constrained or care is denied. In the context of US abortion bans and the existential threat to women's health, self-care is increasingly necessary as a defensive tool. At the same time, messages of taking "control" of one's health through biomedical monitoring build on decades of the social transformation of biomedicine, part of a consumer-surveillance apparatus wherein people have become subjects *and* objects of biomedicine. Self-sampling mediates relationships between companies and consumers, making HPV testing a commodity of care. Evidence of biomedicalization's reach—these commodities reflect a "regime of patienthood" (Joyce and Jeske 2019; Joyce, James, and Jeske 2020) wherein patients signal their concerns, competencies, and compliance. Self-sampling is self-surveillance, part of this regime of patienthood that transforms people into morally good patients and/or self-centered actors. Managing risk, as the historian Ilana Löwy (2010b) argues, capitalizes on the anxiety of healthy (or at least asymptomatic) people, molding them into an established category of "illness" and also into a new category of health consumers. The historian Michelle Murphy (2012) understood these agentic actors as one of the two figures brought forward concurrently in cervical cancer screening technoscience: at-risk populations in need of "mass screening" to prevent death, and at-risk subjects of clinical biomedicine whose fears and worries compel them into enterprise as consumers of health services.

In the US, HPV self-sampling kits are currently available only through direct-to-consumer (DTC) health technology companies. While the Netherlands and Australia have integrated self-sampling into their national cervical screening programs (Arbyn et al. 2018), the US must confront the challenge of making self-sampling available in the context of an opportunistic cervical screening program within a country lacking universal health care. Test kits for HPV sold in the US through DTC companies are fairly similar across the board, each including printed user directions, a cotton swab, a tube for storing biomaterials, and a prepaid envelope for return to a laboratory. Self-testing for HPV in this iteration has been held up as a model by the public health practitioners and policymakers and experts in clinical oncology seeking more (and more effective) screening tools for HPV monitoring. Putting power in the hands of users is not just a formulation for cervical cancer prevention; it is aspirational for detection of all of the other HPV-associated cancers as well (not to mention for developing tests for other viruses that are sexually transmitted and are causally associated with cancer).

Self-testing available for consumer purchase reflects what the sociologist Tressie McMillan Cottom (2018) shows to be part of the false narrative of neoliberal offerings—if you make the right choice, buy the right product, and take personal responsibility for your health, you can avert cancer. A fantasy of control over our lives is enacted by technology apps designed over nearly every area of life, including our health. For Cottom, buying products, making "choices," and directing actions to overcome adversity— e.g., to live near the better hospital, to have the better health insurance, to participate in the best screening modality—uphold the myths of meritocracy while demonstrating the workings of power structures that protect some lives over others. Health care apps, and the health care choices they infer, suggest empowerment and the capacity to control—not the random or unlucky health scare, but the patterned and oppressive structures of protection and vulnerability. There is a presumption that if you have the capacity to do so, if you make the right choice, you will be assured good health and good care, and be deemed a good patient. But there is no amount of researching, choosing, and purchasing (i.e., "shopping") that can overcome the deeply embedded stereotypes and structures of racism and discrimination.

Tech companies use the familiar rhetoric of choice and agency to call for a disruption of business-as-usual medicine, including HPV screening. "Freedom begins here," Nurx asserts, using the company name that implies a new—"nu"—way of issuing prescriptions—"rx". Nurx includes an application platform service that is part of its provision of tele-health care and home delivery of pharmaceutical prescriptions. Founded in 2015, Nurx joined other tech firms offering reproductive and sexual health care services directly to consumers. In the context of right-wing efforts to restrict women's reproductive health care (abortion and contraceptive services) and inclinations to do the same for LGBTQ health, this is a welcome development. Nurx's business model includes the provision of contraceptives and at-home test kits for HPV and other STIs. While the US has no shortage of obstacles to receiving good health care, or in fact any health care at all, these products can (for the right price or with the right insurance) ensure access and care. Prescription services for birth control or the morning-after pill are provided via tele-health appointments (through their app, text messaging, or a video visit); products that do not require a visit, such as home-testing kits for a number of STIs, including chlamydia, gonorrhea, syphilis, hepatitis C, HIV, and HPV, as well as treatments for herpes and other infections can be ordered directly by the consumer. These products are promoted through a discourse of sexual health, made to appeal to consumers who want to take control of their sexual health on their own terms. They promote these offerings by configuring "responsible actors" who are taking charge of their own preventive health needs.

For direct-to-consumer companies in the US, HPV test kits are part of a broader line of health services offered to consumers more than "patients." While business models vary, a shared claim is that these services are "better" and more empowering than traditional options, and offer self-respect in ways traditional health care often does not. There is an ethos of "do it yourself," "test on your terms" (myLAB Box 2020), and "collect . . . in a place of your choosing" (LetsGetChecked 2020b) that underscores this market. HPV self-tests, specifically, can eliminate the discomfort, anxiety, and harms associated with in-person sexual and reproductive health care. From single contact to continuous self-tracking, consumers can monitor bodily changes over time with smartphone apps designed to connect with wearable data technologies into a single streamlined body-monitoring application (LetsGetChecked 2020a), with results shareable to providers, family, and friends. Consumers can subscribe to products—akin to film or music streaming services—to facilitate ongoing body monitoring and supplies of the products they choose (and can earn company loyalty by doing so).

"We're here to fix" the broken system, Nurx (2020a) states on their website. In an interview Graves explained: "You can do the whole thing in text." Nurx refuses to stigmatize or sanitize sex and sexuality, providing products designed to contain the spread (and personal discomfort) of STIs and ensure one's autonomy and privacy in the area of sexual and reproductive health care. Sex and sexuality are life-affirming sites of care. Sexual transmission is neither averted nor tamed in DTC company claims or product offerings, nor do they avert the realities of STIs, including HPV, for sexually active people. In fact, the companies' emergence in the mid-2010s aligns with evidence of high and climbing STI rates in the US (Haelle 2017). HPV is described as a "typically asymptomatic infection for oneself and one's sexual partner(s)": "HPV transmits very easily and often presents no symptoms. Therefore, it's incredibly common. . . . to pass it on. The only sure way to tell if you have HPV is by testing yourself" (SelfCollect 2020). Another company, iDNA (2020), tells their consumers that it's important to test not only "for [one's] own health and safety, [but] to protect the sexual health of [one's] partners, too."

Companies draw on claims about the limitations of and barriers to sexual health care as well as general health care. DTC products are touted as a means to "avoid the stirrups" (Nurx 2020b), to skip the embarrassment that often accompanies STI testing, to be "Responsible not uncomfortable" (SelfCollect 2020). In doing so, these companies at once move the discourse toward and away from Löwy's concern of reigniting stigmatization, in this case through a presumption of shame that can be alleviated only through their own self-determined actions. They instead invoke a good (health) consumer, empowered with the capacity to attend to their own (sexual) health care and (sexual) health promotion.

Not all sexual health providers agreed. Danielle Jones (2019), a clinician and board-certified OBGYN who goes by the online name "Mama Doctor Jones," took to YouTube to speak to would-be consumers about a market creep to women in their twenties who have money and access to social media, and who are vulnerable to the messaging that they are at risk. Mama Doctor Jones warns that the value of risk assessment is questionable: "This is not true. . . . This is not a good thing," she argues. It is "extraordinarily common," she tells viewers, to get a positive HPV test. Yet the companies are not forthcoming; they are "profiting," she says, from young women's worries in the US. "If you get a positive HPV test, so what? It does not matter," she said, adding that "nobody needs an HPV test under thirty unless a doctor prescribed this given your risk." She then concludes by saying, "Yes, home access to STD testing in general, such as for gonorrhea and chlamydia, can be good."

HPV self-tests hold multiple tendencies that include a strategy to ameliorate health inequities and a strategy to enhance the health of those already protected. Self-sampling has the potential to provide needed benefits in contexts of health care insufficiencies and capacities to ensure better and more transparent sexual health care. HPV self-screening tests can serve as the "right tool" to prevent invasive cancer and mortality where cancer rates are highest. The ROSE Solution, an acronym for "Removing Obstacles to cervical ScrEening" (Woo, Ooi, and Saville 2021), serves as an example. Launched in 2017 in Malaysia, the ROSE initiative integrates HPV self-collection and HPV tests with a digital health platform for communications. ROSE was developed and then tested, and proved successful, as a pilot project where screening programs have not been widely implemented, to assess whether this approach could address obstacles to screening.[13] The initiative also reveals the multiple tendencies of biomedicine, here as a public health governance tool and a commodity of care offered in places with spotty health care infrastructure.

Self-sampling also can be a tool of biopower, facilitating and advocating for regular bodily monitoring as a sign of a moral and responsible individual engaging in good science for their own good care. When not followed, self-sampling may signal a shame now reframed as a personal failure, perhaps reinforcing racist and other assumptions about good consumers, good patients, and good medicine.

Sexual Stigma in a New Regime of Cancer Prevention

Sexualizing Cancer has in part picked up where the historian of medicine Ilana Löwy left off in her historical argument for a twentieth-century transformation of cervical cancer beyond its reputation as a well-known "women's disease." I set out to analyze the contemporary ways HPV and HPV-associated cancers are at times infused with sexuality and thus sexualized, and at times held apart from sexuality with the intention of obscuring the connection. How disease is narrated has implications for how it is cared for and prevented. The focus here has been not about the mere presence of sex and sexuality, but about the ways it is mobilized, and specifically normalized or moralized, in narratives of cancer risk and prevention. I followed HPV's manifestation in prevention politics from research conferences to medical offices and into the social disparities in public health policy as well as the cracks in our presumptive "safety net."

This brought my work to a set of puzzles. First, it made me wonder if and how two different specialties—cancer research and oncology, and infectious disease research and its specialties—have converged as each worked on their objects and applied specialized knowledge to prevention and care. And second, it pointed me toward the question of how the presumptions of clinical "me" medicine and collective public health "we" prevention intersected along the way. Löwy (2011) was first among those cautioning that, as a cancer linked explicitly to sexual transmission and an STI, cervical cancer was still at risk of social stigmatization. Here I have examined the "ghostly matters" in the histories of diseases from syphilis to HIV, and the moral presumptions of "good" and "bad" behaviors and people that linger, continuing to reflect cultural claims and finger-pointing that are neither universal nor consistent across and within places and groups. Not only has cancer made the full shift from its former position as random to its current understanding as preventable and calculable disease; that causal association with HPV has also transformed the ways sex, sexuality, and sexual health are conjoined with disease and its prevention.

HPV-associated cancers have one by one taken on new meaning, reconceptualized as sexually transmitted disease—whether that connection was already suspected (in the case of cervical cancer) or took shape as a causal narrative following HPV molecular certainty as oncoviral (in the case of oropharyngeal cancer). They have also produced a new regime of cancer prevention, with its special exigencies for patienthood and responsibility. Is the world now "on alert," as Silja Samerski (2018) has said, as individuals are increasingly brought into new modalities and regimes of screening and monitoring their risk and health? Are some actually protected or better protected by the latest advancements in cancer prevention technology, while others are merely enrolled in surveillance biomedicine?

Each HPV-associated cancer is shaped by prior scientific and sociocultural significations and distinct entanglements with already established notions of risk, riskiness, and health governance. Now that these cancers are shown, epidemiologically, to be both unevenly distributed and associated with sexual transmission, surveillance practices are changing how these cancers are understood and addressed, and in turn how STIs are understood and addressed. A suppression of sex often takes hold: at times through an emphasis on non-infectious cancer and the routinization of epidemiological metrics (such as age of sexual onset, number of partners, and types of activities), and the destigmatization of body parts associated with sex. Yet, as I have shown, controversy and debate, and the ways technologies and approaches are gendered and sexualized, are hard to suppress.

HPV vaccines have followed a path similar to that of pharmaceuticals more generally, producing risk as well as risk markets and offering treatments that resemble not so much the vaccine markets of the early twentieth century as the pharmaceutical markets of the twenty-first century. HPV is part of the regime of cancer prevention technologies shaped in the face of uncertaintainties: infection with oncoviral types is necessary, but *insufficient*, for the development of cancer. Persistence of high-risk viral types is emerging as the scientific cause and object for ongoing screening. Most of those infected with HPVs are asymptomatic, and most HPVs do not develop into cancer; many "high-risk" types are transient, clearing spontaneously; and long latency periods are common from infection to cellular change. It is the interactive social aspects of external life and the internal processes of a virus's replication within its host that come into view.

Early attempts to desexualize HPV vaccination by downplaying the social experience of sex and the sexual transmission of viruses failed to ensure a smooth vaccine acceptance trajectory. The rhetorical strategy of promoting Gardasil as a cancer vaccine may have been chosen to avert the controversies around sex and disease that plagued HIV/AIDS and safe sex campaigns, but it was unable to sidestep the moralizing that often accompanies conversations about youth and sex. The gendered production of HPV and HPV vaccines as a "woman's" risk and cancer prevention strategy ignited familiar tropes of concerns for (heterosexual) promiscuity. When pressure (and evidence) amassed to include boys in what was then a gendered virus and cancer prevention approach for girls, promoting HPV and the HPV vaccine to boys proved to be a hard sell. Genital wart protection, which it was known all along the vaccine could provide, was repositioned as a central object of prevention and a site for renewed and different potential benefit. Given the multizonal nature of HPV's cancer risk, claims to prevent "other" HPV-associated cancers began with adolescent boys turning to cameras inquisitively and asking: "Mom, Dad, did you know?" This inclusion of boys necessitated a re-sexualization and a degendering of HPV and HPV vaccines, as genital warts (a common STI) and other cancers affecting genital areas previously undiscussed, such as cancers of the anus, were brought to the fore with "awareness" campaigns of their own.

Rhetorical and material attempts to normalize HPV as a virus "we all have" punctuated mainstream messaging as the vaccine and HPV itself were "de-gendered" in an attempt to enroll boys and later young men. The risk of anal cancer, rarely discussed openly and already sexualized because of the body part it involved as well as its linkage to sexual acts associated with femininity and homosexuality, would need to be navigated. HPV-anal cancer researchers performed the work of normalizing and desexualizing this viral-cancer association, yet they did so in ways that affirmed sexuality, refusing to erase or sanitize gender and sexual diversity and expression. Clinical trial research from the NIH Multicenter AIDS Cohort Study (MACS) to the more recent ANCHOR and SPANC trials strategically and specifically included gendered, sexual connotations in their recruitment tools. As "evidence-based research" was launched, researchers and clinicians embarked on processes to shift the technology of Pap testing, gendered as a feminine tool, to an all-genders approach that would also resist homo-stereotyping as a tool for screening HIV+ MSM. To do so, they directed normalization processes at the anus itself as a body part we all have. Jurisdictional debates as well as best approaches to prevention unfolded.

HPV-associated oral cancers—and the population group most associated with them, older men—have rarely been construed as associated with increased sexual risk to health (although they have been thought of as threats to others), so they were protected from social stigma, seemingly by their age, gender, and sexuality. Masculine heteronormativity provides a shield, averting stigmatization and sexualization, even as the sex act implicated in this case—cunnilingus, presumably as a solely heterosexual act—is made visible and discussed. Clinicians in oncology who specialize in cancers of the head and neck would find that sex and sexuality entered their clinical offices as they managed sexuality in heterosexual relations when wives momentarily placed blame on their husbands. Finger-pointing accompanied questions of contagion: "Who did I (or he) get this from?" and then "Who did I (or he) give this to?" Quickly, sex and sexuality were pushed into a narrative of the (sexual) past: something that had happened decades ago.

For cervical cancer prevention, vaccination was notably joined by shifts in screening approaches and the ways these gendered and degendered cancer prevention practices: the Pap test already in place, and now the "cancer vaccine." HPV testing needed to avert stigmatization, given that most people knew of an amorphous risk but were largely unaware of a role for sexually transmitted infectious disease in oncogenesis. As Roche developed HPV primary screening, they were keenly aware that they "d[id]n't want women to feel shameful if they g[o]t a positive result." Shame attached to STIs, this book shows, is a lingering association, haunted by past forms of stigma and blame: gendered and racialized presumptions of promiscuity for some women in the case of cervical cancer; the blame and responsibility of sex workers to protect the health of men; and the deviant presumptions about anal or excessive sex that attached to gay men's bodies during the early years of HIV. What also lingers is the relational normative (white) masculine association of being protected from stigma in a normalized rhetoric of sex, drugs, and rock'n'roll as part of their normative youth in the case of oropharyngeal cancer. Yet even these are suppressed, now largely (and more quietly) embedded in the technosciences of biotechnology, biomedicine, and preventive public health.

It was at the International Papillomavirus Conference (IPVC) held in July 2020 that I heard Xavier Bosch, a senior consultant to the Cancer Epidemiology Research Program (CERP) at the Catalan Institute of Oncology in Barcelona, Spain, tell the audience of largely cancer specialists: "We still need to learn from infectious disease." Bosch appealed to experts working on cancer to look toward infectious disease, specifically from hepatitis to HIV, for the needed solutions to preventing HPV-associated cancers. I emailed Bosch and asked for some time together to discuss his brief assertion. Bosch spoke of a "trivialization" of the Pap test and cytology testing in the STD world. He compared the researchers and clinicians—and public health professionals—of the STD world with cancer specialists, describing the differences as "They work with shirts and ties" (referring to cancer specialists), while "the STD guys, they work in t-shirts and jeans." He added that "there is a snob [from cancer guys] in doing routine screening." For the cancer specialists, screening for cancer prevention was an everyday and routine thing that ought to be left in the hands of the lower-status professionals who perform Pap tests and mammography and palpate lymph nodes. STD providers, on the other hand, are familiar with these actions and uphold them as drivers of prevention: the STD guys routinely swab cells for STD checks, so perhaps the Pap test could be brought into their domain. After all, STIs, once called "the grimmest" of gifts by Susan Sontag (1989), were free of stigma and shame in the STI world. STD and HIV medical worlds have largely destigmatized the once metaphorical label of "plague" into a risk to be prevented and a set of viruses to be prevented, tested for, and treated.

While the pharmaceuticalized approach to prevention found in PrEP (Pre-exposure Prophylactic) medication to prevent HIV holds some lingering moral association with promiscuity (or multiple sex partners) and queer intimacies, for many countries and groups this viral prevention has shed its stigma. When Bosch spoke of infectious disease experts, he was also speaking of a long history of expertise to screen and treat for STIs such as gonorrhea and chlamydia. He was asserting that once systems integrated sexual health—and thereby expanded prevention beyond a focus on cancer to include a focus on STI prevention—opportunities would arise to do better for human health. This is not a desexualization, but a recognition of sex and sexuality and its role in transmission of pathogens and, ultimately, risk of infection.

In my interviews I spoke to many who agreed that the question is not which tool is more or less "right" for cancer prevention, but how to move away from these secondary approaches altogether in favor of a vaccine approach for all. For vaccination to gain full acceptability would require that we resist sanitizing and erasing sex and sexuality. Specifically, it was clear in retrospect that eliminating talk of sex and sexuality from messaging directed to adolescents and their parents fell short of the intention. While "it's very difficult for parents to imagine that their kids will be sexually active when they're nine years," Steben told me, and "we saw the backlash from religious people, from school boards, and [these groups] wanting to make sure that vaccines were not given in the school because this was [perceived] as a way to increase promiscuity in kids," it has become clear that "As soon as you start camouflaging the sexual behavior component of HPV, [altering] your capacity to explain properly what that person can do, it diminishes your credibility because inevitably the person will find out." As Steben stated (perhaps with irony), people will "inevitably" find out that HPV is sexually transmitted (as he said, "Google is there"), so why not openly acknowledge this, and by extension, open up more opportunities for cancer prevention?

Infectious disease experts were quick to inform me that "patients in the clinics are fully aware of how they got HPV," and this full disclosure was needed to overcome the hesitancy and "stickiness" of vaccine adoption (Larson 2020). There have been many documented instances in which desexualizing viral life and health needs resulted in misinformation, from myths that monogamy protected adults against HPV-associated cancers today or that youth could remain safe in marriage and get Paps once they became sexually active, as well as the more general contention that HPV vaccination promotes sexual promiscuity. For infectious disease specialists, offering gynecologists a vaccine when they didn't really know how to handle vaccines was a missed opportunity given their expertise in explaining sexual behavior and STIs.

It's been decades since the US Institute of Medicine Report voiced a concern that secrecy and stigma around STDs was contributing to lack of support from government and private organizations for STD prevention activities as a strategy to prevent "STD-related cancers" (Eng and Butler 1997). It has now been more than twenty years since the role of viruses, many of them sexually transmitted, came to be understood as a cause of concern in the world of cancer (Walboomers et al. 1999).[14] Yet an "unwillingness to confront issues regarding sexuality" at times lingers, holding back not just understanding, but public attention and acceptance of the ordinariness of sex (Eng and Butler 1997, 89).

Self-collection direct-to-consumer lab tests are fast appearing on social media threads promoting self-test kits to a generation of US consumers who had most likely already been vaccinated against HPV in their teens. Now in their twenties and thirties, these young people with cervices or without may identify as women, men, genderqueer or expansive, or something else. Yet collectively, they are part of a generation that is calculating and monitoring their bodies and lives in unprecedented ways. No doubt fueled by the stay-at-home orders of the COVID-19 pandemic, product technology companies largely based in Silicon Valley and the San Francisco Bay Area are reaching across digital media spaces into potential customers' homes with the message that, like the girls of Gardasil before them, they can become one less patient-in-waiting: Instead of facing a risky future, they can seize power over their own health. This again may be welcome news in settings constrained by the moralizing of providers and people's lack of control over their own reproductive and sexual health. In a context of public swings to conservative views or public disinvestments, corporate tie-ins are not all bad, but they are reflective of the culture of biomedicalization.

Roche too attempts to normalize HPV infection without dismissing HPV's association with sex for its audience of providers and patients alike. Shame should not be associated with HPV, they now message these groups. "One shouldn't jump to conclusions" if diagnosed with HPV. A provider-patient role play depicts a provider stating "there is no shame in it." HPV, we are told, is "caused by skin to skin contact" instead of the more inflammatory phrasing "sexually transmitted." Roche explains that this is not about sex or lifestyle and should not bring shame. Roche introduces the HPV test as a "modern technology," comparing this "highly accurate laboratory instrument . . . for the [detection of] DNA of high-risk HPV" with "the Pap test [which] does not detect the presence of HPV and is subject to human error," and advises potential customers that "looking for high-risk HPV can determine your risk of cervical cancer."

The linkage of sex with disease and sexuality with health are shown to be entangled objects with a diversity of differently configured meanings and injunctions for different bodies and lives, at times carrying a lingering moral stain and at other times viewed as a positive aspect of health. As increasingly corporatized and commodified health companies and products take up cancer prevention, "health" is able to *sanitize* and legitimize what has so often been the more contentious term "sexual." The materiality and sociality of this linkage has been a generative and uneven process that opens up new biomedical, social, and cultural possibilities—with different ways of imagining being sexually normal or abnormal. STIs are normative and common, yet they create a responsibility to guard against their harm, whether through vaccination, knowledge, or simply a more abstract will to health. Cancer prevention at times provides a particular cover, de-emphasizing and legitimizing the often suppressed acts of sex.

Prevention Politics and the Sexual Future of Viral-Cancer Connections

HPV vaccines have followed a path similar to that of pharmaceuticals more generally, producing risk as well as risk markets, and offering treatments that resemble not so much the vaccine markets of the early twentieth century as the pharmaceutical markets of the twenty-first century. Individual risk, not disease, is the discursive and material object of risk and intervention: the terms upon which immunization practices are deployed.[15]

Reflective of twenty-first-century biomedicalization processes, research, development, and sales are offered by tech start-ups, venture capital firms, and Google health—all for-profit companies looking to gain profitability as they promote "women's empowerment" through pharmaceuticals. A biotechnology company in the San Francisco Bay Area, for example, seeks to produce a topical therapy to treat HPV so that high-risk genotypes do not persist and develop into invasive cancers.[16] Is this good news? Maybe. Technological solutions like these are most often part of the pharmaceuticalization of public health, producing profits for some, arguably protecting those who least need the solution, and excluding the places and people who could benefit most. I am cautiously optimistic, in part because the world still awaits much-needed, available technologies—such as a topical contraceptive that can also prevent the spread of infectious pathogens from HIV, hepatitis C, and other STIs, a tool promised long ago by medical researchers and pharmaceutical companies. Yet I am also aware of the need for change in biomedical care and control to allow and respect agency, whether of providers, organizations, or people. Numerous low-tech, affordable products to protect health, critical to promoting sexual and reproductive health, rights, and justice, have yet to be realized.

Whether such products will continue to destigmatize or to re-sexualize HPV is less certain. Unmoored from politics, linkages among sex and disease will likely linger and continue to demand de-stigmatization and social teaching, activism, and policies to refuse social discrimination and gender and sexual panics reminiscent of the early HIV/AIDS epidemic and present in contemporary abortion politics. Refusing stigmatization is in part what the International Anal Neoplasia Society (IANS) meeting did so well, as attendees and speakers chose to normalize and sanitize sexuality and gender diversity, while also allowing the particular distinctions of sex and sexual cultures to remain in place. The ways sexuality and health intertwine in biomedical and cultural rhetoric are significant for health and health care equity. While sexualization can be culturally stigmatizing, as was the case in some STI-cancer rhetoric and especially with HIV/AIDS, it can also produce recognition of diverse sexual practices and communities and point to sites where intervention is needed.

While the quest for pharmaceutical success of a cancer vaccine (as well as new screening approaches) may have suppressed sex altogether, this goal was not without complications and counter-tendencies. Concerns about HPV and HPV vaccination in the early months of vaccine rollout revolved around the sexualities of teenage girls. Such fears were gradually toned down with a strategy of marketing the vaccine not as STI prevention but as cancer prevention. Persistent processes of desexualization took place as

HPV vaccine technologies expanded, as drug companies sought to ensure their use (Mamo and Epstein 2014). Yet desexualization is uneven and incomplete: as other HPV-related cancer cases have emerged as objects of prevention, declarations of an "epidemic" of oral cancers are being made, and attention and controversy around anal cancer, especially among "high-risk" populations of HIV+ men and women and MSM, percolate. These developments resurrect the symbolic associations between sex, health, and morality as stigma appears to cling to certain bodies and practices.

In highlighting sexual politics—or more specifically, how and when sexualization and desexualization processes unfold and with what social, cultural, and medical biopolitics—the link to infectious disease and the sexualization of this segment of cancer control marks something *new* in the politics of cancer. Discourses of sexuality, when they appear in virus-cancer connections, unfold in ways that re-energize and reveal specific (and sometimes long-standing) cultural linkages of health and disease with risk, sex, and stigma recast in a new language of modern biomedical risk and pharmaceutical possibilities. These developments demonstrate Foucault's (1979) general contention that modern societies are characterized less by simple repression of sexuality than by a proliferation of discourses and practices relating to sexuality, health, and the body aimed at managing populations in the service of numerous social ends. As STI viral-cancer associations are invoked, so too are various conceptions of risk, risky behaviors, and at-risk embodiments that point outward to social explanations of disease causation. The stakes are high, as STIs—part of the ordinariness of intimate relations—will continue to shape health and illness with uneven effects. We will need human rights approaches to prevention that refuse to erase gendered sexual lives. Yet, as these fields of research and prevention are transformed through biomedicalization—for example, through the biomolecular approach of the vaccine "fix" or a molecular test—attempts to desexualize public discourse emerge. The assumption is that preventing sexual transmission simply becomes less important. The suppression of sex and sexuality is an ongoing process and one that in these cases has been accomplished only with difficulty, if at all.

When it comes to HPV cancer prevention, young people are well versed in the links between HPV and various cancers, and many will likely be asking their dentists to check them for early signs of HPV-associated oropharyngeal cancers. Controversy and debate around gender and sexuality will likely play out less in concerns about individual bodies and lives, and more as part of the jurisdictional power of disciplines and capital. This was evident in 2013, for example, when a letter was sent to from the American Board of Obstetrics and Gynecology (ABOG) to gynecologists who were screening "men" for anal cancer demanding that they cease and desist. ABOG announced new guidelines for board certification, stating that certification is limited to those OB-GYNs who "limit their practice to the care of women." When I spoke with Elizabeth Stier, a gynecologist, the day the news broke, she voiced her concern: "What will I tell my patients? Where will they go for needed care?" ABOG was mandating that she and others stop seeing "men" in their clinical practice or risk losing their board certification. As she told me that day, "I don't think the board really cares about a bunch of HIV positive gay men. . . . They're not their patients; who cares?" Gendered sexual politics were unfolding as the ABOG board decision was deemed to be a threat to LGBTQ health, HIV+ health, and the care of transgender people. ABOG was pressuring gynecologists who engage in HIV and STI clinical care of all gender bodies and lives. The board rule was quickly overturned following protest by many professional groups, yet it is evidence to me of the ways HPV-cancer prevention will unevenly and differently produce gendered sexual biopolitics. Many people will find themselves online, ordering DNA-based and other molecular test kits for self-collection of DNA cells to send for direct lab determination of HPV's presence in all areas of their epithelial zones (the mouth, vagina, and anus). I suspect there will be many and various new markets ready to fill these "gaps" with ever-expanding commodities of care. Sadly, with conservative turns in the US and other countries, it will be less clear what markets are needed to fill this care.

Merck released a new (possibly final) advertising campaign for Gardasil 9, now the only HPV vaccine on the US market. In its 2019 approval, the FDA recommended provider-patient co-decision making for the newly allowed indication of a "catch-up" vaccine for people aged twenty-five to forty-nine who may not have received an HPV vaccine. Then, in 2021, Merck released its advertisement, "Help Protect Yourself" (Merck Sharp & Dohme Corp. 2021), aimed at adults. Targeted to mostly men who likely were not vaccinated in their youth, the publicity campaign included a website launch that depicted the same middle-aged white male character who had joined the 5k race in prior ads. The ad claims that Gardasil 9 "helps protect against certain cancers and diseases" linked with nine genomic types, seven of which are associated with cancers and two with non-cancerous genital warts. The protection offered is multizonal—covering the skin zones and risks of cancer formation of the cervix (as well as vulvar and vaginal areas), the anus, and the area deep in the back of the throat, the oropharynx.

In the fifteen years since the public was brought into the conversation, Gardasil has picked up new indications and new target groups for its vaccine approach, demonstrating the ways risk regimes variously incorporate gender, sexuality, and other social categories gradually rendered visible even though their risks were there all along. Shifts unfold at various scales and sites, and with different meanings and contingencies along the way. Some groups are protected, some are over-surveilled, and others are unprotected and under-surveilled, as biomedicine and technology produce some subjects on alert and others without any safety net at all.

In the US, the Centers for Disease Control and Prevention set a vaccination target of 80 percent for adolescents regardless of gender by 2020, yet rates are at 40 percent for girls and 21 percent for boys more than fifteen years after its introduction. Reaching blockbuster status and attracting billions of dollars in funding has proved challenging, as sex stigma and other concerns, from safety to decision-making authority, have hindered the attainment of the multi-billion-dollar sales Merck expected. Other vaccines face challenges as well, as do many non-vaccine efforts to stop viral infectious disease in their tracks. We are losing ground now on long-known pathogens, from polio to mpox to HIV. Microscopic infections, sexually transmitted or otherwise, will likely continue to shape health and disease, from the chronicity of Lyme disease or Epstein-Barr or COVID-19 to life-threatening diseases, including cancers (from STIs). In what ways gender, sexuality, race, class, and place will influence the prevalence, treatment, and prevention of such diseases is not yet fully known.

Today, people are not only patients and objects but also subjects of data generation and reconstruction, as many self-monitor their bodies, navigating their lives "through the grids of potential health threats" (Bauer and Olsén 2009, 125). Self-data collection lends an appearance of empowerment, yet it also transforms people into continuous risk-monitors and "individuals on alert" willing to engage in health management to reduce threat. People, otherwise thought of as patients, consumers, and now users of products and services, are "invited" to adopt a statistical gaze on themselves as they strive for "health," while the risk and danger of these technologies is understated. The multiple tendencies of biomedicine now allow tracking cancer and other risks as easily as one can track one's walking steps, heart rate, and sleep quality. These are not all on the "wrong side" of good care, as some offerings and structures bring care into people's homes or hands as gender and sexual politics continue a relentless attack on the rights of women as well as gender and sexual "minorities." Self-sampling for HPV is part of a potential "right side" for some who may be prohibited or constrained from seeking health care, or rendered without care altogether. All as the social disparities in illness and death persist (as is now even more evident due to the COVID pandemic).

The juxtaposition between the WHO's call for equity in cervical cancer screening and prevention and the ways health apps are commercialized, each with a similar hope to "get to zero" and "eliminate cancer," has brought forward this sociological attention. Commodities of care are one aspect of biomedicalization that produces "citizen consumers" who think they/we can parse everything, from virology to molecular epidemiology. Technoscience has produced a self-reinforcing cycle of fear promotion followed by the marketing of tests and products that promise some means to reassert control over fear. Sex and sexuality continue to be brought into fears and moralizing aspects of control in concerning ways. Sexualizing cancer is a good thing, not one to be effaced nor misconstrued. It is the moralizing, stigmatizing, and exercising of jurisdictional control over whose bodies and what forms of sex are deemed good and in need of protection that require averting and preventing. Viruses, and all of us, are socially connected—we live together in how we play, have sex, and address our health and health care needs.

Acknowledgments

I've been mulling these ideas over for a very long time, in collaboration and as a solo investigator, and especially in the context of a world that often seems to have gone awry. I could not have kept going without the incredible support of my partner, Helen Fitzsimmons, who after her own fatigue from my eight years of travel, anxiety, lack of focus, periodic full immersion in refocusing activities, and general ups and downs came forward in the final months to help me make the word count. Thank you, Helen, for that final push, and even more for all you do to make my life well-lived, loved, and full.

Working at a teaching-intensive university has been harder than I expected. I have been grateful for the unique faculty position to which I was recruited years ago by a faculty committed to creating intellectual and research opportunities in the interdisciplinary social sciences around health and health equity. Many faculty at San Francisco State refuse to give up their research activities, joining in community, conversation, and fun as we toss ideas around. I am especially grateful to the Health Equity Institute and our creation of writing groups, social hours, conferences, peer review, talks, and other activities. The HEI faculty and staff has shifted, yet we continue to function as a little institute that could. I thank Cynthia Gomez, Sonja MacKenzie, Allen Leblanc, Sepideh Modrek, Jessica Wolin, Mirna Vazquez, Emily Mann, and Charmayne Hughes. I also thank Ugo Edu, for her postdoctoral work with me during a crucial fieldwork visit as well as her work on an early grant proposal to the National Science Foundation (NSF).

HEI provided the seed funding to start what is today an almost seven-year science, technology, and society scholars' group (The STS Hub). Martha Kenney willingly contributed her vision, time, and collaborative efforts to build an STS community. We have received some university support and a recent NSF award, but for almost a decade this community has mostly been driven by the efforts of our colleagues who yearn for and are thus willing to join a feminist-oriented "hub" of scholars working at the intersections of sciences, technologies, and society. Ugo Edu contributed as an early co-founder. Over time, Martha and I have established a fellowship program, and I thank the many faculty who have joined our efforts and peer-reviewed some of the pages of this book. Special thanks to Martha Lincoln, Dawn Elissa-Fischer, Chris Hanssmann, and Juliette Hua, as well as all of the STS Hub fellows. I am also grateful for my colleague friends at SF State for supporting me as I continued to work through these ideas: Diane Harris, Emma Sanchez-Vaznaugh, Andreanna Clay (who in the first week of lockdowns joined me in setting a goal of writing), Anoshua Chaudhuri, Carmen Domingo, and Colleen Hoff (who often talked through these ideas with me), as well as my faculty colleagues in public health: Marty, Emma, Lisa, Vivian, Juliana, David, and Supriya.

When I was at the University of Maryland, many of my faculty colleagues and especially PhD students were incredibly supportive of my early excitement to analyze and follow the new HPV vaccine as ads for Gardasil were saturating the media. A small grant gave me some summer funds that enabled me to launch the "Gardasil Working Group" with then graduate students Aleia Clark and Amber Nelson, co-authors and architects of our publication, *Producing and Protecting Risky Girls*. I can't say enough about how grateful I was for those early conversations, their ideas, and the ways they were excited to work together. It was this collaboration that gained me an invitation from Keith Wailoo to a Rutgers University convening where he and Steven Epstein, Julia Livingston, and Robbie Aronowitz were planning a conference and edited volume on the HPV vaccine. I am grateful to Keith and the scholars brought together over two workshops and then into an edited book.

I owe a great deal of gratitude to Steven Epstein for joining me in a collaboration begun in 2015. We overlapped at the Rutgers convening on the HPV vaccine, which led to a collaboration crafted together one day at Café Flore in San Francisco. We agreed to collaborate on the biopolitics of sexual health, a broad title for our overlapping yet also individual interests in the ways sexuality and disease intersected in health, medicine, and society broadly. We tirelessly mapped the emergence of sexual health and sexual cancer, as we referred to it then. I am grateful to Steve for his friendship and great thinking and for co-authoring three papers and giving countless talks before we each set out (as we had agreed) to write our own books. Many ideas from that collaboration appear in the pages of *Sexualizing Cancer*. I am grateful to Steve and to the PhD students that came from Northwestern University and SPAN, and especially for the brilliance of Gemma Mangione, Kellie Owens, Joseph Guisti, and Alka Menon.

Thanks also to the National Science Foundation for funding two grants:

in 2012, "Studying Field Emergence: HPV and the Expanding List of Oncoviruses" (Grant no. SBR-SES 1054024, Award Period September 2012–August 2015); and then in 2018, "Precision Public Health and the Politics of Cancer Prevention" (Award Period September 2018–August 2021). I am indebted to the support of the Science and Society program that funded two grants, each with a component focus on HPV. I thank the program officers at NSF who brought me into the peer-review process or oversaw my awards: Kelly Joyce, Kelly Moore, Wenda Bauchspies, and Fred Kronz.

Along the way I was invited to present my work-in-progress at many institutions. I thank the Yale University history graduate students for coordinating a workshop on Queering Science that allowed me to join Steven Epstein and Cindy Patton in conversation. I am grateful to the conveners of a workshop held at Princeton University and one in Berlin, each of which focused on the history of medicine and vaccines. I thank colleagues at the Center for Research on Women at the University of Michigan for discussing the chapters on anal cancer (and the great audience there!), and I am also grateful to my sociology colleagues for coming to my talks at the American Sociological Association meetings each year.

NSF funds provided time and travel monies; but more importantly, the awards supported research assistance and STS training for students at SF State. I was grateful to receive support from Jesus Gaeta, MPH, Bex MacFife (now a doctoral candidate in sociology), and Lucy Rios (now a doctoral student at University of California Davis), and Josh Calder, the amazing grant administrator at SFSU. Two PhD students in sociology came from the University of California San Francisco to work with me, including Mel Jeske (now at University of Chicago). It is Ashley Pérez to whom I am most indebted for her project leadership on the NSF award focused on cervical cancer screening. Ashley created the database of articles and materials from 2010–2020 on cervical cancer screening, organized files, and supported my work in myriad ways. But most importantly, she developed analytic memos and we co-authored two publications (in *Sociology of Health & Illness* and an edited volume on *Gender, Culture, and the Health of Children*) that shaped some of the ideas in this book. Thank you also to Elena Conis, Sandra Eder, and Aimee Medeiros for inviting our contribution.

While research for this book began in 2012 with the first of two NSF grants and a study of HPV and the other oncoviruses with sexual transmission routes, the story of HPV came to dominate conversations and the social dimensions of health and disease that unfolded for the next eight years. The bulk of my writing for this book took place during COVID-19 shutdowns and in the pandemic that continues to take lives. It was hard not to spend time on the particularities of the social life of COVID-19, another node in the ongoing story of social-cultural viral storms and stark evidence of the ways pandemics, but also risk, follow already established pathways of inequality. I appreciate the many conversations with friends, family, and scholars alike about how the ways we understand, talk about, and respond to health threats have consequences for prevention and care.

This book is entangled with the events and emotions of our present times as much as with the many historians, social scientists, and humanities scholars who remind us of other viral diseases and pandemics, from "Spanish flu" to Zika, SARS, MERS, and now monkeypox outbreaks. Special thanks to Susan Bell and Anne Figert for launching the Zika Social Science Network with me in 2016, and to the participants, especially Ilana Löwy, for joining in this conversation.

I am grateful to the Brocher Foundation on the shore of Lake Geneva, Switzerland for a residency award that kickstarted the idea of a book on HPV. While I had to leave most of the work done there on the editing floor, I was in love with my time and with the kind of intellectual thinking it allowed. I met the wonderful Francois Bayliss, who on long walks with me talked through some of the ideas here.

The hard planning for the book took place during a 2016 sabbatical and a "Wellfleet Fellowship" provided by family and friends through monetary and other supports. During a few amazing months that year and many summers since, I spent time being supported and refreshed by my friends and family as we ate and read and played and swam. Helen made frequent trips across the country to spend time together with me in our new home-place. The Cape allows amazing intellectual and queer communities that include a search for fun. I have been nourished by Susan Reverby, Anne Fausto-Sterling, Sarah Schulman, Jessica Fields, Jen Gilbert, Arlene Stein, Cynthia Chris, Susana Walters, and many artists, thought leaders, and vacationers alike who offer programs and events and make Provincetown and the outer Cape their home in summer or year-round. And it is there on the Cape that most of the sustenance from family also comes: time with Helen and joined by my moms, Ann D'ercole and Linda Brady, and my brothers, David Mamo and Tony Mamo, as well as Helen's sisters and our many nieces and nephews who make their way up to the Cape for summer meals and fun. Thank you all for making the trip! Mom was writing what became a two-volume set, a feminist biography of Clara M. Thompson, during this time, and we shared many adventures of citation, research, and editing along the way.

I must also thank my friends, many of them also academic mates, who have created a life with me. Don Lusty and Raymond Buscemi, Eleanor

Palacios, and Carol Copsy (who very sadly died from cancer midway through this book but left us Ovidio to care for); Jessica Fields and Jen Gilbert, with whom we share so much and plan our retirement together; Beth Marshall, who always helps during those crucial times of writing with sharp wit and a good laugh; Katrina Karkazis, Jennifer Fishman, Jenny Fosket, Kelly Joyce, Susan Bell, Steven Epstein, Anne Pollack, Jennifer Reich, Tony Hatch, Emily Mann, Patrick Grzanka, Jenny Reardon, and the many colleagues who either are part of my everyday life or are there yearly to toast and celebrate our accomplishments and share our struggles. This is what makes an academic life possible.

An extra shout-out to Katrina for introducing me to the amazing Frances Key Philips. It was the editorial direction provided on my first draft that really helped me to continue and to submit the manuscript for review to the university press I most hoped for. Frances, you became a coach as well as an editor, and I am most grateful to you. At University of Chicago Press I thank Karen Darling, Anne Strother, Beth Ina, and the production team for supporting this project and seeing it through, and the anonymous reviewers who championed my early draft.

Finally, I am grateful to the activists and advocates for health equity and justice, many of whom work as researchers and providers and gave time and thoughts to this project. I was not surprised to learn that most are of my generation, and like me came through the HIV/AIDS epidemic that sadly remains unresolved. I have admiration for the activists and people with cancer who have launched organizations or lost their lives. And my thanks to all the people I met who dedicate their work in some part to cancer prevention, especially those who like me share in the understanding that viruses and disease are social and interactive. It is often the discrimination that precedes any "outbreak" that shapes what unfolds in science and medicine, and ultimately among the people who get sick and die. This book is dedicated to a more just world.

Notes

INTRODUCTION

1. The history and continuities of discourse linking cervical cancer and sex as documented by scholars such as Lundy Braun and Nicole Garvey (Braun and Gavey 1999a, b) and Ilana Löwy (Löwy 2010a and b, 2011) provide important references for the arguments of this book about gender, sex, and cancer.

2. Epidemics usually refer to an outbreak confined to a place, while pandemic refers to a disease spread over much of the world. The attribution is not only noteworthy but also important for its stakes—in terms of how and where to mobilize resources, knowledge, prevention, and care.

3. I draw here on the title Samantha Gottlieb chose for her excellent book on the HPV cancer vaccine, *Not Quite a Cancer Vaccine* (Gottlieb 2018).

4. More broadly, virus association with the development of human cancers would be said, scientifically, to be attributable to up to 20 percent of cancers worldwide (Krueger et al. 2010).

5. "Pap test" refers to the Papanicolaou smear developed by George Papanicolaou in 1928. It was in 1941 that this approach entered medical practice with the republication of the Pap method, which spurred epidemiologic studies and screening protocols for cervical cancer. In the US the test was adopted by the American Cancer Society (ACS) and the National Cancer Institute (NCI) in the late 1940s (Swailes, Hossler, and Kesterson 2019). Pap testing became more widespread and institutionalized in the 1960s. For social histories see especially Clarke 1998.

6. The "junky flu" was known among IV drug users who knew something was amiss, yet this was largely subsumed by the early framing of HIV/AIDS.

7. Over time, the framing of the AIDS epidemic—which had ossified around the already stigmatized—would expand and be retold through the experiences of many additional parties, including HIV+ women, health care providers, researchers, and advocates (Hammonds 1997), all of whom coalesced into a formidable coalition of political activism (Schulman 2021). The early symptom presentation of HIV in women's bodies was rendered invisible by the CDC definition until feminists fought for definitional expansion. Similarly, insufficient knowledge and attention to Black sexualities, and a dominant focus on Black women's contraceptive and reproductive lives, shaped omissions and rates of Black AIDS (Fullilove et al. 1990; see also MacKenzie 2013). Activist efforts would shift these invisibilities and omissions (see Schulman 2021). Relatedly, what is referred to as "HIV exceptionalism"—the idea that HIV is an exceptional dis-

ease requiring an exceptional response—has impacted poor countries and by extension the women who reside there, by forcing countries to position themselves as suffering from HIV at the expense of other, often more pressing problems (including cancers) in order to receive the economic and other attention needed from science, medicine, and health and development organizations (Benton 2015; Livingston 2012).

8. The imagery of the inverted pink triangle, chosen to reveal the ghosts and legacy of homophobia and its entanglements with anti-Semitism and the atrocities of murdering Jewish people and others deemed deviant (https://www.poz.com/blog/story-behind-silence-death), was underscored by the bold text: Silence = Death. The message was one of protest over silence, inaction, and overt homophobia. It was a call to see linkage between a sexually transmitted virus, HIV, and its disease manifestations among those who were already marginalized and minoritized as social "deviants" and whom governments, researchers, and the general public already were prone to ignore.

9. I am indebted here to my collaboration with Steven Epstein that set out to analyze the biopolitical linkages between sexuality and health in the expansion and proliferation of the term "sexual health," and through the increased attention to sexually transmitted viruses and cancer. We co-authored numerous presentations as well as three publications (Mamo and Epstein 2014, 2016; Epstein and Mamo 2017). I am grateful for his conversations, support, and insights over those years before we eventually broke off as originally intended to write our own books.

10. I use the gendered terms "girls," "woman," and "women," and "boys," "man," and "men" mostly hewing to what researchers have used in direct quotes, media reports, presentations, and the scientific literature, etcetera. I recognize that genders are varied, multiple, and fluid, but especially constructed in discourse, such as biomedical and other knowledge systems. Given the focus on these products of the systems involved, I only use quotation marks around gendered terms when specifically drawing attention to that construction. I also often choose to use gender neutral and expansive terminology such as "all genders" or "women and people with a cervix" or "men and people with penises" to designate the ways gender does not always adhere to bodies, and thus to bodily risk.

11. Cancer is not only a set of diseases ripe with meaning; it is also widespread: the second leading cause of death and disability around the world, after heart disease. It is referred to as a "global epidemic" that is transnational yet unequal, with varying sets of causes and symptoms that shape the possibilities for diagnosis as well as effective treatment and prevention (Burke and Mathews 2017). It is cancers related to poverty and infection (mainly cervical, liver, and stomach) that are disproportionately represented in the global south, and efforts to prevent these require a broader focus based on combining vaccines with the development of effective means to assist people in both preventing and managing comorbidities like HIV and hepatitis B, as well as more investment in infrastructure and human rights. Incidence is increasing in less developed and economically transitioning countries (mostly in the global south) more than in developed countries (Jemal et al. 2010). Cancers are environmental and economic disorders rooted in material practices which vary among nations arrayed along a continuum from resource rich to resource poor (Burke and Mathews 2017). The association of chemical exposure and cancer causation has received little attention; as S. Lochlann Jain (2013) argues, more cancer could be prevented by reducing environmental exposure than by vaccination and screening. Further, the provision of timely diagnoses and treatments requires infrastructure, workforce, and expertise not

widely available in low- and middle-income countries, where investment would be most effective (Farmer et al. 2010).

12. The unevenness would continue into the twenty-first century. Thirteen thousand women across Europe were dying of cervical cancer annually; 57,000 in the World Health Organization (WHO)'s Africa region; 94,000 in Southeast Asia. In India more than 67,000 women would die each year from cervical cancer (25 percent of deaths among women) (WHO 2020).

13. This book largely focuses on Merck's Gardasil vaccine, which quickly became a dominant player, although much of the analysis applies equally to GSK's Cervarix. While Cervarix is FDA approved in the US, its market share was always low compared to Merck; in 2016, GSK chose to pull out of the US market altogether. The vaccine has 107 regulatory approvals that cover 136 other international markets (Sagonowsky 2016).

14. Research was approved by the Institutional Review Board of San Francisco State University. Due to the professional focus of the interviews, the professionals interviewed were offered the choice of being "on the record" or "off the record" in terms of their names and affiliations. Everyone I spoke with agreed to be "on the record," with one exception who wanted to wait until after I shared my research findings. Unfortunately, I was unable to reestablish connection; therefore I have de-identified this professional in terms of their interview statements, but not their open-source and publicly available research. Those I was able to re-contact at the end of my analysis were able to review the analysis and their quoted material and to confirm their consent. When names appear throughout the book they are either from open-source publications and media reports, from public conferences and professional presentations, or from consented human subject interviews.

15. The names of conferences are used given in their openly available information. Names were not used in observation notes unless these were professional presenters or the organizers asked me to do so. At small scientific meetings like this one, I would be introduced to the room and would make sure to let the audience know I was present and taking notes. For larger meetings, I would introduce myself at all informal exchanges. I am grateful to Fred Wyand and the National Conference Planning Committee for their invitation and their very generous scholarship, which paid for my stay and fieldwork at this important meeting. I am also grateful to Deborah Arrindell, then vice president of the American Sexual Health Association, for the warm welcome, and to all those who serve as NCCC delegates for allowing my presence and speaking with me throughout the meeting. NCCC was founded in 1996 as a grassroots nonprofit organization dedicated to serving women with, or at risk for, cervical cancer and HPV disease. In 2011 NCCC merged with the older American Social Health Association, a nonprofit with a nearly 100-year history and mission to educate and raise awareness on sexual health issues. NCCC has thousands of members around the world, and in the US chapters that make up its membership. A sister organization, the Global Initiative Against HPV and Cervical Cancer, has as its mission to work in low-resource and developing countries; and its own words, the organization serves as a platform to empower people, communities, and societies to reduce the disease burden from HPV and cervical cancers.

16. A large amount of the "data" for the book was generated by a database comprising journal articles, press releases, and media reports in online and newspaper outlets on HPV cancer and HPV screening from 2010 to 2020. I am grateful to Dr. Ashley

Pérez (Sociology, University of California San Francisco), who assembled this database during her role as project lead on the NSF study conducted at San Francisco State University (2018–2021).

17. Rosemary Taylor (1982) first used the phrase "the politics of prevention" when arguing that "prevention" in American health care policy is a contested domain. Different sets of problems and solutions shape this contestation. Which evidence is presented depends on which causal claim one espouses and what strategies one chooses to label as preventive. Taylor was speaking specifically of the 1970s US.political struggle, a contestation in which an ideology of individual self-responsibility moved into health care and preventive medicine. Depending on the causation theory, a different direction of prevention unfolds. Examining why such an ideology took hold in health care, Taylor argues that it is because it is congruent with cultural ideals more generally, the organization of health care, and people's subjective experience of the relationship between their health and aspects of everyday life. Two underlying theories about the causes of illness, she argues, shape the *politics of prevention*: 1) the threats posed by "late capitalism"—stress, toxins, contaminants, and accidents of large scale (oil leaks, etc.) (e.g., exposure to DDT and its causative role in cancer); and 2) the threats posed by individual behaviors, "diseases of civilization"—too much food, the wrong food, too much drinking or drugs, too little exercise, etcetera (e.g., cigarette smoking and its causative link to lung cancer). One is a social theory of the social determinants of disease, and the other is an individualistic theory of responsibility for one's health.

18. Sexuality has often been seen as problematic, something in need of containment and regulation. Aspects typically seen as problematic are mostly non-heteronormative or non-procreative sex, sexual activity within "age-inappropriate" pairings, or commercial transactive sex, as well as practices that transgress boundaries of race or social class (Rubin 2006 [1978]; Nagel 2000). Steven Epstein and I have argued that when the sexual and health are conjoined, the phrase "sexual health" often provides cover and legitimacy and is applied by an ever-expanding store of disciplinary knowledge as well as organizational and social movement groups (Epstein and Mamo 2017; Epstein 2021).

19. The concept of a cancer prevention regime is borrowed from Maren Klawiter's (2008) study of breast cancer. Klawiter shows how depending on the regime, the same diagnosis can be marked by medicalization and biomedicalization.

20. For example, although more than half of new cancer cases and about two-thirds of cancer deaths occur in low- and middle-income countries, about 57 percent and 60 percent respectively, only about 5 percent of global cancer resources are spent there (Beaulieu 2009). This reflects what Adia Benton (2015) described in her ethnography of development through HIV financing and care and its effects in Sierra Leone.

CHAPTER ONE

1. I am indebted to my coauthors Aleia Clark and Amber Nelson for our early collaborations in the Gardasil Working Group. This chapter includes modified and updated ideas from the coauthored chapter published in Wailoo et al. (2010). Aleia Clark wrote an excellent MA thesis at the University of Maryland on the early development of Gardasil as well (Clark 2008).

2. HPV is not a single virus but a group of viral genotypes. There are hundreds of HPV types, each consisting of two strings of DNA enclosed in a hard protein shell. HPVs can infect skin, mucous membranes, and what are referred to as "epithelial

zones"—regions in the body where two different tissues meet—of the soft, often inner linings of human tissue, where they induce what scientists refer to as a "spectrum of proliferative disorders" ranging in severity from warts to cancers.

3. There is a lack of certainty regarding the interactive effects of the virus and the growth and differentiation of the host cell. The immune response to papillomavirus infection is known to affect the degree and duration of disease, yet this contribution (and the social conditions that affect immunity) are less clear. HPVs also clear on their own or "shed" when immune systems produce antibodies, yet some can hide deep in the folds and hidden crevices of these zones and cause persistent infection and disease. It is important to continue to learn about the immune system response to the human papillomavirus if, and as, scientists seek to develop effective vaccines against other viral-associated disease.

4. These cellular changes, when present in the cervix, are what the Pap test screen has been used to identify (histologically, by microscopically examining the characteristics of the tissue cells) for half a century.

5. HSV, the herpes simplex viruses most known for genital and oral herpes, specifically HSV-2, was the first virus suspected in cervical cancer. That association was found to be false. For a history of causal discovery applying HSV and cervical cancer, see Brandon Clarke's dissertation, in which he distinguished three phases of discovery: *suspicion*, when researchers suspect that a new type of cause is at play; *domain finding*, when they detect the kinds of things over which the cause operates; and *making mechanisms*, i.e., constructing a mechanistic model, which is finally *applied* to disease populations (Clarke 2011).

6. zur Hausen's research first focused on the Epstein-Barr virus and its role in the development of Burkitt's lymphoma and nasopharyngeal carcinomas. The DNA technique applied in that research had shifted some of his efforts (with his collaborator, Heinrich Schulte-Holthausen) toward HPV. The suspicion that what was thought of as the genital wart virus, HPV, might also be the causative agent for cervical cancer led zur Hausen and colleagues to research this cause, documenting multiple human papillomaviruses. In 1983 zur Hausen's group, with colleagues Mathias Dürst and Michael Boshart, documented the isolation of HPV-16, and in 1984 the isolation of HPV-18 DNA as oncogenic viral types in cervical cancer biopsies from the HeLa line (from Henrietta Lacks) (Nobel Prize Outreach AB 2008). It was the isolation and characterization of the two most frequent HPV types in cervical cancer and the understanding of the mechanism of HPV-mediated carcinogenesis (cancer causation) that led to the development of a preventive vaccine. zur Hausen was awarded one half of the Nobel Prize for Medicine or Physiology in 2008.

7. The clinical application of this knowledge would come in the form of HPV testing for treatment and as a screening tool for prevention, the focus of chapter 5.

8. The Pap test refers to the Papanicolaou smear test, a procedure that collects cells from the cervix and examines them microscopically for cellular presentations classified as abnormal according to one of several classification systems used around the world (see FN5 Introduction and chapter 5).

9. Other infectious agents, including additional oncoviruses, as well as parasites and bacteria (e.g., *Heliobacter pylori*), are also linked to cancers, and some are transmissible person to person. With the inclusion of *Helicobacter pylori*, the proportion of cancers attributable to infectious agents rises to about 18 percent, or 1.9 million cases worldwide (Krueger et al. 2010: 5).

10. In the early 1990s, several research groups—including one led by Drs. Lowy and Schiller at the US NIH, laboratories supported by National Cancer Institute (NCI) grants at the University of Rochester, Georgetown University, and the University of Queensland (Australia)—independently discovered processes (called VLP) that enabled virus-like protective antibodies, leading to HPV vaccine discovery. The NIH Office of Technology Transfer (OTT) oversaw the patenting of the VLPs invented by Drs. Lowy and Schiller. OTT then sought a suitable company with the necessary resources to license the patent estates toward the end of formulating the vaccine and conducting clinical trials. The technology was licensed to Merck, the maker of Gardasil®. Merck's Gardasil 4 was licensed in the US in 1998 (US Patent No. 7,476,389) ("Vaccines and Immunizations" 2018), and the patent was extended almost a decade later, with Gardasil 9.

11. Patents enable pharmaceutical companies to set prices high and keep them high, requiring price negotiations from purchasers if they hope to reduce costs (or to buy out the patents altogether). Patents also establish "intellectual property" rights to limit competition from manufacturers of generic drugs. They enact barriers to expanding vaccination in low- and middle-income countries unable to afford such prices. One strategy of affording vaccines for low- and middle-income countries (LMIC) is to purchase patents or create "patent pools" by obtaining "voluntary licenses from patent holders and making these licenses available to generic companies in LMICs. Through the MPP, licenses to all patents required to produce a given end product are provided as a package to multiple generic manufacturers on a nonexclusive basis. These manufacturers must meet quality, safety, and efficacy standards, and must have access to markets that are large enough to achieve economies of scale and generate major price reductions. Royalties will be paid to patent holders, and generic licenses will be for use only in LMICs, thereby avoiding infringement upon the main target markets of brand-name manufacturers" (Crager 2018, S416).

12. The length of the patent period, as well as global policies like the Agreement on Trade-Related Aspects of Intellectual Property Rights, enforced since 1995 and administered by the World Health Organization (WHO), create unfair pricing and reduced competition (Chandrasekharan et al. 2015). To protect market monopoly, a common pharmaceutical company strategy is to apply for patents in Brazil, India, and China, in an effort to work around the exceptions built into the TRIPS Agreement for very low-income countries.

13. Between the first patent approval in 1998 and 2010, 81 HPV-vaccine-related patents were granted in the US, of which Merck held 24 (Padmanabhan et al. 2010). In the US, Gardasil patents will fully expire in 2028, given ongoing patent protections for new or extended uses (Songane and Grossmann 2021).

14. Unlike product brand advertisements, unbranded informational ads are more akin to public service announcements. In this case, however, they are produced by privately held and profit-driven pharmaceutical companies. They are also unlike "product claim advertisements," which are also regulated by the FDA and required to provide risk and benefit messaging. Unbranded ads were relatively rare. For Merck, the "Tell Someone" campaign was distinct from Merck's product vaccine advertisements ("Merck's New Gardasil Ads Omit Talk of Transmission" 2006).

15. The FDA is funded in part by commercial manufacturers, with pharmaceutical and biotech companies paying about $1.1 billion, or three-quarters of the agency's annual budget. The 1992 Prescription Drug User Fee Act (PDUFA) established the funding of the FDA in part through "user fees" intended to support the cost of swiftly

reviewing drug applications, thereby moving the FDA away from its earlier model as a fully taxpayer-funded entity (Demasi 2022). The potential for outsized influence is a major critique leveled at the FDA by academics and patient groups alike.

16. Merck won "Brand of the Year" from *Pharmaceutical Executive* in 2007 for their two-part campaign, divided into the unbranded, "disease awareness" effort of 2005 and then the post-approval, branded campaign which finally urged women to "get vaccinated" in 2006 (Herskovits 2007).

17. The elimination discourse and goal of the WHO and others is to reduce cervical cancer to a population threshold that is below 4 cases per 100,000 (World Health Organization 2020).

18. Vaccine effectiveness is a measure of how well vaccines work in the real world. See note 30 on efficacy. Fifty US states require the polio vaccine for students seeking to attend public school.

19. The National Foundation for Infantile Paralysis, better known for its "March of Dimes" campaign, had been in existence since 1939. Along with other charities, it launched "telethons"—the television + marathon fundraisers that produced ideas about illness, prevention, and good citizens as volunteers, charitable actors needed to eradicate disease and disability and provide care for those impacted by them (Longmore 2016). As Paul Longmore described, sex and sexuality were also narrated and produced by these spectacles, which were doing the work to stabilize traditional expectations of gender and sexuality in periods when such narrow norms were in flux.

20. For excellent vaccine histories see especially Conis 2010, 2011, 2013, 2015, 2019; Colgrove 2006, 2010; Colgrove, Abiola, and Mello 2010; Heller 2008; Reich 2018. For histories of HBV vaccine see Muraskin 1995.

21. The National Institutes of Health (NIH) and the NCI launched the US Virus Cancer Program in 1958, with an expert panel on viruses and cancer. Research sought a human cancer virus and ways to develop disease prevention (for a complete history, see Baker 2004; see also Pappas 2009, 962; Kuper, Adami, and Trichopoulos 2000, 172; Yi 2011). This followed the identification of the first "oncovirus," a human cancer virus, discovered in 1958 by Denis Burkitt (Burkitt 1958) and later affirmed in 1964, with the isolation of the Epstein-Barr virus (EBV) and its proven links to a type of lymphoma (see Epstein, Achong, and Barr 1964; see also Krueger et al. 2010, 4). In 1966 Rous was awarded a Nobel Prize for his assertion of RSV, a tumor-inducing virus (Kuper, Adami, and Trichopoulos 2000, 172). By the 1960s, sexual transmission of a virus was firmly established as a possible cause of various cancers, and cancer was rhetorically reconceptualized from unknown "emperor of all maladies" to infectious disease with a potential cure (Mukherjee 2010).

22. By the end of the 1970s, researchers were pursuing the conviction that viruses cause human cancers.

23. See note 24 for US vaccine mandates as of 2021. See Colgrove (2006) for the ways public health goals had to shift over the twentieth century from preventing and addressing serious, life-threatening diseases to promoting a generalized picture of health, particularly for children. To convince the public that these new vaccines were necessary, public health officials pioneered health education, taking cues from the "growth of advertising, marketing, and public relations" at the time in an attempt to integrate with the larger mass culture in the interwar and post–World War II periods (p. 94). Health was seen as a commodity, prompting efforts to effect change in individual behavior as health promotion techniques evolved.

24. As of 2021, according to the Pew Charitable Trust (DeSilver 2021), of the sixteen immunizations the CDC recommends for children and teens, all fifty states (plus the District of Columbia) mandate diphtheria, tetanus, pertussis (whooping cough), polio, measles, rubella, and chickenpox. Every state except Iowa mandates immunization against mumps. The diphtheria, tetanus, and pertussis vaccines are usually given as a single combined shot, as are the measles, mumps, and rubella vaccines. Except for the chickenpox vaccine, available since 1995 in the United States, all those vaccines have been around for fifty years or more. For a discussion of minor consent laws see note 45.

25. These ideas around the pharmaceuticalization of cancer prevention were developed in collaboration with my colleague Steven Epstein and published in the journal article "The Pharmaceuticalization of Sexual Risk: Vaccine Development and the New Politics of Cancer Prevention" (Mamo and Epstein 2014). For histories of hepatitis B vaccination see Mamo and Epstein 2014; Colgrove 2006; Conis 2011; Halpern 2021; Muraskin 1988, 1995. For comparative analysis with HPV and other STIVs as cancer prevention, see Mamo and Epstein 2016.

26. Social ideas concerning what it means to be gendered: a feminine woman or a masculine man is often encoded in and practiced through pharmaceuticalization and biomedicalization. Examples include Seasonale, a birth control pill, which was marketed as a means to maintain one's feminine role (Mamo and Fosket 2009), and the ways women's unhappiness in social relationships could be "treated" with psychopharmaceuticals, once known as "mother's little helpers" (Metzl 2003).

27. There is a vast literature documenting the gendered production of HPV vaccination in different countries that supports this analysis yet shows diversities given contextual particularities: In Austria, Paul (2016; Paul, Wallenburg, and Bal 2018) and colleagues describe how that country promoted the vaccine in ways that disassociated gender from youth sexuality, and Lindén (2017) described how discourse shifted from individual responsibility (individual girl "at risk") to the population level (all children as vaccine recipients). In Australia see Burns and Davies (2015) on the construction of gendered citizenship and Stagg-Taylor (2012) on the medicalization of women's bodies as disease-prone. In Canada see Cayen, Polzer, and Knabe (2016) on the ways female sexuality was deployed to elicit mothers' response; Connel and Hunt (2010), Mishra and Graham (2012), and Rail et al. (2018) on the moralization of health, often the responsibility of mothers; and Mishra and Graham (2012) on the production of a "woman only" discourse and sidelining of gay men as linked with discourses of gendering and racialization as it pertains to the framing of hesitancy (Charles 2013, 2014). In Barbados, Nicole Charles (2021) examines the ways hesitancy is constructed through processes of gender, racialization, and colonial discourse. In Colombia, see Maldonado (2017) on the linkage of state paternalism and gendered subjectivity. In Finland, Virtanen (2019) examined the framing of HPV vaccination as a "girls' thing" through a lens of the "pinkification" of girls. In Sweden, Lisa Lindén (2011, 2013) analyzes the ways girls are constructed as responsible citizens and how those ways are linked to a national discourse of girlhood and sexuality, often by addressing parents (2017). In the US, important early work examined cultural aspects of HPV vaccination, including gendering from both a local and a global perspective, including a volume edited by Wailoo, Epstein, and Livingston (2010) and articles by Carpenter and Casper (2009a, b).

28. The first DTC advertising came in 1981 when Boots Pharmaceuticals used print and television ads to promote Rufen, a prescription pain reliever. The market-

ing strategy was to position Rufen as a cheaper alternative to the leading brand. Merck was the second pharmaceutical company to promote a product directly to consumers, though they did so only through print (due to tighter restrictions). In 1982 Merck began advertising its pneumonia vaccine, Pneumovax, to people over the age of sixty-five in the then popular magazine *Reader's Digest* (Ventola 2011).

29. Meeting the "fair balance" mandate when it came to any "cancer prevention" tool was an easy task; in the case of Gardasil, if the vaccine protected against cancer (however far in the future that cancer might appear), and not just against the proximate and much more mundane and common STI, HPV, then the benefits would be so undeniably great that they would easily outweigh any potential harms from a vaccine.

30. Vaccine efficacy is a measure of how much getting a vaccine lowers the risk of getting sick (compared to not getting vaccinated). It is a measure, based on a clinical trial study, of how many people who got vaccinated developed the "outcome of interest" (usually disease) compared with how many people who got the placebo (no vaccine) developed the same outcome. These two numbers are compared, and a calculation is made about the "relative risk" of getting sick depending on whether or not one is vaccinated. To be approved for use, an efficacy measure of at least 50 percent (and usually much higher) is needed—i.e., a lot fewer people in the group who receive the vaccine get sick than the people in the group who receive the placebo.

31. From 1997 to 2005 when the HPV vaccine began its public launch, the total spending on pharmaceutical promotion had grown from $11.4 billion to $29.9 billion (see Donohue, Cevasco, and Rosenthal 2007).

32. In his book *Drugs for Life* (2012, 17) Dumit applies the concept of "surplus health" as a description of how pharmaceutical companies add medications to our lives by lowering the level of risk required to be "at risk." Dumit documents how thresholds for treatment get pushed ever further back into healthier populations in order to expand the health care market, especially for pharmaceutical companies, with the spurious promise that diseases are being prevented (regardless of the risks of the medications) and mass health improved.

33. Pre-approval marketing of Gardasil was secured through "Make the Connection" and "Make the Commitment" events produced by the Cancer Research and Prevention Foundation (CRPF—see http://preventcancer.org), and the celebrity charity Step Up Women's Network (SUWN—see http://www.suwn.org).

34. Historians of medicine have documented the racist entanglement of health, medicine, and gender in the twentieth century, and much of their work underscores a racist logic of biological difference. See especially Keith Wailoo (2011) on the cancer line, Rima Apple (2006) on "scientific motherhood," and Kristen Gardner (2006) on women's awareness campaigns. These document a message that is simultaneously and symbolically contiguous with twentieth-century messages—often eugenic claims juxtaposing white women's and girls' vulnerability and need for protection from a "white plague" with the scientific racist claims of "Black immunity" that punctuated the twentieth century. Such claims were often entangled with racist immigration policies and claims about racial identity, behaviors, and health (see Molina 2006; Shah 2001). On cancer specifically, see Reagan (1997).

35. A "will to health" (Rose 2001; Rose and Novas 2003) conceives of individuals as possessing a moral imperative to enhance their well-being through reconfigurations of the self and its bio-attributes.

36. I thank Steven Epstein for this point.

37. In a November 2007 issue of *Better Homes and Gardens*, a Gardasil ad reads: "Calling Gardasil a Cervical Cancer Vaccine Is Only the Beginning of the Story."

38. False claims against HPV safety were reported in 2015–2016 in Denmark and Ireland, derailing those programs for a brief time.

39. HPV vaccination requirements passed in 2009 for girls in the District of Columbia, in 2015 for all students in Rhode Island, in 2020 for all students in Hawaii, and in 2021 for all students in Virginia.

40. Other state legislatures across the US have proposed HPV vaccine requirements, with little success; opposition emerged mostly from parents and organizations advancing arguments along the lines of "given the airborne nature of diseases such as whooping cough, you can catch it in the classroom, but you can't catch HPV while at school."

41. New York Senate Bill S298B, act to amend the public health law, in relation to requiring immunization against human papillomavirus (HPV), (Hoylman-Sigal 2019), https://www.nysenate.gov/legislation/bills/2019/S298.

42. The term "anti-vaccination" is an anti-science stance, distinct from hesitancy, that is used to reflect a continuum of concerns for one's own and one's child's safety. One can be reluctant and hold ambiguous feelings about a vaccine without harboring anti-science sentiments or being involved in spreading misinformation (see Reich 2018; Dubé et al. 2021).

43. See also Cook et al. (2018), Zimet, Mays, and Fortenberry (2000), and Vázquez-Otero et al. (2016).

44. These ideas about girls are produced within, and yet stand in contrast to, other outbreak narratives from polio to mumps to SARS, Zika, and mononucleosis. Each holds its own distinct viral imaginaries, shared by the production and interaction of ideas performing the work of containing as well as promoting gendered, racialized, place-based, and sexualized stigma.

45. Minor consent laws in the US are designed to allow clinicians to provide services to young people without parental consent. The terrain is uneven: while most states allow minors to consent independently to STI/HIV testing and treatment, including human papillomavirus vaccination and HIV pre-exposure and post-exposure prophylaxis, the specific criteria applied vary, with many states unclear about confidentiality obligations for clinicians who care for independently consenting minors (Nelson, Skinner, and Underhill 2022). See also analysis by Anny Fenton and colleagues on the role of medical authority and patient perspectives in vaccine acceptance and administration during clinical encounters (Fenton 2019; Fenton et al. 2020).

46. In 2020, the Ad Council unleashed a campaign to overcome COVID-19 vaccine resistance in which the effort was unapologetically brought to the public by big tech companies such as Apple, Google, Facebook, and Salesforce in partnership with state and other non-state organizations. This could be read as a fait accompli, a final step in the "pharmaceuticalizing" of public health where multinational companies and advertising and public relations firms join with regional and federal government actors to promote "awareness" and products over largely privatized and unregulated social media networks well-versed in product placement tie-ins. Given the erosion of public support and financing of public health, this is certainly an important response intended to fill gaps in information.

CHAPTER TWO

1. Lena Dunham is the creator of the popular (albeit controversial) television show, which followed the everyday lives of post-college white and young women coming into (heterosexual) adulthood in Brooklyn, New York. The show is known for its representational politics as a show about "all young women" and the ways these girls are self-absorbed and dripping with white hetero privileged.

2. The episode includes some misinformation, perhaps intentionally. HPV tests were not recommended for or routinely performed on women under thirty in 2012 unless an abnormal Pap test warranted doing so as a triage or secondary information tool used in cervical cancer screening. If it were routinely tested for in this age group, it would not be during an STD panel, which does not include HPV (although some health tech companies are working on this possibility). While the episode implied that "if you have it" you can get treatment, there is no treatment for the virus, although one can screen with a cervical or anal Pap test for early clinical signs of pre-cancer or cancer. Finally, the fact that the vast majority of HPVs are transient, clearing on their own, is only alluded to when Jessa seems fairly comfortable with her "several strains" of HPV.

3. The conceptual understanding of the politics of inclusion emerged in his analysis of claims-making particularly in the 1980s and 1990s and institutionalized at the National Institutes of Health to reduce or ameliorate health disparities, particularly by race, ethnicity, and gender (Epstein 2007a, b).

4. The HPV vaccine is what scientists refer to as a recombinant DNA product composed of "virus-like particles" (VLPs)—specific proteins (55KD) of the L1 class (a self-assemblage of these proteins into a grouping that scientists refer to as a "family"). VLPs are produced by genetic technology to resemble the virus and produce a reaction called an immuno-response (by inducing antibody production) in the absence of the actual biological virus: VLPs contain no DNA; they do not contain the viral genome of "real" HPVs. These virus-like particles imitate the shape and structure of real viruses and mimic the infection that a real virus would ignite, thereby launching an immune response. This engineered vaccine, then, is unlike the majority of previous vaccines that relied on biologics—"natural" organisms such as animals, eggs, serums, and toxins, for example—as the building blocks of the immune response catalyzer. (Two other VLP engineered vaccines exist on the market today, both developed for the hepatitis B virus and promoted as a "cancer vaccine" given HBV's role in liver cancer.) From a manufacturing standpoint, the newer, molecularly engineered VLP process has advantages in terms of safety and efficacy: these engineered materials cannot replicate and do not require cultivation of live viruses. As a result, they do not have a risk for adverse mutations and accidental release. From a business standpoint, they are also more likely to ensure patent protection of the manufacturing processes than older vaccines that relied on biological processes. By the 1980s, vaccines and their potential outsized profits had moved firmly into the arena of tech and big business.

5. HPV vaccines could be designed to cover all of the known high-risk (HR) and oncoviral strains (15 HPV types), yet such a design would be incredibly costly to manufacture. Fewer VLPs made for a simpler, less costly formula. Vaccine development has relied on cross-protection—i.e., they do not explicitly protect against all HPV types, but they offer a significant proportion of cross-protection (Cho, Oh, and Kim 2011).

While none have (yet) been marketed, there are attempts to create "multivalent vaccines" that combine other pathogens. GSK, for example, has patented several vaccine combos—HIV and HPV, HPV and HSV, HPV and hep B—but these have not come to the market nor made media headlines (see Cho, Oh, and Kim 2011).

6. Data for the original FDA application was based on clinical evidence of the efficacy of Gardasil in reducing cervical warts in women ages 16 to 23—or 26, depending on which of the studies conducted from 2001 to 2009 was provided (see Markowitz et al. 2007). Merck had the evidence that Gardasil was effective in the prevention of genital warts in people with cervices (e.g., mostly girls and women). They brought this evidence to the FDA for disease indication. In doing so, Merck elected to immunize against the highest-risk cancer-causing strains, likely thinking the vaccine would therefore appeal to girls and women who would want to lower their risk of cancer. By adding VLPs against the two most prevalent non-carcinogenic strains, they could also appeal to boys (and their parents) who might not see themselves at risk of anal cancer per se but who would want to avoid genital warts. While the choices may have diluted the power of the vaccine's cancer coverage (by selecting only two known cancer-causing types), a less complex multivalent vaccine was cheaper and likely had fewer potential side effects than a vaccine of increased complexity might have had. In Europe, GlaxoSmithKline chose to focus their clinical trials and center their application for approval of Cervarix solely on links to cervical cancer (no surprise, given the name they chose), complicating the potential to expand the application and product market for genital warts. Cervarix was approved for use in the European Union in 2007, and in the US in 2009; it was discontinued in the US in 2015 with GSK citing very low demand (Darby and Kim 2020).

7. When Gardasil was released, pharmaceutical companies had only one example of a single-sex vaccine strategy—for rubella (measles), an airborne virus and respiratory disease that is also spread perinatally from mother to child, the latter vector representing its biggest source of transmission danger to health. The vaccine began as a single-sex strategy but is today most frequently known and administered as a childhood vaccine in the MMR vaccine, which combines protection against measles, mumps, and rubella.

8. The concept of the herd links the ideological values built into most vaccines that confer protection to a "vulnerable body" and/or "the social body" (the community), bound by space (Blume 2017). The "social body" of community had shifted some as lives became increasingly connected and interdependent through transnational flows of relations, migrations, commerce, and product. The concept of the "global" and a "global body" was ever present as COVID-19 ravaged the world, albeit unevenly, with vaccine rollout marked by vast global inequity. Whether immunity is defined as "global good" or "public good," or an "individual good," and for what community, population, or group, reveals its ideological values. The US historiography of HPV vaccination in the early years would indicate that immunity to HPV is not valued as a "public good"; such immunity was neither delivered to all members of the "community" nor delivered freely. This shaped (dis)trust in vaccines.

9. Inclusion in medicine has many social effects: it can provide needed intervention, it can medicalize and stigmatize, and it can also de-marginalize groups previously stigmatized, as these lives are legitimated as a concern for health—what Stefan Ecks (2005) refers to as "re-integrated into the social."

10. The sociologist and bioethicist Jennifer Fishman's research serves as a guide for

how to empirically study and conceptually understand medical technology diffusion. In her examination of sexuo-pharmaceutical drugs and devices (e.g., for erection difficulties and female sexual dysfunctions), she argued that the process of pharmaceutical development and implementation are "multi-directional and located within the drives toward the commodification of goods and services and consumer culture" (Fishman 2004, 210). She highlighted the importance of the *mediating relationships* that academic and other researchers, such as clinical trial investigators, have with pharmaceutical companies and consumers. She argues that to understand the meanings, markets, and diffusion of a technology requires understanding how each is built into multiple phases, from the development of a technology in the laboratory to the diffusion stage once it is approved. At the heart of her analysis is the *in between*, or what she refers to as the "commodification of technologies" before they are available for consumer use (Fishman 2004).

11. This in between is also reflected in the anthropologist Samantha Gottlieb's (2018) analysis of Merck's promotion of Gardasil using the theoretical framework of an anticipatory regime (Adams, Murphy, and Clarke 2009) to describe the ways Merck at once looks forward and backward to imagine the risk-free future and looks from the future of cancer back to what a parent would do.

12. In documents submitted to the FDA, Merck extensively cited a clinical trial underway investigating Gardasil's role in reducing the incidence of anogenital warts in young men, the results of which were subsequently brought to the FDA, in 2008. In a phase III efficacy study, Merck investigators enrolled 4,065 males ages 16–26 years from North America, South America, Europe, Australia, and Asia, excluding men with a history of genital warts or genital lesions (which could be HPV-related) and those with fewer than one, or more than five, lifetime sex partners. The research began collecting human subject data in September 2004, funded exclusively by Merck Sharp & Dohme Corporation (Merck's corporate name in Canada and Europe). For an analysis of the "hyphen-stage" as Merck planned for a vaccine release, see Aleia Clark's (2008) MA thesis, as well as a brief analysis of this stage of development in "The Pharmaceuticalization of Sexual Risk" (Mamo and Epstein 2014).

13. In 2008 Merck Research Laboratories submitted an FDA request for a Biologic License Application supplement (sBLA), with the goal of extending the existing licensing of Gardasil to boys and men 9 through 26 years of age for the prevention of genital warts (condyloma acuminata) caused by HPV types 6 and 11 (FDA 2009).

14. Findings were from the final analysis of the PATRICIA study showing that the HPV-16/18 AS04-adjuvanted vaccine (GlaxoSmithKline) has high efficacy against the pre-cancerous cervical lesions that can eventually lead to cervical cancer. The vaccine also showed cross-protective efficacy against other oncogenic (cancer-causing) HPV types closely related to HPV-16/18 (Paavonen et al. 2009).

15. Manos (2009) noted that the findings from Paavonen et al. (2009) suggest "that vaccination of women with previous HPV 16 or 18 infection might actually increase their risk of high-grade cervical disease." If this is the case and vaccination is contraindicated for those previously infected with HPV, excluding those with a previous infection in developing countries would not be feasible, Manos argued.

16. STDs denote the more than twenty-five infectious organisms transmitted through sexual activity, along with the dozens of clinical syndromes they cause (Eng and Butler 1997). The term has been shown to be symbolically associated with words like "promiscuity," "infidelity," "shame," "divorce," and "embarrassment" (Friedman

and Shepeard 2007). "Sexually transmitted infections" (STIs) is the common usage today to refer to infections caused by intimate relations as bodily fluids are exchanged through rubbing, friction, and various oral, vaginal, penile, and anal penetrations.

17. Keith Wailoo (2011) shows how the American awareness of cancer has been forged in its hidden racial and gender dimensions of the "war on cancer." Cancer took hold medically as a white women's disease affecting a population group in need of protection from their otherwise constructed vulnerability. In the early part of the twentieth century, reproductive cancers occupied nearly all of the focus on cancer as a disease, leading to multiple hypotheses about the relationship between cancer incidence and women's reproductive roles and morals. The observation that African American women experienced lower rates of cancer was understood through the racist lens as evidence that these women remained closer to their "natural" roles. By the 1960s, differences in cancer incidence between racial and ethnic groups drew increasing interest, and epidemiology emerged as a key source and narrative of these differences in cancer rates. These, according to Wailoo, led to environmental and structural possibilities as explanations for the variation. By the 1970s, cancer had effectively crossed the color line. That line would also be responsible for the language and contours of the world of STDs.

18. A series of books on the racism of the research conducted at Tuskegee University, often referred to as the "Tuskegee Study," include the 1993 book by the historian James Jones, *Bad Blood: The Tuskegee Syphilis Experiment*; Alankaar Sharma's (2010) *Diseased Race, Racialized Disease: The Story of the Negro Project of American Social Hygiene Association against the Backdrop of the Tuskegee Syphilis Experiment*; and Susan M. Reverby's *Examining Tuskegee: The Infamous Syphilis Study and Its Legacy* (2009).

19. In her recent political history *Let the Record Show* (2021), Sarah Schulman details how the historiography of AIDS activism continues its own gendered, racist exclusions as discourses of white gay men's heroism and queer failures continue to shroud the coalitional politics of ACT UP as a complicated and messy movement of Black, queer, and gay women, men, and gender activists. STDs and STIs often continue their symbolic adherence to poor women's bodies, driving hyper-surveillance; this exemplifies the ways racism shapes uneven biomedicalization, in this case over-medicalization. This is shown especially well by the legal scholar Khiara Bridges (2011).

20. Palefsky established the Anal Neoplasia Clinic, Research and Education Center (ANCRE). Public-facing UCSF websites describe ANCRE as "the world's first clinic devoted to anal cancer prevention." The clinic serves as the site for most of our HPV-related clinical research studies, and among other areas of interest the laboratory group focuses on developing new biomarkers and HPV-specific approaches to prevention and treatment of HPV-related cancer (ANCRE 2021). Palefsky and colleagues at UCSF were the first research group to publish findings, the only paper at that time, showing that Gardasil prevents anal HPV infection and prevents the very relevant clinical endpoint, anal cancer (or anal squamous intraepithelial lesions—ASIL). This research provided evidence to gain vaccination approval for boys.

21. ACS formed in 1913 as a cancer advocacy organization. The historian of medicine Robin Scheffler's book *A Contagious Cause* (2019) is excellent for its detailed coverage of the rise of viral cancer causation theories and research, and the organizations that supported these efforts, such as the ACS. He details that one of its most important early leaders was Mary Lasker, a fundraiser and lobbyist who helped create what Scheffler describes as the "biomedical settlement" (America's investment in medical research

over universal health care). The passage of the National Cancer Act in 1971 was a penultimate outcome of cancer claims-making by Lasker and others from a mysterious and complex disease beyond state intervention to a "knowable, and curable disease" able to be solved through federal investment in cancer research (Scheffler 2019, 80). Lasker's political and philanthropic efforts (she was a major fundraiser for what was the American Society for the Control of Cancer, ASCC) were part of a larger commitment to federal cancer research, and her efforts led to the funding and authority that allowed the National Cancer Institute (NCI) to grow into the major publicly funded cancer research institute that it is today. By the early 1970s, with the NCI in place, the ASCC (now renamed the American Cancer Society) increasingly turned its attention away from research and toward cancer prevention and education. Operating in alliance with the US government and its moon-shot injections of funding support, the ACS sees its mission as freeing the world from cancer through funding and conducting research, among other activities, including spreading the word about prevention.

22. Research had not yet substantiated an HPV link to oropharyngeal cancer, yet the evidence was accumulating to ultimately prove HPV-16's role in this cancer.

23. Gardasil 9 included protection against five additional HPV types: 31, 33, 45, 52, and 58. This was included in the patent for the processes of VLP incorporation received by the four-variant vaccine (US Patent No. 7,476,389). It would be approved in Europe one year later.

24. ACIP recommended routine vaccination for females 11–12 years old (with start date as early as 9), with "catch-up" recommended through age 26 for those not fully vaccinated or unvaccinated. ACIP's recommendation for Gardasil 9 for males almost mirrored that for girls; the one difference was that the "catch-up" for males was through age 21 or "age 26 years for men who have sex with men (MSM) and for immunocompromised persons (including those with HIV infection) if not vaccinated previously" (Petrosky et al. 2015, 300).

25. The Know HPV campaign "I Knew" segment included an "I Knew: Daughter" version as well.

26. https://www.versedhpv.com/. This website is no longer active as of May 2021. Instead, it has been hyperlinked to an anti-vax page called #unfollowHPV, with a companion Facebook page for this group. No other information has been located about the source.

27. Klick Health is a branding firm with offices in North America. Founded in 1997, the company develops, launches, and supports life sciences brands (Klick Health 2021). Klick's revenue has grown 40 percent every year since its founding, and it has emerged as one of the largest independent digital health agencies (Klick Health 2014).

28. https://www.versedhpv.com/. Website no longer active (see note 26 above).

29. As Beth Snyder Bulik reported, "Versed" generated "3.8 million Snapchat swipe-ups, 374 million impressions on Instagram, 276 million YouTube views, and 4.9 million unique visitors to the campaign within their first year of launch" (Bulik 2019).

30. The YouTube channel was removed during my research period, and I am unable to reconfirm and share these links. The Instagram account is also no longer active.

CHAPTER THREE

1. Rare cancers, according to the National Institutes of Health, affect fewer than 40,000 people per year in the US, and together make up just over a quarter of all

cancers. All HPV-associated cancers, including cervical cancer, are rare by this designation.

2. Abigail C. Saguy (2020) shows how the concept of "coming out" has been used in five distinct contexts: the American LGBTQ+ movement, the fat acceptance movement, the undocumented immigrant youth movement, the plural-marriage family movement among Mormon fundamentalist polygamists, and the #MeToo movement.

3. The Anal Cancer Foundation (ACF) was founded in 2010 by three siblings whose mother, Paulette, died of stage IV HPV-related anal cancer (see https://www .analcancerfoundation.org). The Farrah Fawcett Foundation was founded the same year, in 2010, one year after Fawcett's death (see https://thefarrahfawcettfoundation .org/).

4. Lowy would be named the Acting Director of the National Cancer Institute in 2015. He is best known for his research leading to the development of the HPV vaccine.

5. A repressive force was unleashed in November 2013 when the American Council of Gynecology issued a press release stating that gynecologists could only provide care to women, or they would lose their medical board license. The effect of the statement was that care for men was not approved, including anal cancer screenings performed by gynecologists. That the statement came out during a major meeting on anal cancer research and care was coincidental. Meeting attendees quickly ignited their activist side, making calls and drafting letters about how such a policy would exclude not only trans men and genderqueer patients, but also all men seeking HRA specialists, most of whom are gynecologists. The ABOG definition was overturned after several months of political exchange and pushback from members as well as from professional organizations including ASCCP, IANS, ABOG, most of it on the basis that the new definition was discriminatory toward transgender people and resulted in unequal health care for LGBTQ people (Grady 2013a and b).

6. "Epistemics" refers to knowledge and its formation, specifically relating to how claims are produced, validated, and put into practice. I draw on studies of the classifications used in epidemiology (e.g., race, gender) by Shim (2005) and Wemrell et al. (2016), and in social movements by Epstein (1996), as well as in clinical trials more generally. The concept of epistemic exclusion addresses possible exclusion of older people, women, and ethnic/racial minorities, and is intended to help reduce the unwanted effects of biomedical interventions on clinical research (Epstein 2007a; Rosengarten and Michael 2009; Rosengarten 2009; Will 2009; Will and Moreira 2010).

7. In cancer, for example, these include mammography for breast cancer, Pap testing for cervical cancer, and colonoscopy for colon cancer. In medicine more generally, they include diagnostic tests for viral infections such as HIV and other STIs, COVID-19, and non-viral diseases such as diabetes, for example.

8. Health disparities research focuses on historically produced and systemic health differences in population groups shaped by oppression and inequality. Racism along with other intersectional oppressions such as homophobia are part of the production of health as well as illness, and part of the social movement struggles embodied political efforts to form coalitions (e.g., at the center of much of AIDS activism, for example—see Schulman 2021).

9. The historian of medicine Julie Livingston's (2012) ethnography of an oncology ward argues that such exceptionalism shaped the ways cancers, especially cervical can-

cer, would go unfunded and thus often untreated in low-income countries often reliant on NGOs and the World Health Organization to set a (funding) agenda.

10. As of January 1, 2019, the MACS and Women's Interagency HIV Study (WIHS) combined to form the MACS/WIHS Combined Cohort Study (MWCCS)—see their website: https://aidscohortstudy.org.

11. Anal cytology is usually accompanied by a manual exam called the digital (anal) rectal exam (DRE or DARE), similar to the pelvic exam. DRE is performed using a lidocaine and lubricating jelly. It is performed to detect anal masses or areas of hardness (signs of cancer) and to direct the exam to areas of concern. A lubricated, gloved finger is swept over the entire circumference of the anal canal and used to feel for masses, warty growths, ulcerations, or hard areas. The finger is swept externally to palpate for suspicious external areas.

12. Anoscopy provides a visualization of the anus, anal canal, and lower rectum. The anoscope/anal speculum includes a small plastic disposable cylindrical tube with a light on the end. A cotton swab—thinly wrapped with a single ply 4 x 4 cotton gauze square soaked in 3 percent acetic acid—is inserted through the anoscope, remains in the anus for 1 minute, and is then removed. As the anoscope is slowly withdrawn from the rectum, binoculars of the colposcope are used for visual inspection of the anal epithelium (Palefsky et al. 1997; University of California San Francisco Department of Medicine 2014).

13. Lesions are sized and located with different classification systems (AIN and CIN are two such systems). AIN 1s are smaller lesions with questions as to whether they will regress or recur if removed; they are also challenging to remove. The uncertainty lies with smaller lesions and whether they will regress or progress. Larger lesions (AIN 2 and 3) are removed. See chapter 5 for a longer discussion.

14. Cervical cancer rates and deaths reflect geographic, racial, and socioeconomic disparities. Cervical cancer infrastructures are also uneven. Mortality rates can range from more than 50 per 100,000 in Malawi (Sung et al. 2021) to a low of about 2 per 100,000 in the US (Arbyn et al. 2020).

15. A small percentage (11 percent) of HIV+ gay and bisexual men in health care in the US have received anal Pap smears; moreover, the national average obscures clear regional differentials (Freedman et al. 2016). IANS was, in part, formed to advocate for the health needs of a subset of people who continue to be the objects of health care's biases and structural discrimination.

16. I highlight again that throughout this book not all people with a cervix are women or identify as such.

17. Whether to remove a "pre-cancer" (and those that are ambiguous in classification as opposed to a lesion of clear significance) as a preventive approach has not yet been settled in anal cancer prevention.

18. Scarce was drawing on the important work of cultural critics writing about gay men's health and HIV/AIDS in the 1980s, such as Treichler (1999), Patton (1982, 1985, 1990), and Sontag (1989).

19. An AIDS-defining cancer is defined as a type of cancer that a person infected with human immunodeficiency virus (HIV) is at high risk of developing. If a person with HIV develops one of these cancers, it moves them from having an infectious infection, HIV, to having AIDS. AIDS-defining cancers include KS, certain types of non-Hodgkin lymphoma, and cervical cancer.

20. Another cancer organization in the US focused on lesbian, bisexual, and transgender women with cancer is the Mautner Project in Washington, DC, founded in 1990 (now, since 2013, part of the Whitman Walker Health Clinic). "Respectability politics," coined by Evelyn Brooks Higginbotham in 1993 in her book on Black women's activism in the Baptist church (Higginbotham 1993), refers to the standards and norms of conduct applied especially to Black women. The term was borrowed across marginalized groups, including in feminist and queer theories that advocated that LGBTQ rights were part of respectability politics that rendered sex positivity, non-monogamy, and other aspects of "bad manners" outside of claims for political rights to marriage and family, for example.

21. It was a surprising and important moment of discovery for me when Margolis recognized me as the "not-daughter" of one of those close friends. She knew my second mother, Adria Schwartz, who had then somewhat recently—in January 2003—died of ovarian cancer. Margolis and Adria were avid tennis partners and friends.

CHAPTER FOUR

1. In the US there are many organizations that issue guidelines for cancer screening: American Academy of Family Physicians (AAFP), American College of Obstetrics and Gynecologists (ACOG), American Cancer Society (ACS), American Geriatrics Society (AGS), American Medical Association (AMA), American Society for Clinical Pathology (ASCP), and the American Society for Colposcopy and Cervical Pathology (ASCCP) and US Preventive Services Task Force (USPSTF)—often in combination with the Canadian Task Force (CTFPHC). See also chapter 7.

2. In 2013, Robert Yarchoan's introduction at this fourteenth annual meeting provided some history of the National Cancer Institute (NCI) and the need for a central office to coordinate and prioritize research and reorient HIV funding. In 2007, NCI, under the leadership of John Niederhuber, established the Office of HIV and AIDS Malignancy (OHAM), with Yarchoan as director. Interaction of HPV and HIV was a central component of newly funded research, as was made clear by the sessions at this meeting.

3. Dr. Andrew Grulich was the principal investigator at SPANC.

4. The risk for HIV+ women is less clear. It is estimated that 2 or 3 of every 10 HIV+ women have anal HSIL or pre-cancerous lesions, yet it remains unknown how many HIV+ women will develop anal cancer over their lifetime. Research is, however, developing to show that HIV+ women who have had other HPV-related cancers may be at higher risk. While anal cancer is rare in the general population, for HIV+ people anal cancer incidence is increasing as more people live longer (Silverberg et al. 2012).

5. "About the Study," https://www.anchorstudy.org/about, accessed May 2015.

6. EUROGIN is now referred to as the Multidisciplinary HPV Congress.

7. The SPANC clinical trial research study's goals were: 1) to determine the prevalence, incidence and risk factors for anal HPV genotype detection and associated lesions; 2) to investigate rates of clearance and persistence of anal HPV infection; 3) to investigate rates of progression and regression of intraepithelial anal lesions; and 4) to assess the psychosocial/quality of life (QoL) impact of screening in "homosexual men" (quotes are mine) (Kirby Institute 2021).

8. CIN (Cervical Intraepithelial Neoplasia) is a classification system for Pap test cervical cancer screening results based on thickness of abnormality into the epithelial (skin)

tissue. Each of the three tiers of CIN *may* and *can* become cancer. They are referred to as "precancerous" designations and also simply as "dysplasia." See chapter 5.

CHAPTER FIVE

1. Douglas was diagnosed with tongue cancer, though he initially said (on advice from doctors) it was the less disfiguring throat cancer. Oropharyngeal cancer (OPC) as a diagnostic category includes the back of the tongue. A more recent *New York Times* article states: "He is also a survivor of Stage IV cancer, diagnosed in 2010—a 'large, almond-size tumor at the base of my tongue,' as Douglas described it. 'We made a strategic decision to say that it was throat cancer,' he said, 'because the connotations of having your tongue removed and not being able to speak was not a pretty picture.'" https://www.nytimes.com/2018/11/14/arts/television/michael-douglas-the-kominsky -method-netflix.html.

2. Smoking cigarettes has varied widely over time, undergoing several gendered, racialized, and classed symbolic associations: first attached to men, masculinity, and power; then to upper-class and largely white women's emancipation (Amos and Ha-glund 2000; Brandt 1996); and finally to a shifting racialized class base (Graham 1994; Wailoo 2021b). Evidence of a masculine gendered production of health risk can be found in work by Riska (2002, 2006, 2010) as well as Courtenay (2000) and Rosenfeld and Faircloth (2009). For discussions of the intersectional constructions of masculinity, racialization, and health and illness see Ferber (2007) and Hickey (2006), and for work on the ways medicine and pharmaceuticals construct masculinity, risk, and health see Fishman (2006), Potts (2000), Faro et al. (2013), and Valier (2016).

3. Structural gendered racism is part of health experience, outcomes, and narra-tives, and was revealed (again) in COVID-19 (Laster Pirtle and Wright 2021).

4. The AFA is a Mississippi-based Christian organization and lobbying group founded in 1977 as the National Federation for Decency. AFA is identified by the South-ern Poverty Law Center as one of 838 hate groups across the US.

5. As of 2021 the states with anti-sodomy laws on their legislative books are Alabama, Florida, Idaho, Kansas, Louisiana, Michigan, Mississippi, Missouri, North Carolina, Oklahoma, South Carolina, Texas, Utah, and Virginia.

6. In 1994, Yuan Chang (a pathologist) and Patrick S. Moore (an epidemiologist) isolated DNA fragments from a KS tumor in an AIDS patient and published an article in *Science* reporting what they labeled "KS-associated herpesvirus-like (KSHV) sequences" (Chang et al. 1994). It was in their research at the University of Pittsburgh Medical Center that the findings of KSHV were established in 1984, and Merkel cell polyomavirus (MCV) in 2008. These are two of the seven human viruses to which 20 percent of cancers worldwide and approximately 30 percent of cancer cases in low- and lower-middle-income countries are attributed (Krueger et al. 2010; WHO 2022).

7. For an analysis of the sexualization and desexualization of KS in relation to the other oncoviruses, see Mamo and Epstein (2016).

8. The article reviewed epidemiological findings from the 1990s that had correlated cervical cancers with various UADT cancers, within which the smaller grouping of head and neck squamous cell carcinomas (HNCCs) are included. This cervical-UADT cancer link "tipped off" researchers to a possible HPV-UADT link (see Newell, Kre-menz, and Roberts 1975), which was only reinforced by the absence of any history of tobacco or alcohol use in those diagnosed.

9. Data comprised people who indicated "any heterosexual relationships" who were asked about the lifetime number of opposite-sex partners, whether oral sex had been performed on any opposite-sex partner, and the total number of opposite-sex oral sex partners. Men were asked about sexual orientation since puberty: exclusively heterosexual, primarily heterosexual, heterosexual and homosexual, primarily homosexual, or exclusively homosexual (see Schwartz et al. 1998, 1627).

10. IARC assembled a working group to study HPV's role in oral cancers in 2009, and announced finding in 2012 that 12 types of HPV (2, 3, 6, 11, 13, 16, 18, 31, 33, 35, 52, and 57) found in the oral cavity were associated with malignant lesions (Bouda et al. 2000), with HPV 16 as the most common subtype and HPV 33 accounting for up to 10 percent of cases (Kim et al. 2014; Snow and Laudadio 2010).

11. The evidence presented by cancer treatment specialists that HPV tumors were far more responsive to treatment than those without HPV positivity fueled further research. Other cancers of the throat, as oncologists with specialization in the *treatment* of head and neck cancers knew well, left patients with very debilitating and life-altering side effects.

12. The article was a cautionary and somewhat fearmongering tale for almost all forms of sex, warning that everything is a risk, even "virgins" who engage in open-mouth kissing and sex between those in monogamous relationships.

13. Some may already have been familiar with the well-known chef, Grant Achatz, and his diagnosis in 2007 with tongue cancer. In some reporting, a connection was drawn between this cancer and oral sex, yet the story of Schatz's cancer would be most widely popularized following his book release in 2011 (NPR 2011).

14. Researchers, it was reported, had drawn these conclusions following a study of 4,493 adult men using oral rinses and penile swabs to test for HPV as well as completing a behavioral survey (Hrustic 2017a).

CHAPTER SIX

1. A similar surprise came in a conversation I had at the annual meeting of the National Cervical Cancer Coalition in Atlanta the same year (see Introduction).

2. Risk-assessment tools calculate risk scores and produce the evidence needed to create an intervention program. These tools are part of the biopolitical project of monitoring and shaping risk, health, and disease by defining intervention groups to target for biomedical and pharmaceutical approaches. See Holmberg, Bischof, and Bauer (2013, 401).

3. The risk assessment infographic contrasts with what some refer to as "populationism" tools such as the Breast Cancer Risk Assessment Tool (BCRAT)—which is based on a statistical model known as the Gail Model, named after the physician who developed it (Fosket 2004)—or the diabetes risk score (DRS) model (Holmberg, Bischof, and Bauer 2013, 401).

4. OraGen announced in 2021 that by using a simple oral rinse, their laboratory services can detect the presence of high-risk HPV strains, with genotyping available for the two highest-risk subtypes (HPV 16/18) (Compass Laboratory Services 2021). The company is working to gather results that might someday gain FDA approval and allow them to offer a tool more useful than visual inspection. No new screening has been proven effective, and none have received FDA approval as of October 2022.

5. A field of LGBTQ health, and specifically lesbian health and health disparities,

has been part of social movements for more than thirty years. Yet the vast majority of research compares the same population groups: heterosexual men, gay and MSM men, and women (unspecified and thus presumably heterosexual). There has been some research specifically conducted with lesbian subgroups when it comes to cancer and other health disparities, including Pap smear screening rates and cervical cancer incidence and disparities. Although sexual orientation data is not routinely collected by cancer registries, therefore making it challenging to directly examine population-level cancer rates by sexual orientation, research has confirmed that lesbian, bisexual, and queer women are likely at increased risk of certain cancers due to heightened behavioral risk factors, such as increased rates of smoking and alcohol use (Case et al. 2004), attributable to minority stress and structural discrimination (Krueger, Fish, and Upchurch 2020; Hatzenbuehler et al. 2013). Further, their cancer risk may also be heightened as a result of disparities in sexual health care utilization as well as in use of cancer screening: i.e., lower rates of recent Pap testing among lesbian women, attributable to various factors including lack of health insurance, fear of discrimination, and lower levels of provider recommendation due to assumptions of low risk among lesbian women (Agénor et al. 2014; Matthews et al. 2004; Marrazzo et al. 2001; Cochran et al. 2001). Further, women and those who are part of queer and/or LGBTQ categories are subjects of cervical cancer research as well as its cancer screening apparatus. Researchers have identified barriers for screening among many genderqueer, queer, and LGBT groups, including lesbians (see especially Marrazzo et al. 2001), and disparities among cancers (Brown and Tracy 2008), and health advocacy organizations like Fenway Health and the National LGBT Cancer Network are working to ensure equity in cancer screening and treatment for these groups. It is the world of LGBTQ STI prevention that may be the best place for asking different questions and learning more about how queer and gender diverse people can prevent disease individually as well as collectively.

CHAPTER SEVEN

1. The "annual exam" was replaced by the "wellness exam," a nomenclature and set of recommendations that emerged in the 2000s once the Pap test was no longer the driver for women's clinical office visits (Shulman 2006). The longer interval of three to five years for Pap tests was affirmed in March 2012 by the USPSTF, and came with recommendations for updated nomenclature for office visits by the International Federation of Cervical Pathology and Colposcopy (see a discussion by Rahangdale 2012). The wellness exam and its purpose, frequency, and activities are still unsettled. The usual components of the "well-woman exam" variously include a pelvic exam (with an external genital exam, speculum exam, cervical cancer screen, and bimanual exam) as well as a manual breast exam, which also serves as a prompt to educate patients about how to conduct their own self-exam. According to Harvard Women's Health Watch, this exam would focus on "well-being" and include health education, screening for chronic disease risks, and assessing health concerns from depression to alcohol and drug use to intimate partner and other violence (Cappiello and Levi 2016; American College of Obstetricians and Gynecologists 2018). A "Well-Woman" Chart was launched in 2018 by the Women's Preventive Services Initiative that outlines the preventive service recommendations of the USPSTF, with a separate table of vaccine recommendations from the Advisory for Immunization Practices (https://www.womenspreventivehealth.org/wp-content/uploads/WellWomanChart.pdf).

2. The 2019 ASCCP risk estimator, described in chapter 8, would come to define a risk of having CIN3+ at that moment. This means that in the case of CIN3+, HPV tests offer a "true risk" given various combinations of test results (Demarco et al. 2020). See also asccp.org and the risk estimator clinical application. A full discussion appears in chapter 8.

3. In 2015, Denmark became the first country to include "stand-alone" HPV testing as a primary prevention approach (in lieu of the Pap test) in its cervical cancer screening program; since then many other countries have followed suit. As this chapter and next chapter 8 show, the US, in contrast, began to implement the practice widely in 2018 when the US Preventive Service Task Force (USPSTF) issued guidelines recommending HPV tests alone (or co-test or Pap test alone) as a cervical cancer screening strategy for individuals age thirty to sixty-five. Debate emerged over whether a combination of HPV test and Pap test, the HPV test alone, or the Pap test alone was the best tool for cervical cancer screening. By 2020 this had started to change.

4. Epidemiologically, effectiveness typically refers to the ability of an intervention (e.g., a test) to lead to changes in disease morbidity or mortality, and thus goes beyond the accuracy of a test.

5. The terms "sensitivity" and "specificity" were introduced by the American biostatistician Jacob Yerushalmy in 1947. *Sensitivity* is the extent to which actual positives are not overlooked (false negatives are few and the test correctly detects ill patients who do have the condition), and *specificity* is the extent to which actual negatives are classified as such (false positives are few, the test is able to correctly identify those without the disease). A highly sensitive test rarely overlooks an actual positive; a highly specific test rarely registers a positive classification for anything that is not the target of testing; and a test that is highly sensitive *and* highly specific does both (it "rarely overlooks a thing that it is looking for" *and* it "rarely mistakes anything else for that thing"). Sensitivity, therefore, quantifies the avoidance of false negatives and specificity does the same for false positives. A perfect predictor would be described as 100 percent sensitive, meaning all sick individuals are correctly identified as sick, and 100 percent specific, meaning no healthy individuals are incorrectly identified as sick. In medical diagnoses, for example, if 100 patients known to have a disease are tested, and 43 test positive, then the test has 43 percent sensitivity. If 100 with no disease are tested and 96 return a negative result, then the test has 96 percent specificity.

6. The evidence indicate that test and treat, for example, has evolved as a biomedical approach to prevention and early detection. It was paying off in HIV as viral loads were suppressed with antiviral treatment.

7. For social histories of cancer, see especially Aronowitz 2007; Davis 2007; Wailoo 2011; Mukherjee 2010; Creager and Gaudillière 2001; Löwy 2010a and b, 2011; Timmerman 2013; Creager and Landecker 2009; Landecker 2007; Proctor 1995; and Mei 2009. See also Patterson 1987; for analyses into the invisibility of environmental causes see Jain 2013 and Klawiter 2008. Ilana Löwy, Keith Wailoo, Robbie Aronowitz, and most recently Robin Wolfe Scheffler provide exemplary histories of cancer that each include some part of the convergence told here; I am indebted to their work. See also note 10 below for some histories of gynecological and cervical cancer.

8. Rigoni-Stern's research would displace the previously held presumption of some common biological origin that shaped all cancers and document a protective effect of celibacy in uterine cancers among nuns, thereby prompting the assertion that it must

be the sexual activity among the married that predisposed them to higher rates of cancers (Aviles 2015).

9. The marker event of note is said to be in 1911 when Peyton Rous isolated a cancer-causing virus in animals: the Rous Sarcoma Virus or RSV (zur Hausen 2006, 2). A viral vector (along with a bacterium) took hold in cancer causation. The finding of "horizontal transmission," in this case from bird to bird, was significant in that it provided conceptual proof of possible human-to-human viral transmission, including sexual transmission.

10. Gynecology and obstetrics have shameful pasts of surgical experimentation on Black women's bodies from slavery into the twentieth century. Formed in abuse, professional gynecology was largely a surgical practice. Cancer (shaped as diseases of the womb and reproduction), however, was racialized as a "white disease" and gendered as a "woman's disease." For histories of gynecology and cervical cancer see Murphy 2012; Löwy 2011; McGregor 1989, 1998; Clarke 1998; Roberts 1997; Washington 2008.

11. In the 1970s that screening for breast cancer became a national priority using the mammogram: a radiation tool that can both diagnose illness and screen asymptomatic bodies. Like the Pap smear, this technology was not immediately accepted; it took significant negotiation for the mammogram to become the right tool for the job of breast cancer prevention (Howson 1999; Klawiter 2008; Clarke and Casper 1996; Clarke and Fujimura 1992b).

12. Sexuality has long been part of medicalization and biomedicalization processes and the exercise of power (from nymphomania to homosexuality to infertility), representing a part of a twentieth-century shift from badness to sickness (Conrad and Schneider 1980) and demedicalizing processes moving phenomena from sickness to health (homosexuality). Bringing sex into a connection with health, with the designation of sexual health, has been a legitimizing linkage (Epstein and Mamo 2012, 2017). For a short review of research on the medicalization, demedicalization, and biomedicalization of sex and sexuality see Fishman, Mamo, and Grzanka (2017).

13. Of the 200 HPV types, about 40 genital types are referred to as alpha types and thus as a concern for cancer. The vast majority of these 200 HPV types are considered "beta" and/or "gamma" and infect other types of skin or epithelium (e.g., types that cause common skin warts).

14. A surrogate marker or endpoint is used in clinical trials when the clinical outcome—in this case invasive cancer—might take a long time to find expression and thus provide the study with a result. Some clinical endpoints are "validated," meaning the connection between the surrogate marker and the disease is well understood—e.g., the amount of HIV and the occurrence of AIDS.

15. Histories of epidemics (Prescott 2000; Dubos and Dubos 1987; Rosenberg 1962; Briggs and Mantini-Briggs 2004; Leavitt 1997; Rogers 1992; Hammonds 1999) are instrumental here as well, specifically those that are transmitted in part or exclusively through sexual means. These are especially important for the ways they explicitly brought scientific and public claims of risk and responsibility and stigma and blame into play that, in turn, influenced how states, science, and medicine responded to and shaped disease. Historians have shown the ways such productions—sexual in connotation—reinforced and produced homophobia, racism, and the visibility and/or invisibility of women. For social histories of the STDs see especially Jones 1993; Treichler 1999; Altman 1986; Cohen 1999; and Brandt 1985. In turn, approaches to

global governance of disease were shaped by xenophobia and racism. For excellent histories of racialization and governance of disease see especially Shah 2001; Gamble 1997; Reverby 2009; and Molina 2006. And see the recent review titled "Epidemic Inequities" (Wailoo 2021a).

16. Frequent screening can lead to unnecessary tests (colposcopy) and harms (stress, emotional and physical discomfort) and trigger additional diagnostics in search of either confirming or disconfirming diagnostic knowledge.

17. Roche is the common use name of "Roche Molecular," a subdivision of the large Swiss pharmaceutical and diagnostic firm Hoffman-La Roche formed in 1991. Roche was formerly F. Hoffman-La Roche AG, founded in 1896 in Switzerland. For a history of Roche and molecular cancer see the historian of science and medicine Carsten Timmerman's book, *Moonshots at Cancer: The Roche Story* (2019), which focuses on therapeutics but also includes a brief section on diagnostics.

18. Roche acquired the worldwide marketing rights to PCR from Cetus Corporation in 1991.

19. DNA target amplification is a laboratory-based procedure that duplicates DNA fragments from a target sequence of a gene, thus providing concentrated samples of a specific genetic sequence. Several types of DNA target amplification technologies exist; however, PCR is the most commonly employed in HPV detection. PCR is a standard laboratory procedure that can be adapted for the detection and typing of HPV (Malloy, Sherris, and Herdman 2000).

20. In 1983, at zur Hausen's lab in Germany, Reid's in Michigan, and Manos's at Cetus (Reid 1983).

21. The results were published in the journal *Applied Pathology* in 1987 (zur Hausen 1987). When BLT first started their research into HPV, they found that many cervical tumors were not infected with HPV types 16 and 18, compelling them to change their focus from developing an HPV test for those viral types to instead identifying other HPV genomic types associated with cancer. The lead researcher, Lorincz, and others patented their discoveries. BLT gained approval for the first HPV test in 1988; the test was not commercially successful, and in 1990 BLT sold its molecular diagnostics division to Digene. It was Digene that took a tool to the FDA (see Hogarth, Hopkins, and Rodriguez 2012; Hogarth, Hopkins, and Rotolo 2015).

22. Molecular techniques can be broadly divided into those that are not amplified, such as nucleic acid probe tests, and those that utilize amplification, such as polymerase chain reaction (PCR). Amplification techniques include: (1) *target amplification*, in which the assay amplifies the target nucleic acids (for example, PCR); (2) *signal amplification*, in which the signal generated from each probe is increased by a compound-probe or branched-probe technology; and (3) *probe amplification*, in which the probe molecule itself is amplified (for example, ligase chain reaction). To date, target and signal amplification techniques, in addition to non-amplified techniques, have been applied to the detection of HPV (Malloy, Sherris, and Herdman 2000).

23. HC is an assay test, an analytic test to detect nucleic acid targets directly, using signal amplification. The first HC test was patented in 1992 and approved by the FDA in late April 1995 as ViraType Plus HPV DNA No. 890064 S003. Digene would be acquired by QIAGEN in 2007.

24. The nine types are: 16, 18, 31, 33, 35, 45, 51, 52, and 56.

25. A second-generation hybrid-capture technology, HCII, added four additional

"high risk" (hr) HPV genotypes—39, 58, 59, and 68—and was approved by the FDA in March 1999 (approval no. P890064; Malloy, Sherris, and Herdman 2000).

26. The first publication using the technique came out in 1989 (Manos, Ting, Wright, et al. 1989). See the website https://www.michelemanos.com/about-michele .html to learn more about Manos in this history as well as science studies research by Hogarth, Hopkins, and Rotolo (2015, 95) and Shibata, Arnheim, and Martin (1988).

27. While accounts vary, Cetus was started in about 1971 (according to Roy D. Merrill it was in 1973) and is regarded as the first biotech company. Kary Mullis, a Cetus employee, received the 1993 Nobel Prize in chemistry for inventing the PCR method. Cetus sold their PCR process, the most important discovery in biotechnology of the twentieth century, to Hoffman-La Roche in the early 1990s. Hoffman-La Roche then later renamed itself Roche and has made tens of billions of dollars leveraging the PCR method into a diagnostics company. "Roche," as the company is now commonly known, is a publicly traded company with a reported 2019 market capitalization (the total dollar market value of a company's outstanding shares) of more than $200 billion. Along with technological processes, Roche acquired many smaller companies as it grew into this multibillion-dollar company, including the (originally) San Francisco Bay–area startup Genentech (Engineering and Technology History Wiki [ETHW] 2021).

28. Hogarth and I met through my prior research examining the set of STI viruses associated with cancers that include and yet also lie "beyond HPV."

29. The Bethesda System for Reporting Cervical Cytology (Bethesda System) was introduced in 1988 and revised in 1991 and then 2001 when ASCUS was added as a reporting category of interpretation of results based on morphological criteria of shape and size of cells. See note 32 below on classification systems. The terminology of ASCUS changed to ASC-US following an update to the Bethesda System. I use the second version throughout this book.

30. LB Cytology was developed by Cytec in 1996 and later trademarked as "Thin-Prep" (Hologic would later acquire Cytec); a similar tool, "Sure Path," developed by Autocyte, would later be acquired by BD.

31. A particularly American concern were the increases in legal liability (and need for medical malpractice insurance) from false negative results that were later followed by diagnoses of cervical cancer or, ultimately, death. For providers and health systems, this liability was an unwelcome economic exposure. Overcompensating for ambiguity with referral or more testing was a reasonable accommodation, even though it added costs.

32. Three Pap test classification systems coexist, each with their own ambiguities: 1) the WHO and Pan American Health Organization (PAHO) system of mild, moderate, and severe dysplasia; 2) the Richart system (largely used by colposcopists), with three tiers (or stages) of intraepithelial neoplasia: CIN1, CIN2, CIN3; and 3) the Bethesda System, largely used by cytopathologists and cytotechnicians, that differentiates between low- and high-grade squamous intraepithelial lesions (L-SIL to HSIL, including ASC-US as the ambiguity). Another system, most often used in German-speaking countries, differentiates cytology results using a scale of low, moderate, and severe dysplasia as categorized by levels of "cervical intraepithelial neoplasia" or CIN. CIN categorization is a histological grade system of CIN 1, 2, and 3 (Kainz et al. 1995). While CIN1 was once aligned with LSIL, and CIN2 and CIN3 with HSIL, these have

diverged and differences have emerged in how to classify disease using this system, depending on the HPV type or biomarkers (Waxman et al. 2012; American College of Obstetricians and Gynecologists 2011; see also Löwy 2011 and Jug and Bean 2020).

33. Examples of new *pre-disease* states (pre-diabetic, pre-bone density, etc.) reflect processes by which individuals previously considered healthy are now categorized in an at-risk of disease state and clinical diagnoses of preexisting disease are extended to "earlier" points in a disease's natural history.

CHAPTER EIGHT

1. Two significant studies examining the Hybrid Capture (HC) tools are by Schiffman et al. (2000) and Wright et al. (2000), both using the HC2.

2. Roche is the common use name "Roche Molecular," which is a subdivision of the large Swiss pharmaceutical and diagnostic firm Hoffman-la-Roche formed in 1991.

3. BD is the common use name for Becton, Dickinson and Co., a New Jersey–based global medical technology company.

4. CIN is a three-tier classification, CIN-1, CIN-2, and CIN-3, with each classification determined by the microscopic visual inspection of cells from colposcopy. CIN-1 and CIN-2 carry the greatest uncertainty, and are often considered "not cancer"; however, any sample classified CIN, especially 3, *may* and *can* become cancer. See chapter 7, note 32 on the various classification systems, specifically the Bethesda and Richart.

5. https://www.thinprep.com.au/thinprep-pap-test-for-hcps, accessed July 21, 2020; by September 4, 2021 it had become passcode protected.

6. Digene Corporation (now QIAGEN) sought US FDA approval in 2000 for a four-in-one-sample assay to concurrently test for HPV, *Neisseria gonorrhoeae, Chlamydia trachomatis*, and herpes simplex virus using the procedure (Malloy, Sherris, and Herdman 2000).

7. Sponsorship of an article in EmpowerHER include a website link to www.theHPVTest.com, a site that is no longer active; hits on that site were diverted to a company site called HerQIAGEN (https://herqiagen.com/hpv/), accessed on August 23, 2021.

8. Groups opposing primary testing ranged from patient advocacy organizations such as Cervivor to professional associations such as the National Association of Nurse Practitioners in Women's Health, the National Black Nurses Association, and the National Hispanic Medical Association. All of these groups wrote or co-authored letters in support of USPSTF's recommendation to retain co-testing as an option, and not to shift to primary HPV screening.

9. Melnikow and colleagues conducted a meta-analysis (performed and reviewed by the USPSTF) of eight RCTs, 5 cohort studies, and their own individual participant data meta-analysis that was published in the flagship journal of the American Medical Association, *JAMA* (Melnikow et al. 2018). The evidence showed that HPV testing led to greater decreases in cervical cancer than cytology alone. The largest clinical trials had triaged everyone with a positive HPV test to colposcopy (something never done in the US) in an effort to increase detection and treatment of CIN3+ and thus lead to decreases in cancers.

10. The 2003 FDA approval of Digene's Hybrid Capture 2 High Risk HPV DNA Test (Digene would later be acquired by QIAGEN in 2007) was the first FDA-approved test. It was followed by four others: In 2009 Hologic received FDA clearance for two HPV

assays. In 2011 Roche and Gen-Probe (acquired by Hologic) received FDA approvals for their tests. Each of these tests works differently and is approved for different uses. Hybrid Capture shows the presence or absence of the genetic (DNA) material from the human papillomavirus (HPV), and then DNA probe molecules are added that can differentiate HPV types. This test is used only in conjunction with Pap testing (Medical Laboratory Observer staff 2012). A description of these can be found on the Medical Laboratory Observer site: https://www.mlo-online.com/home/article/13004462/the -five-fdaapproved-hpv-assays.

11. DNA is isolated from cervical cells, and mixed in reaction wells with primers and probes that specifically recognize and amplify HPV DNA. A reaction produces fluorescence, which is then measured to determine the presence of HPV in the cervical sample.

12. HPV 31, 33, 35, 39, 45, 51, 52, 56, 58, 59, 66, and 68.

13. Other recommendations include referring a normal Pap result and a positive HPV test result to genotyping for HPV 16 and 18, or repeating both the Pap and HPV tests in one year. The proposed guideline recommends against immediate colposcopy; women having a mildly abnormal Pap result (called ASC-US) and a negative HPV test result should be monitored by either HPV testing plus Pap or HPV testing alone at intervals of three years or longer. The guidelines did not recommend or oppose primary screening and reasserted screening for people who have been vaccinated against HPV.

14. See Docket No. FDA–2014–N–0001.

15. Submitted under P100020/S008.

16. "Nonpregnant US women ≥ 21 years of age presenting for routine cervical cancer screening (n = 47,208) were enrolled in this observational study between May 2008 and August 2009. . . . This study is registered with ClinicalTrials.gov (NCT00709891) and was completed in December 2012" (Wright et al. 2015, 190).

17. Roche also produces histology and cytology tests (CINtec® Histology and CINtec® PLUS Cytology). "The CINtec® Histology test is the only 510(k) p16 biomarker for clinical/IVD use in the evaluation of cervical biopsy specimens" (Roche 2021). This test can be used by pathologists to increase the sensitivity and specificity of cervical precancer diagnoses. The CINtec® PLUS Cytology was approved in the US in 2020, joining earlier guidelines already in place in France, Germany, Hong Kong, South Africa, Portugal, and Spain. The test can also be used as a "biomarker test" to triage cervical cytology results; to triage cervical cytology-negative/HPV+ results; and as an "HPV+ screening" tool. The claim in support of this tool, similar to what I began hearing for HPV testing in general, was to avoid unnecessary colposcopy following abnormal Pap or combination results of some kind (Roche 2020).

18. The letter was sent by the following cosigners: American Medical Student Association, American Medical Women's Association, American Public Health Association, Annie Appleseed Project, Cancer Prevention and Treatment Fund, Community Catalyst, Connecticut Center for Patient Safety, Consumers Union, Jacobs Institute of Women's Health, National Alliance of Hispanic Health, National Consumers League, National Organization for Women, National Physicians Alliance, Our Bodies Ourselves, The TMJ Association, Women Advocating Reproductive Safety, and Woody Matters, as well as the following individuals: Benjamin A. Gitterman, MD, Nancy S. Hardt, MD, Vivian W. Pinn, MD, FCAP, John H. Powers, MD, Alexandra Stewart, JD, and Duchy Trachtenberg, MSW, with contact Information: Anna Mazzucco, PhD. On April 24, in response to the coalition letter, the FDA wrote a letter announcing that the

HPV test had been approved for primary use. (As of August 2021, the response letter is no longer on the Stop Cancer website; it may be accessed via the FDA archives.)

19. This was the position of the National Women's Health Network (2015).

20. The cobas test platform was unchanged: it provides pooled results on known high-risk HPV genotypes (31, 33, 35, 39, 45, 51, 52, 56, 58, 59, 66, and 68) and individual results on the two highest-risk types, HPV 16 and HPV 18.

21. Along the way, in 2020 BD Onclarity had received FDA approval for its HPV Assay as a primary test, making it the second HPV test to gain primary approval (it is also approved for co-testing and triage use). BD Onclarity Assay was extended from its 2006 original use as a triage tool (see note 25).

22. Nancy G. Brinker, who wrote the opinion piece in *USA Today*, is an adviser to Hologic.

23. A Facebook post also flagged that the financial connection between Hologic and ASCP poses a conflict of interest: "Let me understand this, Hologic doesn't have a primary screen test, owns the majority of the reference lab business, and they fund this e-policy letter discouraging primary screen—that's a problem. All reference labs have to do is acquire the technology to offer primary screen, but that would be from a company OTHER than Hologic."

24. This is referred to as "populationism" by the German researchers Cristine Holmberg, Christine Bishof, Susanne Bauer, and Marc Parascandola (Holmberg, Bischof, and Bauer 2013; Holmberg and Parascandola 2010), where individual-level information is aggregated to the population level in order to inform risk stratification and cervical cancer screening schema.

25. In 2006, BD had submitted their own (and first) pre-market application to the US FDA for the BD Onclarity™ HPV Assay, their HPV test, to be used with their own trademarked Pap tests and automation system in a total solution similar to QIAGEN's. The original request and evidence was for referral to colposcopy for ASC-US results. This was extended to primary testing in 2020.

CHAPTER NINE

1. It is well documented that gynecology and reproductive medicine are sites of misogynoir (gendered racism), with a history of abuse of Black women's bodies in the name of science and medicine (Murphy 2012, Roberts 1997, Washington 2008). Scholars have examined the extraction of women's reproductive labor as part of racial capitalism (Weinbaum 2019), rendering visible the coerced experimentations on Black and enslaved women (Owens 2017, Morgan 2011) as well as the continued inequities that follow from racist claims about bodily difference (Kapsalis 1997, Owens 2017). Angela Davis, Faye Ginsburg and Rayna Rapp, Evelynn Hammonds, Dorothy Roberts, Deidre Owens Cooper, Harriet Washington, Laura Briggs, Sydney A. Halpern, and others have shown a history of exploitative and extractive research in the name of science, often perpetrated within a logic of US imperialism. Twentieth-century examples include unethical clinical trials such as the Tuskegee trial for the study of syphilis (Reverby 2009), the Willowbrook study of hepatitis B and its vaccine research (Halpern 2021), studies of the birth control pill in Puerto Rico and among "mentally ill" people in Massachusetts, and the Uganda HIV trials. See also the Guatemalan syphilis study and the ways John Cutler obtained the cooperation of the PHS, the Guatemalan government, and the Pan American Sanitary Bureau. See https://publichealth.jhu.edu/2020/leadership

-on-syphilis-studies-for-better-and-for-worse; and *Health and Humanity: A History of the Johns Hopkins Bloomberg School of Public Health, 1935–1985* by Karen Kruse Thomas (2016). See also: Interview with Dr. Heller: https://history.nih.gov/display/history/Heller%2C+John+R.+1964; and https://aquila.usm.edu/cgi/viewcontent.cgi?article=1242&context=ojhe.

2. In *Dear Science and Other Stories*, Katherine McKittrick (2021) illustrates the ways scientific knowledge systems, as harms, are consistently interrupted by Black writers, scholars, creative artists, and storytelling more generally with powerful interventions against legacies and continuities of anti-Black science. "Rebellious methodologies," McKittrick asserts, "are needed to live outside of oppressive knowledge systems that continue to render the lives of Black and other marginalized people as dispossessed." Black feminist scholars such as Karla Holloway, Evelynn Hammonds, Alondra Nelson, Dorothy Roberts, Christina Sharpe, and McKittrick shed historical and social light on the way scientific knowledge systems perpetuate assumptions that some bodies and lives matter more than others.

3. The WHO cervical cancer elimination plan is based on a 90–70–90 plan to vaccinate 90 percent of girls age 15; to ensure that 70 percent of women are screened with a "high performance test" by age thirty-five and again by age forty-five; and to ensure that 90 percent of women with pre-cancer are treated and 90 percent of women with invasive cancer are managed (WHO 2020).

4. The Henrietta Lacks Foundation was founded in 2010 by members of the Lacks family with a mission to honor Lacks's memory by collaborating with other organizations focused on medical injustice and providing funding and grants to family members and young people pursuing education.

5. The anthropologist and historian of science and medicine Hannah Landecker's book, *Culturing Life*, emphasized the transformation of biology into capital (biocapital—Landecker 2007). Chapter 4 of Landecker's book examined the HeLa cell line as part of this story of the ways cells became technologies, being cultured and reproduced in lab dishes and ultimately made into components used to transform what she describes as the immutable building blocks of individual bodies into the flexible and malleable resources of biotechnology, and of life itself.

6. Joseph Earle Moore headed the Johns Hopkins syphilis clinic and "Department L" at Johns Hopkins (see Reverby 2009, 8, 136). The historian Susan M. Reverby is the source for the findings in the Moore papers, which she described in her 2009 book and in personal communications.

7. While syphilis is not associated with the onset of any cancer, it is part of how ideas about sex and disease entangle socially and medically. Reverby has written extensively on what is often referred to as the Tuskegee Trial, infamous for its known racist logic and intent: the Black men with syphilis in the clinical trial study were knowingly denied treatment either with the (ineffective) heavy metals that were in standard use at the time, or with penicillin even after it was known to be an effective treatment. Instead, public health researchers and medical providers followed the "natural history of the disease," allowing undue suffering for the men in the study who had this disease, as well as for the family members who were subsequently infected and/or were witness to the men's often terminal suffering.

8. See "The Miracle of 'Hela,'" 1976, https://libguides.cfcc.edu/c.php?g=321640&p=2151431, accessed October 10, 2021.

9. Parham spoke of the young women in their twenties, thirties, and forties who are

dying premature deaths from what he called a preventable disease. Those women leave young people behind in the poorest and harshest environments, where "deep poverty, starvation and communicable diseases are biting at their heels on a daily basis." Parham cites research by IARC (the research arm of WHO) showing that across the continent of Africa, for every 100 young women who die of cervical cancers, up to thirty children under age ten will also die. These people and places cannot access or purchase the treatments that are available in high-income countries.

10. These include discourses of scientific racism, sexism, and assumptions of normative heterosexuality, as well as the intersectional racism and homophobia proclaiming Black men's bodies to be hypersexual and "risky" for white women, a biopolitical trope used for repression, containment, and criminalization from colonial times to the present (Brandt 1985, Jones 1993).

11. In 2006, the same year Gardasil entered the US market, the FDA authorized DTC advertisements for genetic testing (Curnutte and Testa 2012), and a panoply of companies moved into this domain of consumer-directed marketing to sell IVDs that had until then been exclusively used in clinical care and medical research.

12. Steben may have been referring to a systematic review conducted by the WHO in 2018 finding that "HPV self-sampling can increase cervical cancer screening uptake compared with standard of care" (Yeh et al. 2019).

13. ROSE was partially funded by the Compass trial for which self-sample kits and partial funding came from Roche (and for which kits were donated by Seegene, Cepheid, BD [Becton Dickinson], Abbott, AusDiagnostics, and Atila Biosystems for research purposes). Investigator-initiated study grants also came from Roche and Merck, Sharp, and Dohme, and the University Malaya has also received kits from Cepheid, Roche, and Becton Dickinson for study purposes. See https://www.hpvworld.com/media/29/media_section/4/4/3344/hpvworld-177.pdf.

14. The set of six viruses, with some degree of sexual transmission, that are now said to accounted for up to 20 percent of the cancers diagnosed around the world (Krueger et al. 2010). These other viral-cancer connections—HHV-8 and the cancer Kaposi's sarcoma; hepatitis B (HBV) and hepatitis C (HCV) and liver cancer; human T-lymphotropic virus (HTLV) and adult T-cell leukemia/lymphoma; and the Epstein-Barr virus and lymphoma—are also part of the long, newly reinvigorated search for a contagious cause of human cancer. See Mamo and Epstein (2016) for the ways each held distinct sexualization and desexualization processes as they moved from pre-AIDS to the new millennium.

15. Hepatitis B vaccine success also hinged on the suppression, management, or "taming" of sexual dynamics related to the risk of infection. Desexualization was accomplished by construing the vaccine as a tool of cancer prevention and by working to move the vaccine target from adults (with the messy and complex politics surrounding their sexual identities and practices) to newborns, who by virtue of their age are free from such associations (Mamo and Epstein 2014).

16. See the press release on the Antiva company website: http://www.antivabio.com/news/2021/110221.php, accessed November 3, 2021.

Bibliography

Abraham, John. 2010. "Pharmaceuticalization of Society in Context: Theoretical, Empirical and Health Dimensions." *Sociology* 44 (4): 603–22.

Adams, Vincanne, Michelle Murphy, and Adele E. Clarke. 2009. "Anticipation: Technoscience, Life, Affect, Temporality." *Subjectivity* 28 (1): 246–65. https://doi.org/10.1057/sub.2009.18.

Agénor, Madina, Nancy Krieger, S. Bryn Austin, Sebastien Haneuse, and Barbara R. Gottlieb. 2014. "Sexual Orientation Disparities in Papanicolaou Test Use among US Women: The Role of Sexual and Reproductive Health Services." *American Journal of Public Health* 104 (2): e68–e73. https://doi.org/10.2105/AJPH.2013.301548.

Altman, Dennis. 1986. *AIDS in the Mind of America.* New York: Anchor Press.

Altman, Lawrence K. 1982. "New Homosexual Disorder Worries Health Officials." *New York Times*, May 11, 1982.

American Cancer Society. 2005. *Cancer Prevention and Early Detection: Facts and Figures.* Atlanta, GA: American Cancer Society.

American Cancer Society. 2014. *Anal Cancer: Key Statistics.* Atlanta, GA: American Cancer Society.

American Cancer Society. 2020. "Cancer Facts for Lesbian and Bisexual Women." Last modified July 30, 2020, accessed March 22, 2021. https://www.cancer.org/healthy/cancer-facts/cancer-facts-for-lesbian-and-bisexual-women.html.

American Cancer Society. 2021. *Cancer Facts & Figures 2021.* Atlanta, GA: American Cancer Society.

American College of Obstetricians and Gynecologists. 2011. "Frequently Asked Questions: Understanding Abnormal Pap Test Results." Accessed January 16, 2023. https://www.acog.org/womens-health/faqs/abnormal-cervical-cancer-screening-test-results.

American College of Obstetricians and Gynecologists. 2018. "ACOG Committee Opinion No. 755: Well-Woman Visit." *Obstetrics & Gynecology* 132 (4): e181–e186. https://doi.org/10.1097/aog.0000000000002897.

American Society of Clinical Oncology. 2021. *With Strong Screening & Vaccination Guidelines, Cervical Cancer Rates Drop; Other HPV-Related Cancers Are On the Rise.* Alexandria, VA: American Society of Clinical Oncology.

Amos, Amanda, and Margaretha Haglund. 2000. "From Social Taboo to 'Torch of Freedom': The Marketing of Cigarettes to Women." *Tobacco Control* 9 (1): 3. https://doi.org/10.1136/tc.9.1.3.

ANCRE. 2021. "Anal Neoplasia Clinic, Research and Education (ANCRE) Center."

UCSF Health, University of California San Francisco. Accessed July 2, 2021. https://www.ucsfhealth.org/clinics/anal-neoplasia-clinic-research-and-education-ancre-center.

Aninye, Irene O., Michael J. Berry-Lawhorn, Paul Blumenthal, Tamika Felder, Naomi Jay, Janette Merrill, Jenna B. Messman, Sarah Nielsen, Rebecca Perkins, Tami Rowen, Debbie Saslow, Connie Liu Trimble, and Karen Smith-McCune. 2021. "Gaps and Opportunities to Improve Prevention of Human Papillomavirus-Related Cancers." *Journal of Women's Health* 30 (12): 1667–72. https://doi.org/10.1089/jwh.2021.0507.

Apple, Rima D. 2006. *Perfect Motherhood: Science and Childrearing in America.* New Brunswick, NJ: Rutgers University Press.

Arbyn, Marc, Silvia de Sanjose, and Elisabete Weiderpass. 2019. "HPV-based Cervical Cancer Screening, Including Self-Sampling, versus Screening with Cytology in Argentina." *The Lancet Global Health* 7 (6): e688–e689.

Arbyn, Marc, Sara B. Smith, Sarah Temin, Farhana Sultana, and Philip Castle. 2018. "Detecting Cervical Precancer and Reaching Underscreened Women by Using HPV Testing on Self Samples: Updated Meta-analyses." *BMJ* 363 (December 5). https://10.1136/bmj.k4823/.

Arbyn, Marc, Elisabete Weiderpass, Laia Bruni, Silvia de Sanjosé, Mona Saraiya, Jacques Ferlay, and Freddie Bray. 2020. "Estimates of Incidence and Mortality of Cervical Cancer in 2018: A Worldwide Analysis." *The Lancet Global Health* 8 (2): e191–e203. https://doi.org/10.1016/S2214-109X(19)30482-6.

"Are Pap Smears on the Way Out?" 2014. Editorial, *New York Times*, May 4. https://www.nytimes.com/2014/05/05/opinion/are-pap-smears-on-the-way-out.

Aronowitz, Robert A. 2007. *Unnatural History: Breast Cancer and American Society.* Cambridge and New York: Cambridge University Press.

Aronowitz, Robert A. 2009. "The Converged Experience of Risk and Disease." *The Millbank Quarterly* 87 (2): 417–42.

Aronowitz, Robert A. 2010. "Gardasil: A Vaccine against Cancer and a Drug to Reduce Risk." In *Three Shots at Prevention: The HPV Vaccine and the Politics of Medicine's Simple Solutions*, edited by Keith Wailoo, Julie Livingston, Steven Epstein, and Robert Aronowitz, 21–38. Baltimore, MD: Johns Hopkins University Press.

"ASCP Articulates Serious Concerns with ACS Cervical Cancer Guidelines." 2020. *ASCP ePolicy News*, August 28. https://www.ascp.org/content/news-archive/news-detail/2020/08/28/ascp-articulates-serious-concerns-with-acs-cervical-cancer-guidelines#.

Aviles, Natalie B. 2015. "The Little Death: Rigoni-Stern and the Problem of Sex and Cancer in 20th-Century Biomedical Research." *Social Studies of Science* 45 (3): 395–415. https://doi.org/10.1177/0306312715584402.

Bakalar, Nicholas. 2008. "Oral Cancer in Men Associated with HPV." *New York Times*, May 13, 2008, Health. https://www.nytimes.com/2008/05/13/health/13canc.html.

Baker, Carl. 2004. *An Administrative History of the National Cancer Institute's Viruses and Cancer Programs, 1950–1972.* Washington, DC: National Institute of Health, Office of History.

Baltzer, Nicholas, Karin Sundström, Jan F. Nygård, Joakim Dillner, and Jan Komorowski. 2017. "Risk Stratification in Cervical Cancer Screening by Complete Screening History: Applying Bioinformatics to a General Screening Population." *International Journal of Cancer* 141 (1): 200–209. https://doi.org/10.1002/ijc.30725.

Banerjee, Dwaipayan. 2020. *Enduring Cancer: Life, Death, and Diagnosis in Delhi*. Durham, NC: Duke University Press.

Barrett, Thomas J., John D. Silbar, and James P. McGinley. 1954. "Genital Warts—A Venereal Disease." *Journal of the American Medical Association* 154 (4): 333–34.

Bauer, Susanne, and Jan Eric Olsén. 2009. "Observing the Others, Watching Over Oneself: Themes of Medical Surveillance in Society." *Surveillance & Society* 6 (2): 116–27.

Bean, Anna. 2012. "Let's Hear It for the Girls!" *BUST*, April 4, 2012.

Bell, Susan E. 2009. *DES Daughters: Embodied Knowledge and the Transformation of Women's Health Politics*. Philadelphia, PA: Temple University Press.

Bell, Susan E., and Ann E. Figert. 2012. "Medicalization and Pharmaceuticalization at the Intersections: Looking Backward, Sideways and Forward." *Social Science & Medicine* 75 (5): 775–83. https://doi.org/10.1016/j.socscimed.2012.04.002.

Benard, Vicki B., Cheryll C. Thomas, Jessica King, Greta M. Massetti, V. Paul Doria-Rose, and Mona Saraiya. 2014. "Vital Signs: Cervical Cancer Incidence, Mortality, and Screening—United States, 2007–2012." *MMWR: Morbidity and Mortality Weekly Report* 63 (44): 1004.

Benjamin, Ruha. 2016. "Racial Fictions, Biological Facts: Expanding the Sociological Imagination through Speculative Methods." *Catalyst: Feminism, Theory, Technoscience* 2 (2): 1–28.

Benton, Adia. 2015. *HIV Exceptionalism: Development through Disease in Sierra Leone*. Minneapolis: University of Minnesota Press.

Berghom, Jennifer L. 2007. "Valley Reactions Mixed to Perry's HPV Vaccine Mandate." *Tribune Business News* (Tacoma, WA), February 7, 2007, 1.

Bharti, Nishtha, and Sergio Sismondo. 2022. "Political Prescriptions: Three Pandemic Stories." *Science, Technology, & Human Values* 0. https://doi.org/10.1177/01622439221123831.

Biehl, João. 2006. "Pharmaceutical Governance." In *Global Pharmaceuticals: Ethics, Markets, Practices*, edited by Adriana Petryna, Andrew Lakoff, and Arthur Kleinman. Durham, NC: Duke University Press.

Blum, Linda M. 2007. "Mother-Blame in the Prozac Nation: Raising Kids with Invisible Disabilities." *Gender & Society* 21 (2): 202–26.

Blume, Stuart. 2017. *Immunization: How Vaccines Became Controversial*. London: Reaktion Books.

Bosch, F. X., C. Robles, M. Díaz, M. Arbyn, I. Baussano, C. Clavel, G. Ronco, J. Dillner, M. Lehtinen, K. U. Petry, M. Poljak, S. K. Kjaer, C. J. Meijer, S. M. Garland, J. Salmerón, X. Castellsagué, L. Bruni, S. de Sanjosé, and J. Cuzick. 2016. "HPV-FASTER: Broadening the Scope for Prevention of HPV-related Cancer." *National Review of Clinical Oncology* 13 (2): 119–32. https://doi.org/10.1038/nrclinonc.2015.146.

Bosman, Fred T. 2019. "Anal Cancer: Pathology and Genetics." In *Encyclopedia of Cancer*, edited by Paolo Boffetta and Pierre Hainaut. Cambridge, MA: Academic Press.

Bouda, Martha, Vassilis G. Gorgoulis, Nikos G. Kastrinakis, Athina Giannoudis, Efthymia Tsoli, Despina Danassi-Afentaki, Periklis Foukas, Aspasia Kyroudi, George Laskaris, C. Simon Herrington, and Christos Kittas. 2000. "'High Risk' HPV Types Are Frequently Detected in Potentially Malignant and Malignant Oral Lesions, but Not in Normal Oral Mucosa." *Modern Pathology* 13 (6): 644–53. https://doi.org/10.1038/modpath01.3880113.

Bouvard, V., R. Baan, K. Straif, Y. Grosse, B. Secretan, F. El Ghissassi, L. Benbrahim-

Tallaa, N. Guha, C. Freeman, L. Galichet, V. Cogliano, and the IARC Working Group on the Evaluation of Carcinogenic Risks to Humans. 2009. "A Review of Human Carcinogens—Part B: Biological Agents." *Lancet Oncology* 10 (4): 321–2. https://doi.org/10.1016/s1470-2045(09)70096-8.

Bowker, Geoffrey C., and Susan Leigh Star. 1999. *Sorting Things Out: Classification and Its Consequences*. Cambridge, MA: MIT Press.

Bowker, Geoffrey C., and Susan Leigh Star. 2000. "Categorical Work and Boundary Infrastructures: Enriching Theories of Classification." In *Sorting Things Out: Classification and Its Consequences*, chapter 9. Cambridge: MIT Press.

Brandle, Lars. 2015. "Iron Maiden's Bruce Dickinson Blames Oral Sex for His Throat Cancer." *Billboard*, September 6, 2015. https://www.billboard.com/articles/news/6685962/iron-maiden-bruce-dickinson-throat-cancer-oral-sex/.

Brandt, Allan M. 1996. "Recruiting Women Smokers: The Engineering of Consent." *Journal of the American Medical Women's Association* 51 (1–2): 63–66.

Brandt, Allan M. 1978. "Racism and Research: The Case of the Tuskegee Syphilis Study." *The Hastings Center Report* 8 (6): 21–29. https://doi.org/10.2307/3561468.

Brandt, Allan M. 1985. *No Magic Bullet: A Social History of Venereal Disease in the United States since 1880*. New York: Oxford University Press.

Braun, Lundy, and Ling Phoun. 2010. "HPV Vaccination Campaigns: Masking Uncertainty, Erasing Complexity." In *Three Shots at Prevention: The HPV Vaccine and the Politics of Medicine's Simple Solutions*, edited by Keith Wailoo, Julie Livingston, Steven Epstein, and Robert Aronowitz, 39–60. Baltimore, MD: Johns Hopkins University Press.

Braun, Virginia, and Nicola Gavey. 1999a. "'Bad Girls' and 'Good Girls'? Sexuality and Cervical Cancer." *Women's Studies International Forum* 22 (2): 203–13. https://doi.org/10.1016/S0277-5395(99)00007-2.

Braun, Virginia, and Nicola Gavey. 1999b. "'With the Best of Reasons': Cervical Cancer Prevention Policy and the Suppression of Sexual Risk Factor Information." *Social Science & Medicine* 48 (10): 1463–74. https://doi.org/10.1016/S0277-9536(98)00451-1.

Brenner, Barbara. 2016. *So Much to Be Done: The Writings of Breast Cancer Activist Barbara Brenner*. Edited by Barbara Sjoholm. Minneapolis: University of Minnesota Press.

Bridges, Khiara. 2011. *Reproducing Race: An Ethnography of Pregnancy as a Site of Racialization*. Berkeley: University of California Press.

Brier, Jennifer. 2009. *Infectious Ideas: US Political Responses to the AIDS Crisis*. Chapel Hill: University of North Carolina Press.

Briggs, Charles L., and Clara Mantini-Briggs. 2004. *Stories in the Time of Cholera: Racial Profiling during a Medical Nightmare*. Berkeley: University of California Press.

Bright, Beckey. 2006. "Majority of Americans Back HPV Vaccine, Poll Shows." *Wall Street Journal*, August 8. http://online.wsj.com/article/SB115464198706026167.html.

Britton, Luke Morgan. 2015. "Iron Maiden's Bruce Dickinson Says Oral Sex Gave Him Tongue Cancer." *New Musical Express*, September 3, 2015.

Brown, Jessica P., and J. Kathleen Tracy. 2008. "Lesbians and Cancer: An Overlooked Health Disparity." *Cancer Causes & Control* 19 (10): 1009. https://doi.org/10.1007/s10552-008-9176-z.

Bruni, Laia, Mireia Diaz, Leslie Barrionuevo-Rosas, Rolando Herrero, Freddie Bray,

F. Xavier Bosch, Silvia de Sanjosé, and Xavier Castellsagué. 2016. "Global Estimates of Human Papillomavirus Vaccination Coverage by Region and Income Level: A Pooled Analysis." *The Lancet Global Health* 4 (7): e453–e463. https://doi.org/10.1016/S2214-109X(16)30099-7.

Bulik, Beth Snyder. 2019. "Social Media: 'Versed on HPV.'" *FiercePharma*, November 4, 2021.

Bunton, Robin, and Alan Petersen. 1997. *Foucault, Health and Medicine*. New York: Routledge.

Burke, Nancy J., and Holly F. Mathews. 2017. "Returning to Earth: Setting a Global Agenda for the Anthropology of Cancer." *Medical Anthropology* 36 (3): 179–86.

Burkitt, Denis. 1958. "A Sarcoma Involving the Jaws in African Children." *The British Journal of Surgery* 46 (197): 218–23.

Burns, Kellie, and Cristyn Davies. 2015. "Constructions of Young Women's Health and Wellbeing in Neoliberal Times: A Case Study of the HPV Vaccination Program in Australia." In *Rethinking Youth Wellbeing: Critical Perspectives*, edited by Katie Wright and Julie McLeod, 71–89. Singapore: Springer Singapore.

Busfield, Joan. 2006. "Pills, Power, People: Sociological Understandings of the Pharmaceutical Industry." *Sociology* 40 (2): 297–314.

Canales, Christie V. 2009. "HPV Vaccination Requirement for Female Immigrants: An Example of Discrimination." *Journal of Gender, Race, and Justice* 13: 779.

Cancer Prevention & Treatment Fund et al. 2014. "Coalition Letter to FDA Commissioner Hamburg about Approving Cobas HPV Test Alone (Without Pap Smear) and FDA Response." National Center for Health Research, April 11. http://www.center4research.org/coalition-letter-fda-commissioner-hamburg-approving-cobas-hpv-test-alone-without-pap-smear-fda-response/.

Cappiello, J., and A. Levi. 2016. "The Annual Gynecologic Examination Updated for the 21st Century." *Nurs Women's Health* 20 (3): 315–19. https://doi.org/10/1016/j.nwh.2016.03.006/.

Carpenter, Laura M., and Monica J. Casper. 2009a. "Global Intimacies: Innovating the HPV Vaccine for Women's Health." *WSQ: Women's Studies Quarterly* 37 (1/2): 80–100.

Carpenter, Laura M., and Monica J. Casper. 2009b. "A Tale of Two Technologies: HPV Vaccination, Male Circumcision, and Sexual Health." *Gender & Society* 23 (6): 790–816.

Case, Patricia, S. Bryn Austin, David J. Hunter, Joann E. Manson, Susan Malspeis, Walter C. Willett, and Donna Spiegelman. 2004. "Sexual Orientation, Health Risk Factors, and Physical Functioning in the Nurses' Health Study II." *Journal of Women's Health* 13 (9): 1033–47.

Casper, Monica J., and Laura M. Carpenter. 2008. "Sex, Drugs, and Politics: The HPV Vaccine for Cervical Cancer." *Sociology of Health & Illness* 30 (6): 886–99.

Casper, Monica J., and Adele E. Clarke. 1998. "Making the Pap Smear into the 'Right Tool' for the Job: Cervical Cancer Screening in the USA, circa 1940–95." *Social Studies of Science* 28 (2): 255–90.

Cayen, Laura, Jessica Polzer, and Susan Knabe. 2016. "Tween Girls, Human Papillomavirus (HPV), and the Deployment of Female Sexuality in English Canadian Magazines." In *Neoliberal Governance and Health: Duties, Risks, and Vulnerabilities, edited by Jessica Polzer and Elaine Power*, 82. Kingston, Ont.: McGill-Queen's University Press.

"Cervical Cancer Statistics." 2021. Centers for Disease Control and Prevention. Last modified June 8, 2021, accessed June 25, 2021. https://www.cdc.gov/cancer/cervical/statistics/index.htm.

Chandrasekharan, Subhashini, Tahir Amin, Joyce Kim, Eliane Furrer, Anna-Carin Matterson, Nina Schwalbe, and Aurélia Nguyen. 2015. "Intellectual Property Rights and Challenges for Development of Affordable Human Papillomavirus, Rotavirus and Pneumococcal Vaccines: Patent Landscaping and Perspectives of Developing Country Vaccine Manufacturers." *Vaccine* 33 (46): 6366–70. https://doi.org/10.1016/j.vaccine.2015.08.063.

Chang, Yuan, Ethel Cesarman, Melissa S. Pessin, Frank Lee, Janice Culpepper, Daniel M. Knowles, and Patrick S. Moore. 1994. "Identification of Herpesvirus-like DNA Sequences in AIDS-associated Kaposi's Sarcoma." *Science* 266 (5192): 1865–69.

Charles, Nicole. 2013. "Mobilizing the Self-Governance of Pre-Damaged Bodies: Neoliberal Biological Citizenship and HPV Vaccination Promotion in Canada." *Citizenship Studies* 17 (6/7): 770–84. https://doi.org/10.1080/13621025.2013.834128.

Charles, Nicole. 2014. "Injecting and Rejecting, Framing and Failing: The HPV Vaccine and the Subjectification of Citizens' Identities." *Feminist Media Studies* 14 (6): 1071–89. https://doi.org/10.1080/14680777.2014.882855.

Charles, Nicole. 2021. *Suspicion: Vaccines, Hesitancy, and the Affective Politics of Protection in Barbados.* Durham, NC: Duke University Press.

Chaturvedi, Anil K., Eric A. Engels, Ruth M. Pfeiffer, Brenda Y. Hernandez, Weihong Xiao, Esther Kim, Bo Jiang, Marc T. Goodman, Maria Sibug-Saber, and Wendy Cozen. 2011. "Human Papillomavirus and Rising Oropharyngeal Cancer Incidence in the United States." *Journal of Clinical Oncology* 29 (32): 4294.

Chiao, Elizabeth Y., Thomas P. Giordano, Joel M. Palefsky, Stephen Tyring, and Hashem El Serag. 2006. "Screening HIV-Infected Individuals for Anal Cancer Precursor Lesions: A Systematic Review." *Clinical Infectious Diseases* 43 (2): 223–33.

Chitale, Radha. 2009. "Doctors Say 'Wait And See' before Prescribing Gardasil in Boys." *ABC News*, September 11. https://abcnews.go.com/Health/MensHealthNews/gardasil-boys/story?id=8541892.

Cho, Hee-Jeong, Yu-Kyoung Oh, and Young Bong Kim. 2011. "Advances in Human Papilloma Virus Vaccines: A Patent Review." *Expert Opinion on Therapeutic Patents* 21 (3): 295–309. https://doi.org/10.1517/13543776.2011.551114.

Cichocki, Mark. 2008. "The Dangers of Anal Cancer—The Silent Killer in Men with HIV." University of Michigan HIV/AIDS Treatment Program.

Clark, Aleia Yvonne 2008. "Biomedical Innovation and the Politics of Scientific Knowledge: A Case Study of Gardasil." Master's thesis, Sociology, University of Maryland.

Clarke, Adele E. 1998. *Disciplining Reproduction: Modernity, American Life Sciences, and "The Problems of Sex."* Berkeley: University of California Press.

Clarke, Adele E. 2005. *Situational Analysis: Grounded Theory after the Postmodern Turn.* Thousand Oaks, CA: Sage Publications.

Clarke, Adele E., and Monica J. Casper. 1996. "From Simple Technology to Complex Arena: Classification of Pap Smears." *Medical Anthropology Quarterly* 10: 601–23.

Clarke, Adele E., and Joan H. Fujimura. 1992a. "What Tools? Which Jobs? Why Right?" In *The Right Tools for the Job: At Work in Twentieth-Century Life Sciences*, edited by Adele E. Clarke and Joan H. Fujimura, 1–49. Princeton, NJ: Princeton University Press.

Clarke, Adele E., and Joan H. Fujimura. 1992b. *The Right Tools for the Job: At Work in Twentieth-Century Life Sciences*. Princeton, NJ: Princeton University Press.

Clarke, Adele E., Laura Mamo, Jennifer Fishman, Jennifer Fosket, and Janet Shim, eds. 2010. *Biomedicalization: Technoscience, Health, and Illness in the US*. Durham, NC: Duke University Press.

Clarke, Adele E., Janet Shim, Laura Mamo, Jennifer R. Fosket, and Jennifer R. Fishman. 2003. "Biomedicalization: Theorizing Technoscientific Transformations of Health, Illness, and U.S. Biomedicine." *American Sociological Review* 68 (2): 161–94.

Clarke, Brendan. 2011. *Causality in Medicine with Particular Reference to the Viral Causation of Cancers*. Doctoral thesis, University College London.

Cochran, Susan D., Vickie M. Mays, Deborah Bowen, Suzann Gage, Deborah Bybee, Susan J. Roberts, Robert S. Goldstein, Ann Robison, Elizabeth J. Rankow, and Jocelyn White. 2001. "Cancer-related Risk Indicators and Preventive Screening Behaviors among Lesbians and Bisexual Women." *American Journal of Public Health* 91 (4): 591–97. https://doi.org/10.2105/ajph.91.4.591.

Cohen, Cathy J. 1999. *The Boundaries of Blackness: AIDS and the Breakdown of Black Politics*. Chicago: University of Chicago Press.

Colgrove, James. 2006. *State of Immunity: The Politics of Vaccination in Twentieth-Century America*. Berkeley: University of California Press.

Colgrove, James. 2010. "The Coercive Hand, the Beneficent Hand: What the History of Compulsory Vaccination Can Tell Us about HPV Vaccine Mandates." In *Three Shots at Prevention: The HPV Vaccine and the Politics of Medicine's Simple Solutions*, edited by Keith Wailoo, Julie Livingston, Steven Epstein, and Robert Aronowitz, 3–20. Baltimore, MD: Johns Hopkins University Press.

Colgrove, James, Sara Abiola, and Michelle M. Mello. 2010. "HPV Vaccination Mandates—Lawmaking amid Political and Scientific Controversy." *New England Journal of Medicine* 363 (8): 785–91. https://doi.org/10.1056/NEJMsr1003547.

Collins, Patricia Hill. 2004. *Black Sexual Politics: African Americans, Gender, and the New Racism*. New York: Routledge.

Compass Laboratory Services. 2021. "Compass Laboratory Services Introduces OraGen HPV, a New Method to Detect High-Risk HPV Strains in the Oral Cavity." Press release, Cision PRNewswire, February 24.

Conis, Elena. 2010. "Calling the Shots: A Social History of Vaccination in the US, 1968–2008." PhD diss., History of Health Sciences, University of California San Francisco.

Conis, Elena. 2011. "'Do We Really Need Hepatitis B on the Second Day of Life?' Vaccination Mandates and Shifting Representations of Hepatitis B." *Journal of Medical Humanities* 32: 155–66.

Conis, Elena. 2013. "A Mother's Responsibility: Women, Medicine, and the Rise of Contemporary Vaccine Skepticism in the United States." *Bulletin of the History of Medicine* 87 (3): 407–35.

Conis, Elena. 2015. *Vaccine Nation: America's Changing Relationship with Immunization*. Chicago: University of Chicago Press.

Conis, Elena. 2019. "Measles and the Modern History of Vaccination." *Public Health Reports* 134 (2): 118–25. https://doi.org/10.1177/0033354919826558.

Connel, Erin, and Alan Hunt. 2010. "The HPV Vaccination Campaign: A Project of Moral Regulation in an Era of Biopolitics." *Canadian Journal of Sociology / Cahiers canadiens de sociologie* 35 (1): 63–82.

Conrad, Peter. 1975. "The Discovery of Hyperkinesis: Notes on the Medicalization of Deviant Behavior." *Social Problems* 23 (1): 12–21.

Conrad, Peter. 1992. "Medicalization and Social Control." *Annual Review of Sociology* 18: 209–32.

Conrad, Peter, and Joseph W. Schneider. 1980. *Deviance and Medicalization*. St. Louis: The C. V. Mosby Co.

Cook, Erin E., Atheendar S. Venkataramani, Jane J. Kim, Rulla M. Tamimi, and Michelle D. Holmes. 2018. "Legislation to Increase Uptake of HPV Vaccination and Adolescent Sexual Behaviors." *Pediatrics* 142 (3): e20180458.

Cooper Owens, Deirdre. 2017. *Medical Bondage: Race, Gender, and the Origins of American Gynecology*. Athens: University of Georgia Press.

Cottom, Tressie McMillan. 2018. *Thick, and Other essays*. New York: The New Press.

Courtenay, Will H. 2000. "Constructions of Masculinity and Their Influence on Men's Well-Being: A Theory of Gender and Health." *Social Science & Medicine* 50 (10): 1385–1401. https://doi.org/10.1016/S0277-9536(99)00390-1.

Crager, Sara Eve. 2018. "Improving Global Access to New Vaccines: Intellectual Property, Technology Transfer, and Regulatory Pathways." *American Journal of Public Health* 108 (S6): S414–S420. https://doi.org/10.2105/AJPH.2014.302236r.

Crawford, Robert. 1980. "Healthism and the Medicalization of Everyday Life." *International Journal of Health Services* 10 (3): 365–88.

Crawford, Robert. 2006. "Health as a Meaningful Social Practice." *Health* 10 (4): 401–20.

Creager, Angela N. H., and Jean-Paul Gaudillière. 2001. "Experimental Platforms and Technologies of Visualization: Cancer as Viral Epidemic, 1930–1960." In *Heredity and Infection: The History of Disease Transmission*, edited by Jean-Paul Gaudillière and Ilana Löwy. London: Routledge.

Creager, Angela N. H., and Hannah Landecker. 2009. "Technical Matters: Method, Knowledge and Infrastructure in Twentieth-Century Life Science." *Nature Methods* 6 (10): 701–5. https://doi.org/10.1038/nmeth1009-701.

Crosswell, Laura, and Lance Porter. 2018. *Politics, Propaganda, and Public Health: A Case Study in Health Communication and Public Trust*. Lanham, MD: Lexington Books.

Curnutte, Margaret, and Giuseppe Testa. 2012. "Consuming Genomes: Scientific and Social Innovation in Direct-to-Consumer Genetic Testing." *New Genetics and Society* 31 (2): 159–181. https://doi.org/10.1080/14636778.2012.662032.

Curtis, C. Robinette, Christina Dorell, David Yankey, Jenny Jeyarajah, Harrell Chesson, Mona Saraiya, Rebecca Gold, Eileen F. Dunne, Shannon Stokley, and Centers for Disease Control and Prevention. 2014. "National Human Papillomavirus Vaccination Coverage among Adolescents Aged 13–17 Years—National Immunization Survey-Teen, United States, 2011." *MMWR Surveillance Summary* 63 (suppl. 2): 61–70.

Cvejic, Erin, Isobel Mary Poynten, Patrick J. Kelly, Fengyi Jin, Kirsten Howard, Andrew E. Grulich, David J. Templeton, Richard J. Hillman, Carmella Law, Jennifer M. Roberts, and Kirsten McCaffery. 2019. "Psychological and Utility-Based Quality of Life Impact of Screening Test Results for Anal Precancerous Lesions in Gay and Bisexual Men: Baseline Findings from the Study of the Prevention of Anal Cancer." *Sexually Transmitted Infections* 96 (3): 177–83. https://doi.org/10.1136/sextrans-2019-054098.

D'Souza, Gypsyamber, Aimee R. Kreimer, Raphael Viscidi, Michael Pawlita, Carole Fakhry, Wayne M. Koch, William H. Westra, and Maura L. Gillison. 2007. "Case-

Control Study of Human Papillomavirus and Oropharyngeal Cancer." *New England Journal of Medicine* 356 (19): 1944–56.

D'Souza, Gypsyamber, T. S. McNeel, and Carol Fakhry. 2017. "Understanding Personal Risk of Oropharyngeal Cancer: Risk-Groups for Oncogenic Oral HPV Infection and Oropharyngeal Cancer." *Annals of Oncology* 28 (12): 3065–69. https://doi.org/10.1093/annonc/mdx535.

Daling, Janet R., Noel S. Weiss, T. Gregory Hislop, Christopher Maden, Ralph J. Coates, Karen J. Sherman, Rhoda L. Ashley, Marjorie Beagrie, John A. Ryan, and Lawrence Corey. 1987. "Sexual Practices, Sexually Transmitted Diseases, and the Incidence of Anal Cancer." *New England Journal of Medicine* 317 (16): 973–77.

Daling, Janet R., Noel S. Weiss, Larry L. Klopfenstein, Leah E. Cochran, Wong H. Chow, and Richard Daifuku. 1982. "Correlates of Homosexual Behavior and the Incidence of Anal Cancer." *JAMA, Journal of the American Medical Association* 247: 1988–90. https://doi.org/10.1001/jama.247.14.1988.

Darby, Alexis, and Grace Kim. 2020. "Cervarix HPV Vaccination Series." In *The Embryo Project Encyclopedia*. Tempe: The Embryo Project at Arizona State University.

Davis, Devra. 2007. *The Secret History of the War on Cancer*. New York: Basic Books.

de Sanjosé, S., B. Serrano, X. Castellsagué, M. Brotons, J. Muñoz, L. Bruni, and F. X. Bosch. 2012. "Human Papillomavirus (HPV) and Related Cancers in the Global Alliance for Vaccines and Immunization (GAVI) Countries. A WHO/ICO HPV Information Centre Report." *Vaccine* 30, Suppl. 4: D1–83, vi. https://doi.org/10.1016/s0264-410x(12)01435-1.

Deeken, John F., and Liron Pantanowitz. 2019. "HIV Infection and Malignancy: Epidemiology and Pathogenesis." *UptoDate*, edited by David M. Aboulafia and Sonali Shah. https://www.uptodate.com/contents/hiv-infection-and-malignancy-epidemiology-and-pathogenesis.

Dehn, Donna, Kathleen C. Torkko, and Kenneth R. Shroyer. 2007. "Human Papillomavirus Testing and Molecular Markers of Cervical Dysplasia and Carcinoma." *Cancer Cytopathology* 111 (1): 1–14. https://doi.org/10.1002/cncr.22425.

Demarco, Maria, Didem Egemen, Tina R. Raine-Bennett, Li C. Cheung, Brian Befano, Nancy E. Poitras, Thomas S. Lorey, Xiaojian Chen, Julia C. Gage, Philip E. Castle, Nicolas Wentzensen, Rebecca B. Perkins, Richard S. Guido, and Mark Schiffman. 2020. "A Study of Partial Human Papillomavirus Genotyping in Support of the 2019 ASCCP Risk-Based Management Consensus Guidelines." *Journal of Lower Genital Tract Disease* 24 (2): 144–47. https://doi.org/10.1097/lgt.0000000000000530.

Demasi, Maryanne. 2022. "From FDA to MHRA: Are Drug Regulators for Hire?" *BMJ* 377 (June 29): o1538. https://doi.org/10.1136/bmj.o1538.

Deshmukh, Ashish A., Jagpreet Chhatwal, Elizabeth Y. Chiao, Alan G. Nyitray, Prajnan Das, and Scott B. Cantor. 2015. "Long-Term Outcomes of Adding HPV Vaccine to the Anal Intraepithelial Neoplasia Treatment Regimen in HIV-Positive Men Who Have Sex with Men." *Clinical Infectious Diseases* 61 (10): 1527–35. https://doi.org/10.1093/cid/civ628.

Deshmukh, Ashish A., Elizabeth Chiao, Jagpreet Chhatwal, and Scott B. Cantor. 2017. "How the Anal Cancer Epidemic in Gay and Bi HIV-Positive Men Can Be Prevented." *The Conversation*, September 26. http://theconversation.com/how-the-anal-cancer-epidemic-in-gay-and-bi-hiv-positive-men-can-be-prevented-80358.

Deshmukh, Ashish A., Ryan Suk, Meredith S. Shiels, Kalyani Sonawane, Alan G. Nyitray, Yuxin Liu, Michael M. Gaisa, Joel M. Palefsky, and Keith Sigel. 2020. "Recent

Trends in Squamous Cell Carcinoma of the Anus Incidence and Mortality in the United States, 2001–2015." *JNCI: Journal of the National Cancer Institute* 112 (8): 829–38. https://doi.org/10.1093/jnci/djz219.

DeSilver, Drew. 2021. "States Have Mandated Vaccinations since Long Before COVID-19." Fact-Tank, Pew Research Center, October 8. https://www.pew research.org/fact-tank/2021/10/08/states-have-mandated-vaccinations-since-long -before-covid-19/.

Dickenson, Donna. 2013. *Me Medicine vs. We Medicine: Reclaiming Biotechnology for the Common Good.* New York: Columbia University Press.

Dillner, J., M. Elfström, and I. Baussano. 2021. "The EVEN FASTER Concept for Cervical Cancer Elimination." *HPVW* 182 (November). https://www.hpvworld.com/ articles/the-even-faster-concept-for-cervical-cancer-elimination/.

Division of Cancer Prevention. 2021. "The ASCUS/LSIL Triage Study for Cervical Cancer (ALTS)." National Cancer Institute. Accessed August 17, 2021. https:// prevention.cancer.gov/clinical-trials/landmark-trials/ascuslsil-triage-study.

Donohue, Julie M., Marisa Cevasco, and Meredith B. Rosenthal. 2007. "A Decade of Direct-to-Consumer Advertising of Prescription Drugs." *New England Journal of Medicine* 357 (7): 673–81. https://doi.org/10.1056/NEJMsa070502.

Dubé, Ève, Jeremey K. Ward, Pierre Verger, and Noni E. MacDonals. 2021. "Vaccine Hesitancy, Acceptance, and Anti-Vaccination: Trends and Future Perspectives of Public Health." *Annual Review of Public Health* 42: 175–91.

Dubos, Jean, and René Dubos. 1987. *The White Plague: Tuberculosis, Man and Society.* New Brunswick, NJ: Rutgers University Press.

Dumit, Joseph. 2012. *Drugs for Life: How Pharmaceutical Companies Define Our Health.* Durham, NC: Duke University Press.

Ecks, Stefan. 2005. "Pharmaceutical Citizenship: Antidepressant Marketing and the Promise of Demarginalization in India." *Anthropology & Medicine* 12 (3): 239–54.

Economist Intelligence Unit. 2009. *Breakaway: The Global Burden of Cancer— Challenges and Opportunities.* New York: Economist Intelligence Unit. https://www .livestrong.org/sites/default/files/what-we-do/reports/globaleconomicimpact.pdf.

Eng, Thomas R., and William T. Butler, eds. 1997. *The Hidden Epidemic: Confronting Sexually Transmitted Diseases.* Edited by Institute of Medicine Committee on Prevention and Control of Sexually Transmitted Diseases. Washington, DC: National Academy Press.

Engineering and Technology History Wiki (ETHW). 2021. "First-Hand: Starting Up Cetus, the First Biotechnology Company—1973 to 1982." Last modified March 4, 2015, accessed July 3, 2021. https://ethw.org/First-Hand:Starting_Up_Cetus,_the _First_Biotechnology_Company_-_1973_to_1982.

Epstein, M. A., B. G. Achong, and Y. M. Barr. 1964. "Virus Particles in Cultured Lymphoblasts from Burkitt's Lymphoma." *The Lancet* 1 (7335): 702–3.

Epstein, Steven. 1996. *Impure Science: AIDS, Activism, and the Politics of Knowledge.* Berkeley: University of California Press.

Epstein, Steven. 2007a. *Inclusion: The Politics of Difference in Medical Research.* Chicago Studies in Practices of Meaning. Chicago: University of Chicago Press.

Epstein, Steven. 2007b. "Patient Groups and Health Movements." In *New Handbook of Science and Technology Studies,* edited by Edward J. Hackett, Olga Amsterdamska, Michael Lynch, and Judy Wajcman, 499–540. Cambridge, MA: MIT Press.

Epstein, Steven. 2008. "The Rise of 'Recruitmentology': Clinical Research, Racial

Knowledge, and the Politics of Inclusion and Difference." *Social Studies of Science* 38 (5): 801–32. https://doi.org/10.1177/0306312708091930.

Epstein, Steven. 2010. "The Great Undiscussable: Anal Cancer, HPV, and Gay Men's Health." In *Three Shots at Prevention: The HPV Vaccine and the Politics of Medicine's Simple Solution*, edited by Keith Wailoo, Julie Livingston, Steven Epstein, and Robert Aronowitz, 61–90. Baltmore, MD: Johns Hopkins University Press.

Epstein, Steven, and Laura Mamo. 2012. "Sexual Health as Buzzword: Beyond 'Normal' vs 'Deviant.'" Paper presented at the American Sociological Association Conference, Denver, Colorado, August 17–20.

Epstein, Steven, and Laura Mamo. 2017. "The Proliferation of Sexual Health: Diverse Social Problems and the Legitimation of Sexuality." *Social Science & Medicine* 188: 176–90. https://doi.oirg/10.1016/j.socscimed.2017.06.033.

Fan, Elsa. 2021. *Commodities of Care: The Business of HIV testing in China*. Minneapolis: University of Minnesota Press.

Farmer, Paul, Julio Frenk, Felicia M. Knaul, Lawrence N. Shulman, George Alleyne, Lance Armstrong, Rifat Atun, Douglas Blayney, Lincoln Chen, and Richard Feachem. 2010. "Expansion of Cancer Care and Control in Countries of Low and Middle Income: A Call to Action." *The Lancet* 376 (9747): 1186–93.

Faro, Livi, Lilian Chazan, Fabiola Rohden, and Jane Russo. 2013. "Man with Capital 'M': Masculinity Ideals Reconstructed in Pharmaceutical Marketing." *Cadernos Pagu* 40: 287–321.

Faulkner, Alex. 2012. "Resisting the Screening Imperative: Patienthood, Populations and Politics in Prostate Cancer Detection Technologies for the UK." *Sociology of Health & Illness* 34 (2): 221–233. https://doi.org/10.1111/j.1467-9566.2011.01385.x.

FDA. 2009. "Clinical Review of Biologics License Application Supplement STN# 125126/1297.0—Male Indication for GARDASIL." Edited by Office of Vaccines Research and Review Center for Biologics Evaluation and Research, Division of Vaccines and Related Product Applications, Food and Drug Administration. https://www.fda.gov/media/77941/download.

FDA. 2014. "PMA P100020/S008: FDA Summary of Safety and Effectiveness Data." Accessed August 18, 2021. https://www.accessdata.fda.gov/cdrh_docs/pdf10/p100020s008b.pdf.

Fenton, Anny T. 2019. "Abandoning Medical Authority: When Medical Professionals Confront Stigmatized Adolescent Sex and the Human Papillomavirus (HPV) Vaccine." *Journal of Health and Social Behavior* 60 (2): 240–56. https://doi.org/10.1177/0022146519849895.

Fenton, Anny T. H. R., Terresa J. Eun, Jack A. Clark, and Rebecca B. Perkins. 2020. "Calling the Shots? Adolescents' Influence on Human Papillomavirus Vaccine Decision-Making during Clinical Encounters." *Journal of Adolescent Health* 66 (4): 447–54. https://doi.org/10.1016/j.jadohealth.2019.10.020.

Ferber, Abby L. 2007. "The Construction of Black Masculinity: White Supremacy Now and Then." *Journal of Sport and Social Issues* 31 (1): 11–24. https://doi.org/10.1177/0193723506296829.

Ferguson, Roderick A. 2003. *Aberrations in Black: Toward a Queer of Color Critique*. Durham, NC: Duke University Press.

Ferlay, J., F. Bray, and P. Pisani. 2004. *GLOBOCAN 2002: Cancer Incidence, Mortality and Prevalence Worldwide*. Lyon, France: IARC.

Fernandez, Elizabeth. 2021. "Treating Anal Cancer Precursor Lesions Reduces Cancer

Risk for People with HIV: Groundbreaking National Clinical Trial Halted Due to Therapy's High Success Rates." *UCSF Health*, October 8. https://www.ucsf.edu/news/2021/10/421591/treating-anal-cancer-precursor-lesions-reduces-cancer-risk-people-hiv

Fields, Jessica. 2008. *Risky Lessons: Sex Education and Social Inequality*. Childhood Studies. New Brunswick, NJ: Rutgers University Press.

Fishman, Jennifer R. 2004. "Manufacturing Desire: The Commodification of Female Sexual Dysfunction." *Social Studies of Science* 34 (2): 187–218.

Fishman, Jennifer R. 2006. "Making Viagra: From Impotence to Erectile Dysfunction." In *Medicating Modern America*, edited by Andrea Tone and Elizabeth Siegel Watkins, 229–52. New York: New York University Press.

Fishman, Jennifer R., Laura Mamo, and Patrick R. Grzanka. 2017. "Sex, Gender, & Sexuality in Biomedicine." In *The Handbook of Science and Technology Studies*, edited by U. Felt, R. Fouché, C. Miller, and L. Smith-Doerr, 379–405. Cambridge, MA: MIT Press.

Fontham, Elizabeth T. H., Andrew M. D. Wolf, Timothy R. Church, Ruth Etzioni, Christopher R. Flowers, Abbe Herzig, Carmen E. Guerra, Kevin C. Oeffinger, Ya-Chen Tina Shih, Louise C. Walter, Jane J. Kim, Kimberly S. Andrews, Carol E. DeSantis, Stacey A. Fedewa, Deana Manassaram-Baptiste, Debbie Saslow, Richard C. Wender, and Robert A. Smith. 2020. "Cervical Cancer Screening for Individuals at Average Risk: 2020 Guideline Update from the American Cancer Society." *CA: A Cancer Journal for Clinicians* 70 (5): 321–46. https://doi.org/10.3322/caac.21628.

Forastiere, Arlene, Wayne Koch, Andrew Trotti, and David Sidransky. 2001. "Head and Neck Cancer." *New England Journal of Medicine* 345 (26): 1890–1900. https://doi.org/10.1056/NEJMra001375.

Fosket, Jennifer. 2004. "Constructing 'High-Risk Women': The Development and Standardization of a Breast Cancer Risk Assessment Tool." *Science, Technology, & Human Values* 29 (3): 291–313. https://doi.org/10.1177/0162243904264960.

Fosket, Jennifer Ruth. 2010. "Breast Cancer Risk as Disease: Biomedicalizing Risk." In *Biomedicalization: Technoscience, Health and Illness in the U.S.*, edited by Adele Clarke, Laura Mamo, Jennifer R. Fishman, Jennifer Ruth Fosket, and Janet Shim. Durham, NC: Duke University Press.

Foucault, Michel. 1979. *Discipline and Punish*. New York: Vintage Books.

Foucault, Michel. 1980. *The History of Sexuality: An Introduction, Volume I*. New York: Vintage Books.

France, Lisa Respers. 2019. "Marcia Cross Says Her Anal Cancer Is Linked to HPV and Husband's Throat Cancer." *CNN Entertainment*, June 7. https://www.cnn.com/2019/06/06/entertainment/marcia-cross-husband-cancer-trnd.

Franceschi, Silvia, Nubia Muñoz, Xavier F. Bosch, Peter J. Snijders, and Jan M. Walboomers. 1996. "Human Papillomavirus and Cancers of the Upper Aerodigestive Tract: A Review of Epidemiological and Experimental Evidence." *Cancer Epidemiology Biomarkers & Prevention* 5 (7): 567.

Frank, Arthur W. 2013 [1995]. *The Wounded Storyteller: Body, Illness, and Ethics*. Chicago: University of Chicago Press.

Freedman, Mark, John Weiser, Linda R. Beer, and R. Luke Shouse. 2016. "Anal Cancer Screening in Men Who Have Sex with Men in Care for HIV Infection, United States, 2009–2012." *Open Forum Infectious Diseases* 3 (suppl. 1): 855. https://doi.org/10.1093/ofid/ofw194.62.

Friedman, Allison L., and Hilda Shepeard. 2007. "Exploring the Knowledge, Attitudes, Beliefs, and Communication Preferences of the General Public Regarding HPV: Findings from CDC Focus Group Research and Implications for Practice." *Health Education & Behavior* 34 (3): 471–85. https://doi.org/10.1177/1090198106292022.

Fullilove, Mindy Thompson, Robert E. Fullilove, Katherine Haynes, and Shirley Gross. 1990. "Black Women and AIDS Prevention: A View toward Understanding the Gender Rules." *Journal of Sex Research* 27 (1): 47–64.

Gabriel, Trip, and Denise Grady. 2011. "In Republican Race, a Heated Battle over the HPV Vaccine." *New York Times*, September 13, 2011, Politics. https://www.nytimes.com/2011/09/14/us/politics/republican-candidates-battle-over-hpv-vaccine.html.

Gamble, Vanessa Northington. 1997. "Under the Shadow of Tuskegee: African Americans and Health Care." *American Journal of Public Health* 87 (11): 1773–78.

Gardner, Kristen. 2006. *Early Detection: Women, Cancer and Awareness Campaigns in the Twentieth-Century United States*. Chapel Hill: University of North Carolina Press.

Gaudillière, Jean-Paul, and Ilana Löwy, eds. 1998. *The Invisible Industrialist: Manufacturers and the Construction of Scientific Knowledge*. London and New York: Macmillan and St. Martin's Press.

GAVI. 2021. "Human Papillomavirus Vaccine Support." Gavi, the Vaccine Alliance. Accessed May 12, 2021. https://www.gavi.org/types-support/vaccine-support/human-papillomavirus.

Gillison, Maura L., Tatevik Broutian, Robert K. L. Pickard, Zhen-yue Tong, Weihong Xiao, Lisa Kahle, Barry I. Graubard, and Anil K. Chaturvedi. 2012. "Prevalence of Oral HPV Infection in the United States, 2009–2010." *JAMA* 307 (7): 693–703. https://doi.org/10.1001/jama.2012.101.

Gillison, Maura L., Wayne M. Koch, Randolph B. Capone, Michael Spafford, William H. Westra, Li Wu, Marianna L. Zahurak, Richard W. Daniel, Michael Viglione, David E. Symer, Keerti V. Shah, and David Sidransky. 2000. "Evidence for a Causal Association between Human Papillomavirus and a Subset of Head and Neck Cancers." *JNCI: Journal of the National Cancer Institute* 92 (9): 709–20. https://doi.org/10.1093/jnci/92.9.709.

Gillison, Maura L., Wayne M. Koch, and Keerti V. Shah. 1999. "Human Papillomavirus in Head and Neck Squamous Cell Carcinoma: Are Some Head and Neck Cancers a Sexually Transmitted Disease?" *Current Opinion in Oncology* 11 (3): 191.

Giuliano, Anna R., and Daniel Salmon. 2008. "The Case for a Gender-Neutral (Universal) Human Papillomavirus Vaccination Policy in the United States: Point." *Cancer Epidemiology, Biomarkers & Prevention* 17 (4): 805–8.

Goodwyn, Wade. 2011. "In Texas, Perry's Vaccine Mandate Provoked Anger." *All Things Considered*, September 16. https://www.npr.org/2011/09/16/140530716/in-texas-perrys-vaccine-mandate-provoked-anger.

Gordon, Avery. 2008. *Ghostly Matters: Haunting and the Sociological Imagination*. Minneapolis: University of Minnesota Press.

Gottlieb, Samantha D. 2018. *Not Quite a Cancer Vaccine: Selling HPV and Cervical Cancer*. New Brunswick, NJ: Rutgers University Press.

Grady, D. 2013a. "Gynecology's Gender Question." *New York Times*, December 24. https://www.nytimes.com/2013/12/24/health/gynecologys-gender-question.html.

Grady, D. 2013b. "Gynecologists May Treat Men, Board Says in Switch." *New York*

Times, November 27. https://www.nytimes.com/2013/11/27/health/gynecologists
-may-treat-men-board-says-in-switch.html.

Grady, Denise, and Jan Hoffman. 2018. "HPV Vaccine Expanded for People Ages 27 to
45." *New York Times*, October 5, 2018, Health. https://www.nytimes.com/2018/10/
05/health/hpv-virus-vaccine-cancer.html.

Graham, Hilary. 1994. "Surviving by Smoking." In *Women and Health: Feminist Perspectives*, edited by Sue Wilkinson and Celia Kitzinger, 102–23. London: Taylor &
Francis.

Greaves, Lorraine. 1996. *Smoke Screen: Women's Smoking and Social Control*. Halifax,
NS: Fernwood Publishing.

Gresko, Jessica. 2011. "Farrah Fawcett's Red Swimsuit Goes to Smithsonian." *Washington Times*, February 2. https://www.washingtontimes.com/news/2011/feb/2/farrah
-fawcetts-red-swimsuit-going-smithsonian/.

Groopman, Jerome. 1999. "Contagion." *The New Yorker*, September 13.

Guyon, Janet. 2005. "The Coming Storm over a Cancer Vaccine." *Fortune* 152 (9): 123–
24, 126, 128.

Haelle, Tara. 2017. "You Can Order a Dozen STD Tests Online—But Should You?"
Shots: Health News from NPR, August 13. https://www.npr.org/sections/health
-shots/2017/08/13/536905120/you-can-order-a-dozen-std-tests-online-but-should
-you.

Halpern, Sydney A. 2021. *Dangerous Medicine: The Story behind Human Experiments
with Hepatitis*. New Haven, CT: Yale University Press.

Hammonds, Evelynn M. 1990. "Missing Persons: African American Women, AIDS,
and the History of Disease." *Radical America* 24 (2): 7–23.

Hammonds, Evelynn M. 1997. "Seeing AIDS: Race, Gender, and Representation."
In *The Gender Politics of HIV/AIDS in Women: Perspectives on the Pandemic in the
United States*, edited by Nancy Goldstein, 113–26. New York: New York University
Press.

Hammonds, Evelynn M. 1999. *Childhood's Deadly Scourge: The Campaign to Control
Diphtheria in New York City, 1880–1930*. Baltimore, MD: Johns Hopkins University
Press.

Hammonds, Evelynn M., and Rebecca M. Herzig. 2009. *The Nature of Difference:
Sciences of Race in the United States from Jefferson to Genomics*. Cambridge, MA: The
MIT Press.

Haraway, Donna J. 1991. *Simians, Cyborgs, and Women: The Reinvention of Nature*. New
York: Routledge.

Haraway, Donna J. 1997. *Modest_Witness@Second_Millennium.FemaleMan©_Meets
_Onco Mouse: Feminism and Technoscience*. New York: Routledge.

Harris, Gardiner. 2012. "Can Oral Sex Cause Cancer?" *Men's Journal*, August 9. https://
www.mensjournal.com/health-fitness/can-oral-sex-cause-cancer-20120809/.

Hart, Lianne. 2007. "Uproar over HPV Vaccine Order." *Los Angeles Times*, February 25,
2007. https://www.latimes.com/archives/la-xpm-2007-feb-25-na-vaccine25-story
.html.

Hatzenbuehler, Mark L., Hee-Jin Jun, Heather L. Corliss, and S. Bryn Austin. 2013.
"Structural Stigma and Cigarette Smoking in a Prospective Cohort Study of Sexual
Minority and Heterosexual Youth." *Annals of Behavioral Medicine* 47 (1): 48–56.
https://doi.org/10.1007/s12160-013-9548-9.

Hauck, Grace. 2020. "Are Pap Smears 'Obsolete'? There's a Better Option for Cervical Cancer Screening, American Cancer Society Says." *USA Today*, July 30, 2020, Health. https://www.usatoday.com/story/news/health/2020/07/30/cervical -cancer-american-cancer-society-updates-screening-guidelines/5538424002/.

Heck, Julia E., Julien Berthiller, Salvatore Vaccarella, Deborah M. Winn, Elaine M. Smith, Oxana Shan'gina, Stephen M. Schwartz, Mark P. Purdue, Agnieszka Pilarska, Jose Eluf-Neto, Ana Menezes, Michael D. McClean, Elena Matos, Sergio Koifman, Karl T. Kelsey, Rolando Herrero, Richard B. Hayes, Silvia Franceschi, Victor Wünsch-Filho, Leticia Fernández, Alexander W. Daudt, Maria Paula Curado, Chu Chen, Xavier Castellsagué, Gilles Ferro, Paul Brennan, Paolo Boffetta, and Mia Hashibe. 2009. "Sexual Behaviours and the Risk of Head and Neck Cancers: A Pooled Analysis in the International Head and Neck Cancer Epidemiology (INHANCE) Consortium." *International Journal of Epidemiology* 39 (1): 166–81. https://doi.org/10.1093/ije/dyp350.

Heller, Jacob. 2008. *The Vaccine Narrative*. Nasvhille, TN: Vanderbilt University Press.

Herrero, Rolando, Xavier Castellsagué, Michael Pawlita, Jolanta Lissowska, Frank Kee, Prabda Balaram, Thangarajan Rajkumar, Hema Sridhar, Barbara Rose, Javier Pintos, Leticia Fernández, Ali Idris, María José Sánchez, Adoración Nieto, Renato Talamini, Alessandra Tavani, F. Xavier Bosch, Ulrich Reidel, Peter J. F. Snijders, Chris J. L. M. Meijer, Raphael Viscidi, Nubia Muñoz, and Silvia Franceschi, for the IARC Multicenter Oral Cancer Study Group. 2003. "Human Papillomavirus and Oral Cancer: The International Agency for Research on Cancer Multicenter Study." *JNCI: Journal of the National Cancer Institute* 95 (23): 1772–83. https://doi.org/10 .1093/jnci/djg107.

Herskovits, Beth. 2007. "Brand of the Year." *Pharmaceutical Executive* 27 (2): 58–60.

Hess, David. 2004. "Medical Modernisation, Scientific Research Fields and the Epistemic Politics of Health Social Movements." *Sociology of Health and Illness* 26 (6): 695–709.

Hickey, Ann Marie. 2006. "The Sexual Savage: Race Science and the Medicalization of Black Masculinity." In *Medicalized Masculinities*, edited by Dana Rosenfeld and Christopher A. Faircloth, 165–82. Philadelphia, PA: Temple University Press.

Higginbotham, Evelyn Brooks. 1993. *Righteous Discontent: The Women's Movement in the Black Baptist Church, 1880–1920*. Cambridge, MA: Harvard University Press.

Hogarth, Stuart, Michael M. Hopkins, and Victor Rodriguez. 2012. "A Molecular Monopoly? HPV Testing, the Pap Smear and the Molecularisation of Cervical Cancer Screening in the USA." *Sociology of Health and Illness* 34 (2): 234–50.

Hogarth, Stuart, Michael Hopkins, and Daniele Rotolo. 2015. "Technological Accretion in Diagnostics: HPV Testing and Cytology in Cervical Cancer Screening." In *Medical Innovation: Science, Technology and Practice*, edited by Davide Consoli, Andrea Mina, Richard R. Nelson, and R. Ramlogan, 88–116. London and New York: Routledge and Taylor & Francis Group.

Holland, Janet, Caroline Ramazanoglu, Sue Sharpe, and Rachel Thomson. 1994. "Power and Desire: The Embodiment of Female Sexuality." *Feminist Review* 46 (1): 21–38.

Holmberg, Christine, Christine Bischof, and Susanne Bauer. 2013. "Making Predictions: Computing Populations." *Science, Technology, & Human Values* 38 (3): 398–420. https://doi.org/10.1177/0162243912439610.

Holmberg, Christine, and Mark Parascandola. 2010. "Individualised Risk Estimation and the Nature of Prevention." *Health, Risk & Society* 12 (5): 441–52. https://doi .org/10.1080/13698575.2010.508835.

Holmes, King K., John M. Karon, and Joan Kreiss. 1990. "The Increasing Frequency of Heterosexually Acquired AIDS in the United States, 1983–88." *American Journal of Public Health* 80 (7): 858–63. https://doi.org/10.2105/ajph.80.7.858.

hooks, bell. 2004. *We Real Cool: Black Men and Masculinity.* New York: Psychology Press.

Hoppe, Trevor. 2017. *Punishing Disease: HIV and the Criminalization of Sickness.* Berkeley: University of California Press.

"How Many Cancers Are Linked with HPV Each Year?" 2020. Division of Cancer Prevention and Control, Centers for Disease Control and Prevention. Last modified September 3, 2020, accessed March 24, 2021. https://www.cdc.gov/cancer/hpv/ statistics/cases.htm.

Howson, Alexandra. 1999. "Cervical Screening, Compliance and Moral Obligation." *Sociology of Health & Illness* 21 (4): 401–25. https://doi.org/10.1111/1467–9566.00164.

Hrustic, Alisa. 2017a. "1 in 9 Men Have This Cancer-Causing STD." *Men's Health,* October 17.

Hrustic, Alisa. 2017b. "Here's How Oral Sex Can Give You Cancer." *Men's Health,* August 31.

IARC Working Group on the Evaluation of Carcinogenic Risks to Humans. 2012. *A Review of Human Carcinogens. Part B: Biological Agents.* Lyon, France: International Agency for Research on Cancer.

iDNA. 2020. "Frequently Asked Questions." Accessed August 25, 2020. https://idna .com/faq.

International Agency for Research on Cancer. 1995. "Human Papillomaviruses." In *IARC Monographs on the Evaluation of Carcinogenic Risks to Humans.* Lyon, France: International Agency for Research on Cancer.

Irvine, Janice M. 2006. *Talk about Sex: The Battles over Sex Education in the United States.* Berkeley: University of California Press.

Jain, S. Lochlann. 2013. *Malignant: How Cancer Becomes Us.* Berkeley: University of California Press.

Jasanoff, Sheila, and Sang-Hyun Kim, eds. 2015. *Dreamscapes of Modernity: Sociotechnical Imaginaries and the Fabrication of Power.* Chicago: University of Chicago Press.

Javier, R. T., and J. S. Butel. 2008. "The History of Tumor Virology." *Cancer Research* 68 (19): 7693–7706. https://doi.org/10.1158/0008–5472.Can-08–3301.

Jemal, A., M. M. Center, C. DeSantis, and E. M. Ward. 2010. "Global Patterns of Cancer Incidence and Mortality Rates and Trends." *Cancer Epidemiology, Biomarkers & Prevention* 19 (8): 1893–1907. https://doi.org/10.1158/1055–9965.Epi-10–0437.

Jemal, Ahmedin, Edgar P. Simard, Christina Dorell, Anne-Michelle Noone, Lauri E. Markowitz, Betsy Kohler, Christie Eheman, Mona Saraiya, Priti Bandi, Debbie Saslow, Kathleen A. Cronin, Meg Watson, Mark Schiffman, S. Jane Henley, Maria J. Schymura, Robert N. Anderson, David Yankey, and Brenda K. Edwards. 2013. "Annual Report to the Nation on the Status of Cancer, 1975–2009, Featuring the Burden and Trends in Human Papillomavirus (HPV)-Associated Cancers and HPV Vaccination Coverage Levels." *Journal of the National Cancer Institute* 105 (3): 175– 201. https://doi.org/10.1093/jnci/djs491.

Jones, Danielle. 2019. "HPV Testing at HOME?! . . . plus Human Papillomavirus &

Pap Smear General Review." MamaDoctorJones, YouTube video, 14:27. Accessed December 3, 2021. https://www.youtube.com/watch?v=a5sDTEjTTjU.

Jones, James H. 1993. *Bad Blood: The Tuskegee Syphilis Experiment.* 2nd ed. New York: The Free Press.

Jordan, Miriam. 2008. "Gardasil Requirement for Immigrants Stirs Backlash." *Wall Street Journal,* October 1, 2008. https://www.wsj.com/articles/SB122282354408892791.

Joyce, Kelly, Jennifer E. James, and Melanie Jeske. 2020. "Regimes of Patienthood: Developing an Intersectional Concept to Theorize Illness Experiences." *Engaging Science, Technology & Society* 6: 185–92.

Joyce, Kelly, and Melanie Jeske. 2019. "Revisiting the Sick Role: Performing Regimes of Patienthood in the 21st Century." *Sociological Viewpoints* 33 (1): 70–90.

Jug, Rachel, and Sarah M. Bean. 2020. "Cervix Cytology: Bethesda System." PathologyOutlines.com, Inc. Last modified 2021, accessed November 18, 2021. https://www.pathologyoutlines.com/topic/cervixcytologybethesda.html.

Kainz, C., C. Tempfer, D. Bancher, G. Sliutz, G. Breitenecker, and A. Reinthaller. 1995. "[The Bethesda System—An Improvement in Classification of Cervix Cytology?]" *Geburtshilfe Frauenheilkd* 55 (8): 435–40. https://doi.org/10.1055/s-2007-1022816.

Kapsalis, Terri. 1997. *Public Privates: Performing Gynecology from Both Ends of the Speculum.* Durham, NC: Duke University Press.

Kasting, Monica L., Gilla K. Shapiro, Zeev Rosberger, Jessica A. Kahn, and Gregory D. Zimet. 2016. "Tempest in a Teapot: A Systematic Review of HPV Vaccination and Risk Compensation Research." *Human Vaccines & Immunotherapeutics* 12 (6): 1435–50.

Keim-Malpass, Jessica, Emma M. Mitchell, Pamela B. DeGuzman, Mark H. Stoler, and Christine Kennedy. 2017. "Legislative Activity Related to the Human Papillomavirus (HPV) Vaccine in the United States (2006–2015): A Need for Evidence-based Policy." *Risk Management and Healthcare Policy* 10: 29.

Kenney, Martha, and Laura Mamo. 2020. "The Imaginary of Precision Public Health." *Medical Humanities* 46 (3): 192–203. https://doi.org/10.1136/medhum-2018-011597/.

Kim, Kwang Sung, Shin Ae Park, Kyung-Nam Ko, Seokjae Yi, and Yang Je Cho. 2014. "Current Status of Human Papillomavirus Vaccines." *Clinical and Experimental Vaccine Research* 3 (2): 168–75.

Kimbol, Anne S. 2008. "HPV Vaccine Debate Meets the International Stage." *Health Law Perspectives,* October. https://www.law.uh.edu/healthlaw/perspectives/2008/(AK)%20HPV%20imm.pdf.

King, Samantha. 2008. *Pink Ribbons, Inc.: Breast Cancer and the Politics of Philanthropy.* Minneapolis: University of Minnesota Press.

Kirby Institute. 2021. "Study of the Prevention of Anal Cancer (SPANC)." University of New South Wales Sydney. Accessed May 5, 2021. https://kirby.unsw.edu.au/project/spanc.

Klahr Coey, Sharon. 2021. "Merck Rolls First Gardasil TV Commercial That Pushes HPV Vaccines for Adults." FiercePharma, February 25. https://www.fiercepharma.com/marketing/merck-encourages-adults-to-get-vaccinated-against-hpv-to-protect-against-certain-cancers.

Klawiter, Maren. 2008. *The Biopolitics of Breast Cancer: Changing Cultures of Disease and Activism.* Minneapolis: University of Minnesota Press.

Klick Health. 2014. "The Decoded Company." Klick Inc. Accessed May 2, 2021. https://www.klick.com/health/news/blog/strategy/the-decoded-company/.

Klick Health. 2021. "Commercialization Partnership." Klick Inc. Accessed April 21, 2021. https://www.klick.com/different-thinking.

Kreimer, Aimee R., Gary M. Clifford, Peter Boyle, and Silvia Franceschi. 2005. "Human Papillomavirus Types in Head and Neck Squamous Cell Carcinomas Worldwide: A Systematic Review." *Cancer Epidemiology Biomarkers & Prevention* 14 (2): 467. https://doi.org/10.1158/1055–9965.EPI-04–0551.

Krueger, Evan A., Jessica N. Fish, and Dawn M. Upchurch. 2020. "Sexual Orientation Disparities in Substance Use: Investigating Social Stress Mechanisms in a National Sample." *American Journal of Preventive Medicine* 58 (1): 59–68. https://doi.org/https://doi.org/10.1016/j.amepre.2019.08.034.

Krueger, Hans, Richard Gallagher, Gavin Stuart, Jon Kerner, and Dan Williams. 2010. *HPV and Other Infectious Agents in Cancer: Opportunities for Prevention and Public Health.* New York: Oxford University Press.

Kuper, H., H. O. Adami, and D. Trichopoulos. 2000. "Infections as a Major Preventable Cause of Human Cancer." *Journal of Internal Medicine* 248 (3): 171–83.

Ladson, Gwinnett. 2021. "Co-testing a Helpful Tool for Women of Color in Their Fight against Cervical Cancer." *The Tennessean,* March 9, 2021, Opinion. https://www.tennessean.com/story/opinion/2021/03/09/concerning-health-disparities-regarding-cervical-cancer-women-color/4630548001/.

Landecker, Hannah. 2007. *Culturing Life: How Cells Became Technologies.* Cambridge, MA: Harvard University Press.

Lareau, Annette. 2003. *Unequal Childhoods: Class, Race, and Family Life.* Berkeley: University of California Press.

Larson, Heidi J. 2020. *Stuck: How Vaccine Rumors Start—and Why They Don't Go Away.* London: Oxford University Press.

Laster Pirtle, Whitney N., and Tashelle Wright. 2021. "Structural Gendered Racism Revealed in Pandemic Times: Intersectional Approaches to Understanding Race and Gender Health Inequities in COVID-19." *Gender & Society* 35 (2): 168–79. https://doi.org/10.1177/08912432211001302.

Lawson, Kimberly. 2017. "Oral Sex and the Alarming Rise of HPV-Related Throat Cancer in Men." *Vice,* April 27. https://www.vice.com/en/article/9k9aqd/oral-sex-and-the-alarming-rise-of-hpv-related-throat-cancer-in-men.

Leavitt, Judith Walzer. 1997. *Typhoid Mary: Captive to the Public's Health.* Boston: Beacon Press.

LetsGetChecked. 2020a. Accessed August 25. https://www.letsgetchecked.com/us/en/.

LetsGetChecked. 2020b. "How It Works." Accessed August 25. https://www.letsgetchecked.com/us/en/how-it-works/.

Lindén, Lisa. 2011. "Producing 'Healthy' Girl Subjectivities—Pharmaceutical Advertising of the HPV Vaccine in Sweden." Master's thesis, Department of Sociology, University of Gothenburg.

Lindén, Lisa. 2013. "'What Do Eva and Anna Have to Do with Cervical Cancer?' Constructing Adolescent Girl Subjectivities in Swedish Gardasil Advertisements." *Girlhood Studies: An Interdisciplinary Journal* 6 (2): 83. https://doi.org/10.3167/ghs.2013.060207.

Lindén, Lisa. 2017. "You Will Protect Your Daughter, Right?" In *Gendering Drugs:*

Feminist Studies of Pharmaceuticals, edited by Ericka Johnson, 107–26. Cham, Switzerland: Palgrave Macmillan.

Lindén, Lisa. 2021. "Initiators, Controllers, and Influencers: Enacting Patient Advocacy Roles in Cervical Cancer Screening Policy Practices." In *Healthcare Activism: Markets, Morals, and the Collective Good*, edited by Susi Geiger, 140–64. Oxford: Oxford University Press.

Livingston, Julie. 2012. *Improvising Medicine: An African Oncology Ward in an Emerging Cancer Epidemic*. Durham, NC: Duke University Press.

Longmore, Paul K. 2016. *Telethons: Spectacle, Disability, and the Business of Charity*. Oxford: Oxford University Press.

Löwy, Ilana. 2010a. "HPV Vaccination in Context: A View from France." In *Three Shots at Prevention: The HPV Vaccine and the Politics of Medicine's Simple Solutions*, edited by Keith Wailoo, Julie Livingston, Steven Epstein, and Robert Aronowitz, 270–92. Baltimore, MD: Johns Hopkins University Press.

Löwy, Ilana. 2010b. *Preventive Strikes: Women, Precancer, and Prophylactic Surgery*. Baltimore, MD: Johns Hopkins University Press.

Löwy, Ilana. 2011. *A Woman's Disease: The History of Cervical Cancer*. Oxford: Oxford University Press.

Luttmer, Roosmarijn, Maaike G. Dijkstra, Peter J. F. Snijders, Ekaterina S. Jordanova, Audrey J. King, Divera T. M. Pronk, Carlo Foresta, Andrea Garolla, Peter G. A. Hompes, Johannes Berkhof, Maaike C. G. Bleeker, John Doorbar, Daniëlle A. M. Heideman, and Chris J. L. M. Meijer. 2015. "Presence of Human Papillomavirus in Semen of Healthy Men Is Firmly Associated with HPV Infections of the Penile Epithelium." *Fertility and Sterility* 104 (4): 838–44.e8. https://doi.org/https://doi.org/10.1016/j.fertnstert.2015.06.028.

Mackenzie, Sonja. 2013. *Structural Intimacies: Sexual Stories in the Black AIDS Epidemic*. New Brunswick, NJ: Rutgers University Press.

Madhivanan, Purnima, Dudith Pierre-Victor, Soumyadeep Mukherjee, Prasad Bhoite, Brionna Powell, Naomie Jean-Baptiste, Rachel Clarke, Tenesha Avent, and Karl Krupp. 2016. "Human Papillomavirus Vaccination and Sexual Disinhibition in Females: A Systematic Review." *American Journal of Preventive Medicine* 51 (3): 373–83.

Madzima, Tina R., Mandana Vahabi, and Aisha Lofters. 2017. "Emerging Role of HPV Self-Sampling in Cervical Cancer Screening for Hard-to-Reach Women: Focused Literature Review." *Canadian Family Physician / Medecin de famille canadien* 63 (8): 597–601.

Maldonado, Oscar Javier. 2017. "Evidence, Sex and State Paternalism: Intersecting Global Connections in the Introduction of HPV Vaccines in Colombia." In *Gendering Drugs: Feminist Studies of Pharmaceuticals*, edited by Ericka Johnson, 129–58. Cham, Switzerland: Palgrave Macmillan.

Malloy, Curt, Jacqueline Sherris, and Cristina Herdman. 2000. "HPV DNA Testing: Technical and Programmatic Issues for Cervical Cancer Prevention in Low-Resource Settings." Alliance for Cervical Cancer Prevention, IARC PATH, December. https://screening.iarc.fr/doc/HPV-DNA-Testing-Issues.pdf.

Mammas, I. N., and D. A. Spandidos. 2015. "Four Historic Legends in Human Papillomaviruses Research." *JBUON* 20 (2): 658–61.

Mamo, Laura, and Steven Epstein. 2014. "The Pharmaceuticalization of Sexual Risk:

Vaccine Development and the New Politics of Cancer Prevention." *Social Science & Medicine* 101: 155–65.

Mamo, Laura, and Steven Epstein. 2016. "The New Sexual Politics of Cancer: Oncoviruses, Disease Prevention, and Sexual Health Promotion." *BioSocieties* 12 (3): 367–91. https://doi.org/10.1057/biosoc.2016.10.

Mamo, Laura, and Jennifer Fosket. 2009. "Scripting the Body: Pharmaceuticals and the (Re)Making of Menstruation." *Signs: Journal of Women in Culture and Society*, [special issue on reproductive technologies] 34 (4): 925–50.

Mamo, Laura, Amber Nelson, and Aleia Clark. 2010. "Producing and Protecting Risky Girlhoods." In *Three Shots at Prevention: The HPV Vaccine and the Politics of Medicine's Simple Solutions*, edited by Keith Wailoo, Julie Livingston, Steven Epstein, and Robert Aronowitz, 121–45. Baltimore, MD: Johns Hopkins University Press.

Mamo, Laura, and Ashley E. Pérez. 2021. "Chapter 11: Gender and HPV Vaccination: Responsible Boyhood or Responsible Girls and Women?" In *Pink and Blue: Gender, Culture, and the Health of Children*, edited by Amy Medeiros, Elena Conis, and Sandra Eder. New Brunswick, NJ: Rutgers University Press.

Manos, M. Michele. 2009. "Appropriate Human Papillomavirus Vaccination Strategies." *The Lancet* 374 (9698): 1328.

Manos, M. M., Y. Ting, D. K. Wright, A. J. Lewis, T. R. Broker, and S. M. Wolinsky. 1989. "Use of Polymerase Chain Reaction Amplification for the Detection of Genital Human Papillomaviruses." *Molecular Diagnostics of Human Cancer* 7: 209–14.

Manos, M. M., D. K. Wright, Y. Ting, T. R. Broker, and S. M. Wolinsky. 1989. "Detection of the Human Papillomavirus by the Polymerase Chain Reaction." International patent application PCT/US1989/003747, filed August 29, 1989, and issued January 20, 1994.

Mara, Miriam. 2010. "Spreading the (Dis)ease: Gardasil and the Gendering of HPV." *Feminist Formations* 22 (2): 124–43.

Marcus, E. N. 2015. "Putting Your Bottom at the Top of Your List—The Pap Smear That's Not Just for Women." HuffPost, April 27. https://www.huffpost.com/entry/anal-cancer-test_b_7099662 2015.

Margolies, Liz, and Bill Goeren. 2009. "Anal Cancer, HIV, and Gay/Bisexual Men." *GMHC Treatment Issues*, Gay Men's Health Crisis Center newsletter, September. https://img.thebody.com/gmhc/pdfs/ti_0909.pdf.

Markowitz, Lauri. 2019. "Overview and Background." PowerPoint presentation, Advisory Committee on Immunization Practices, February 27, 2019.

Markowitz, Lauri E., Eileen F. Dunne, Mona Saraiya, Herschel W. Lawson, Harrell Chesson, and Elizabeth R. Unger. 2007. "Quadrivalent Human Papillomavirus Vaccine: Recommendations of the Advisory Committee on Immunization Practices (ACIP)." *MMWR Recommendations and Reports* 56 (Rr-2): 1–24.

Marrazzo, Jeanne M., Laura A. Koutsky, Nancy B. Kiviat, Jane M. Kuypers, and Kathleen Stine. 2001. "Papanicolaou Test Screening and Prevalence of Genital Human Papillomavirus among Women Who Have Sex with Women." *American Journal of Public Health* 91 (6): 947–52. https://doi.org/10.2105/ajph.91.6.947.

Marshall, Sarah, Mandana Vahabi, and Aisha Lofters. 2019. "Acceptability, Feasibility and Uptake of HPV Self-Sampling among Immigrant Minority Women: A Focused Literature Review." *Journal of Immigrant and Minority Health* 21 (6): 1380–93. https://doi.org/10.1007/s10903-018-0846-y.

Masur, Henry, Jonathan E. Kaplan, and King K. Holmes. 2002. "Guidelines for Preventing Opportunistic Infections among HIV-Infected Persons—2002: Recommendations of the U.S. Public Health Service and the Infectious Diseases Society of America." *Annals of Internal Medicine* 137 (5, Part 2): 435–78. https://doi.org/10.7326/0003-4819-137-5_Part_2-200209031-00002.

Matthews, Alicia K., Dana L. Brandenburg, Timothy P. Johnson, and Tonda L. Hughes. 2004. "Correlates of Underutilization of Gynecological Cancer Screening among Lesbian and Heterosexual Women." *Preventive Medicine* 38 (1): 105–13. https://doi.org/10.1016/j.ypmed.2003.09.034.

Mbembe, Achille. 2003. "Necropolitics." *Public Culture* 15 (1): 11–40.

McCook, A. 2017. "BMJ Journal Yanks Paper on Cancer Screening in India for Fear of Legal Action." *Retraction Watch*, May 30. http://retractionwatch.com/2017/05/30/bmj-journal-yanks-paper-cancer-screening-india-fear-legal-action/.

McGinley, Laurie. 2016. "Do the New Merck HPV Ads Guilt-Trip Parents or Tell Hard Truths? Both." *Washington Post*, August 12, 2016.

McGregor, Deborah Kuhn. 1989. *Sexual Surgery and the Origins of Gynecology: J. Marion Sims, His Hospital, and His Patients*. New York: Garland Publishing, Inc.

McGregor, Deborah Kuhn. 1998. *From Midwives to Medicine: The Birth of American Gynecology*. New Brunswick, NJ: Rutgers University Press.

McKay, Betsy. 2016. "New Approach to Promoting HPV Vaccinations: Pediatricians Talk about Cancer Risk, Not Sex, in an Effort to Get More Boys and Girls Vaccinated against HPV." *Wall Street Journal*, October 17.

McKittrick, Katherine. 2021. *Dear Science and Other Stories*. Durham, NC: Duke University Press.

Medical Care Criteria Committee. 2007. "Anal Dysplasia and Cancer Guideline: Screening and Diagnosis." New York State Department of Health, AIDS Institute. Accessed May 6, 2019. https://www.hivguidelines.org/hiv-care/anal-dysplasia-cancer/#tab_2.

Medical Laboratory Observer staff. 2012. "The Five FDA-Approved HPV Assays." *Medical Laboratory Observer* (MLO), July 1, 2012. https://www.mlo-online.com/home/article/13004462/the-five-fdaapproved-hpv-assays.

MedLine Plus. 2012. "Anoscopy." Accessed November 11, 2014. http://www.nlm.nih.gov/medlineplus/ency/article/003890.htm.

Mei, Leyla. 2009. "The Color of Cancer: Disease and the Measure of Race in the United States from the 1920s to the 1990s." PhD diss., History, City University of New York (304857117).

Meisal, Roger, Trine Rounge, Irene Christiansen, Alexander Eieland, Merete Worren, Tor Molden, Oyvind Kommedal, Eivind Hovig, Truls Leegaard, and Ole Ambur. 2017. "HPV Genotyping of Modified General Primer-Amplicons Is More Analytically Sensitive and Specific by Sequencing than by Hybridization." *PLoS ONE* 12. https://doi.org/10.1371/journal.pone.0169074.

Mello, Michelle M., Sara Abiola, and James Colgrove. 2012. "Pharmaceutical Companies' Role in State Vaccination Policymaking: The Case of Human Papillomavirus Vaccination." *American Journal of Public Health* 102 (5): 893–98. https://doi.org/10.2105/AJPH.2011.300576.

Mello, Vickie, and Renee K. Sundstrom. 2021. "Cervical Intraepithelial Neoplasia." *StatPearls* [internet]. Treasure Island, FL: StatPearls Publishing.

Melnikow, Joy, Jillian T. Henderson, Brittany U. Burda, Caitlyn A. Senger, Shauna Durbin, and Meghan S. Weyrich. 2018. "Screening for Cervical Cancer with High-

Risk Human Papillomavirus Testing: Updated Evidence Report and Systematic Review for the US Preventive Services Task Force." *JAMA* 320 (7): 687–705. https://doi.org/10.1001/jama.2018.10400.

Memorial Sloan Kettering Cancer Center. 2021. "Low-Dose Radiation a Possible 'Game Changer' for Treating HPV-Positive Throat Cancer." https://www.mskcc.org/news/low-dose-radiation-possible-game-changer-treating-hpv-positive-head-and-neck.

Menezes, Lynette J., Lianet Vazquez, Chilukuri K. Mohan, and Charurut Somboonwit. 2019. "Eliminating Cervical Cancer: A Role for Artificial Intelligence." In *Global Virology III: Virology in the 21st Century*, edited by Paul Shapshak, Seetharaman Balaji, Pandjassarame Kangueane, Francesco Chiapelli, Charurut Somboonwit, Lynette J. Menezes, and John T. Sinnott, 405–22. Cham: Springer Nature Switzerland.

Merck & Co., Inc. 2007. "The Power to Help Prevent Cervical Cancer Is in Your Hands. And on Your Daughter's Arm." *Ebony*, February 2007, 106.

Merck & Co., Inc. 2020a. "FDA Approves Merck's GARDASIL 9 for the Prevention of Certain HPV-Related Head and Neck Cancers." News release, June 12. https://www.merck.com/news/fda-approves-mercks-gardasil-9-for-the-prevention-of-certain-hpv-related-head-and-neck-cancers/.

Merck & Co., Inc. 2020b. "Merck TV Spot, 'Get in Its Way.'" Ispot.tv.Accessed May 14, 2021. https://www.ispot.tv/ad/nBEB/know-hpv-get-in-its-way.

Merck & Co., Inc. 2021a. "GARDASIL®9." Merck Sharp & Dohme Corp. Accessed April 21, 2021. https://www.gardasil9.com/.

Merck & Co., Inc. 2021b. "Not My Child." Merck Sharp & Dohme, Corp. Accessed May 14, 2021. https://www.hpv.com/.

Merck & Co. Inc. 2021c. "Cost Information." Merck Sharp & Dohme Corp. Accessed May 12, 2021. https://www.gardasil9.com/adults/cost/.

Merck Sharp & Dohme Corp. 2021. "Information about GARDASIL 9." Accessed April 21. https://www.gardasil9.com/adults/.

"Merck's New Gardasil Ads Omit Talk of Transmission." 2006. *Medical Marketing and Media*, November 15. https://www.mmm-online.com/home/channel/mercks-new-gardasil-ads-omit-talk-of-transmission/.

Messaris, Paul. 1997. *Visual Persuasion: The Role of Images in Advertising*. Newbury Park, CA: Sage.

Metzl, Jonathan M. 2003. "'Mother's Little Helper': The Crisis of Psychoanalysis and the Miltown Resolution." *Gender & History* 15 (2): 228–55. https://doi.org/10.1111/1468-0424.00300.

Michels, Karin B., and Harald zur Hausen. 2009a. "Author's Reply." *The Lancet* 374: 1328–29.

Michels, Karin B., and Harald zur Hausen. 2009b. "HPV Vaccine for All [Commentary]." *The Lancet* 374 (9686): 268–70. https://doi.org/10.1016/S0140-6736(09)61247-2.

Mills, C. Wright. 1959. *The Sociological Imagination*. London: Oxford University Press.

"The Miracle of 'HeLa.'" 1976. *Ebony*, June 1976, 93–98.

Mishra, Amrita, and Janice E. Graham. 2012. "Risk, Choice and the 'Girl Vaccine': Unpacking Human Papillomavirus (HPV) Immunisation." *Health, Risk & Society* 14 (1): 57–69. https://doi.org/10.1080/13698575.2011.641524.

Mol, Annemarie. 2003. *The Body Multiple: Ontology in Medical Practice*. Durham, NC: Duke University Press.

Molina, Natalie. 2006. *Fit to Be Citizens: Public Health and Race in Los Angeles, 1879–1939*. Berkeley: University of California Press.

Moran, Jeffrey P. 2000. *Teaching Sex: The Shaping of Adolescence in the 20th Century*. Cambride, MA: Harvard University Press.

Morgan, Jennifer. 2011. *Laboring Women: Reproduction and Gender in New World Slavery*. Philadelphia: University of Pennsylvania Press.

Moynihan, Ray. 2006. "Caution! Diagnosis Creep." *Australian Prescriber* 39 (2): 30–31. https://doi.org/10.18773/austprescr.2016.021.

Mukherjee, Siddhartha. 2010. *The Emperor of All Maladies: A Biography of Cancer*. New York: Scribner.

Mundell, E. J. 2008. "Experts Debate Giving HPV Vaccine to Boys." ABC News, March 23. https://abcnews.go.com/Health/Healthday/story?id=4507166&page=1.

Muñoz, Nubia, Xavier Castellsagué, Amy Berrington de González, and Lutz Gissmann. 2006. "Chapter 1: HPV in the Etiology of Human Cancer." *Vaccine* 24: S1–S10. https://doi.org/10.1016/j.vaccine.2006.05.115.

Muraskin, William. 1988. "The Silent Epidemic: The Social, Ethical and Medical Problems Surrounding the Fight against Hepatitis B." *Journal of Social History* 22: 277–98.

Muraskin, William. 1995. *The War against Hepatitis B: A History of the International Task Force on Hepatitis B Immunization*. Philadelphia: University of Pennsylvania Press.

Murphy, Michelle. 2012. *Seizing the Means of Reproduction: Entanglements of Feminism, Health, and Technoscience*. Experimental Futures. Durham, NC: Duke University Press.

Murphy, Michelle. 2017. *The Economization of Life*. Durham, NC: Duke University Press.

myLAB Box. 2020. "About myLAB Box." Accessed August 25, 2020. https://www.mylabbox.com/about/.

Nagel, Joane. 2000. "Ethnicity and Sexuality." *Annual Review of Sociology* 26 (1): 107–33. https://doi.org/10.1146/annurev.soc.26.1.107.

Nathan, Mayura, Naveena Singh, Nigel Garrett, Nicola Hickey, Teresa Prevost, and Michael Sheaff. 2010. "Performance of Anal Cytology in a Clinical Setting When Measured against Histology and High-Resolution Anoscopy Findings." *AIDS* 24 (3): 373–79.

National Cancer Institute. 2014. "SEER Cancer Statistics Factsheets: Anal Cancer." Accessed January 16, 2023. https://seer.cancer.gov/statfacts/html/anus.html,.

National Cancer Institute. 2017. "NCI and the Precision Medicine Initiative°." Last modified July 24, 2017, accessed August 17, 2021. https://www.cancer.gov/research/areas/treatment/pmi-oncology.

National Cancer Institute. 2021. "How Cancer Research Led to AIDS Breakthroughs." National Institutes of Health. Last modified August 26, 2021, accessed December 13, 2021. https://www.cancer.gov/about-nci/organization/oham/hiv-aids-research/how-cancer-research-led-to-aids-breakthroughs.

National Conference of State Legislatures. 2018. "HPV Vaccine: State Legislation and Statutes." Accessed February 28, 2019. http://www.ncsl.org/research/health/hpv-vaccine-state-legislation-and-statutes.aspx.

National Institutes of Health. 1996. "Cervical Cancer." *NIH Consensus Statement* 43 (1): 1–38.

National LGBT Cancer Network. 2021. "Behind Closed Drawers." Accessed May 2, 2021. https://cancer-network.org/programs/behind-closed-drawers/.

National Women's Health Network. 2015. "Less Safe and More Expensive: The FDA Approves New Use of the HPV Test." Accessed April 7, 2021. https://nwhn.org/less-safe-and-more-expensive-the-fda-approves-new-use-of-the-hpv-test/.

Navin, Mark. 2015. "HPV and the Ethics of CDC's Vaccination Requirements for Immigrants." *Kennedy Institute of Ethics Journal* 25 (2): 111–32.

Nayar, Ritu, and David C. Wilbur, eds. 2015. *The Bethesda System for Reporting Cervical Cytology Definitions, Criteria, and Explanatory Notes.* 3rd edition. Berlin: Springer International Publishers.

"A Necessary Vaccine." 2007. Editorial, *New York Times*, February 26. https://www.nytimes.com/2007/02/26/opinion/26mon1.html.

Nelson, Alondra. 2011. *Body and Soul: The Black Panther Party and the Fight against Medical Discrimination.* Minneapolis: University of Minnesota Press.

Nelson, Kimberly M., Alexandra Skinner, and Kristen Underhill. 2022. "Minor Consent Laws for Sexually Transmitted Infection and HIV Services." *JAMA* 328 (7): 674–76. https://doi.org/10.1001/jama.2022.10777.

New York State Department of Health AIDS Institute. 2007. "NYS Guidelines Recommendations on Anal Pap Smears." National AIDS Treatment Advocacy Project. Last modified July 2007, accessed May 4, 2021. https://www.natap.org/2010/HIV/032510_01.htm.

Newell, Guy R., Edward T. Kremenz, and Jane D. Roberts. 1975. "Excess Occurrence of Cancer of the Oral Cavity, Lung, and Bladder Following Cancer of the Cervix." *Cancer* 36: 2155–58.

Nichols, James. 2014. "'Behind Closed Drawers': Raising Awareness about Anal Cancer." *Huffington Post*, December 21. https://www.huffpost.com/entry/behind-closed-drawers-anal-cancer_n_6357212.

Nobel Prize Outreach AB. 2008. "Harald zur Hausen—Biographical." NobelPrize.org. Accessed December 9, 2020. https://www.nobelprize.org/prizes/medicine/2008/hausen/biographical/.

Nolte, Karen. 2008. "Carcinoma Uteri and 'Sexual Debauchery': Morality, Cancer and Gender in the Nineteenth Century." *Social History of Medicine* 21 (1): 31–46.

NPR. 2011. "Grant Achatz: The Chef Who Lost His Sense of Taste." *Fresh Air*, March 3. https://www.npr.org/2011/03/03/134195812/grant-achatz-the-chef-who-lost-his-sense-of-taste.

Nurx. 2020a. "About Us." Accessed August 24, 2020. https://www.nurx.com/team/.

Nurx. 2020b. "At Home HPV Testing." Accessed August 24, 2020. https://www.nurx.com/hpv-screening/.

"Oropharynx." 2020. ADAM Medical Encyclopedia, edited by Linda J. Vorvick, David Zieve, Brenda Conaway, and ADAM Editorial Team. Johns Creek, GA: Ebix, Inc., ADAM.

Ortman, Emily. 2020. "Women with Anal Cancer: 'The Invisible Victims of HPV.'" Society for Women's Health Research, Blog, June 22. https://swhr.org/women-with-anal-cancer-the-invisible-victims-of-hpv/.

Oudshoorn, Nelly. 2003. *The Male Pill: A Biography of a Technology in the Making.* Durham, NC: Duke University Press.

Paavonen, J., P. Naud, J. Salmerón, C. M. Wheeler, S. N. Chow, D. Apter, H. Kitchener, X. Castellsagué, J. C. Teixeira, S. R. Skinner, J. Hedrick, U. Jaisamrarn, G. Limson, S. Garland, A. Szarewski, B. Romanowski, F. Y. Aoki, T. F. Schwarz, W. A. J. Poppe, F. X. Bosch, D. Jenkins, K. Hardt, T. Zahaf, D. Descamps, F. Struyf, M. Lehtinen, and G. Dubin. 2009. "Efficacy of Human Papillomavirus (HPV)-16/18 AS04-Adjuvanted Vaccine against Cervical Infection and Precancer Caused by Oncogenic HPV Types (PATRICIA): Final Analysis of a Double-Blind, Randomised Study in Young Women." *The Lancet* 374 (9686): 301–14. https://doi.org/10.1016/S0140-6736(09)61248-4.

Padmanabhan, Swathi, Tahir Amin, Bhaven Sampat, Robert Cook-Deegan, and Subhashini Chandrasekharan. 2010. "Intellectual Property, Technology Transfer and Manufacture of Low-Cost HPV Vaccines in India." *Nature Biotechnology* 28 (7): 671–78. https://doi.org/10.1038/nbt0710–671.

Palefsky, Joel M. 2010. "Human Papillomavirus-Related Disease in Men: Not Just a Women's Issue." *Journal of Adolescent Health* 46 (4, Supplement): S12–S19. https://doi.org/10.1016/j.jadohealth.2010.01.010.

Palefsky, Joel M., Anna R. Giuliano, Stephen Goldstone, Edson D. Moreira Jr., Carlos Aranda, Heiko Jessen, Richard Hillman, Daron Ferris, Francois Coutlee, Mark H. Stoler, J. Brooke Marshall, David Radley, Scott Vuocolo, Richard M. Haupt, Dalya Guris, and Elizabeth I. Garner. 2011. "HPV Vaccine against Anal HPV Infection and Anal Intraepithelial Neoplasia." *New England Journal of Medicine* 365 (17): 1576–85. https://doi.org/10.1056/NEJMoa1010971.

Palefsky, Joel M., John Gonzales, Ruth M. Greenblatt, David K. Ahn, and Harry Hollander. 1990. "Anal Intraepithelial Neoplasia and Anal Papillomavirus Infection among Homosexual Males with Group IV HIV Disease." *Journal of the American Medical Association* 263 (21): 2911–16. https://doi.org/10.1001/jama.1990.0344021006103.

Palefsky, Joel M., Elizabeth A. Holly, Charissa J. Hogeboom, J. Michael Berry, Naomi Jay, and Teresa M. Darragh. 1997. "Anal Cytology as a Screening Tool for Anal Squamous Intraepithelial Lesions." *Journal of Acquired Immune Deficiency Syndromes & Human Retrovirology* 14 (5): 415–22.

Palefsky, Joel M., Jeannette Y. Lee, Naomi Jay, Stephen E. Goldstone, Teresa M. Darragh, Hillary A. Dunlevy, Isabella Rosa-Cunha, Abigail Arons, Julia C. Pugliese, Don Vena, Joseph A. Sparano, Timothy J. Wilkin, Gary Bucher, Elizabeth A. Stier, Maribel Tirado Gomez, Lisa Flowers, Luis F. Barroso, Ronald T. Mitsuyasu, Shelly Y. Lensing, Jeffrey Logan, David M. Aboulafia, Jeffrey T. Schouten, Juan de la Ossa, Rebecca Levine, Jessica D. Korman, Michael Hagensee, Thomas M. Atkinson, Mark H. Einstein, Bernadette M. Cracchiolo, Dorothy Wiley, Grant B. Ellsworth, Cristina Brickman, and J. Michael Berry-Lawhorn. 2022. "Treatment of Anal High-Grade Squamous Intraepithelial Lesions to Prevent Anal Cancer." *New England Journal of Medicine* 386 (24): 2273–82. https://doi.org/10.1056/NEJMoa2201048.

Pantanowitz, Liron, and Bruce J. Dezube. 2010. "The Anal Pap Test as a Screening Tool." *AIDS* 24 (3): 463–65.

Pantanowitz, Liron, Hans P. Schlecht, and Bruce J. Dezube. 2006. "The Growing Problem of Non-AIDS-Defining Malignancies in HIV." *Current Opinion in Oncology* 18 (5): 469–78.

Pappas, G. 2009. "Infectious Causes of Cancer: An Evolving Educational Saga." *Clinical Microbiology and Infection* 15 (11): 961–63.

Patterson, James T. 1987. *The Dread Disease: Cancer and Modern American Culture.* Cambridge, MA: Harvard University Press.

Patton, Cindy. 1982. "Lesbian and Gay Health Care: Moving into the '80s." *Gay Community News* 9 (September): 7.

Patton, Cindy. 1985. *Sex and Germs: The Politics of AIDS.* Montréal, PQ: South End Press.

Patton, Cindy. 1990. *Inventing AIDS.* New York and London: Routledge.

Patton, Cindy. 1994. *Last Served: Gendering the HIV Pandemic.* Edited by Peter Aggleton. Social Aspects of AIDS. London: Taylor & Francis.

Paul, Katharina T. 2016. "'Saving Lives': Adapting and Adopting Human Papilloma Virus (HPV) Vaccination in Austria." *Social Science & Medicine* 153: 193e–200.

Paul, Katharina T., Iris Wallenburg, and Roland Bal. 2018. "Putting Public Health Infrastructures to the Test: Introducing HPV Vaccination in Austria and the Netherlands." *Sociology of Health & Illness* 40 (1): 67–81. https://doi.org/10.1111/1467-9566.12595.

Perkins, Rebecca B., Richard S. Guido, Philip E. Castle, David Chelmow, Mark H. Einstein, Francisco Garcia, Warner K. Huh, Jane J. Kim, Anna-Barbara Moscicki, Ritu Nayar, Mona Saraiya, George F. Sawaya, Nicolas Wentzensen, and Mark Schiffman, for the ASCCP Risk-Based Management Consensus Guidelines Committee. 2020. "2019 ASCCP Risk-Based Management Consensus Guidelines for Abnormal Cervical Cancer Screening Tests and Cancer Precursors." *Journal of Lower Genital Tract Disease* 24 (2): 102–31. https://doi.org/10.1097/lgt.0000000000000525.

Petrosky, Emiko, Joseph A. Bocchini, Susan Hariri, Harrell Chesson, C. Robinette Curtis, Mona Saraiya, Elizabeth R. Unger, and Lauri E. Markowitz. 2015. "Use of 9-Valent Human Papillomavirus (HPV) Vaccine: Updated HPV Vaccination Recommendations of the Advisory Committee on Immunization Practices." *Morbidity and Mortality Weekly Report* 64 (11): 300–304.

Petryna, Adriana, and Arthur Kleinman. 2006. "The Pharmaceutical Nexus." In *Global Pharmaceuticals: Ethics, Markets, Practices,* edited by Adriana Petryna, Andrew Lakoff, and Arthur Kleinman, 1–32. Durham, NC: Duke University Press Books.

Pflanzer, Lydia Ramsey. 2016. "A Shocking New Ad Is Shaming Parents for Not Giving Their Children This Unpopular Vaccine." *Business Insider,* July 15, 2016.

PharmaTimes. 2007. "Merck's Profits Rise on Back of Gardasil." *PharmaTimes,* April 20.

Pollack, Andrew. 2014. "Alternative to Pap Test Is Approved by F.D.A." *New York Times,* April 24, 2014. https://www.nytimes.com/2014/04/25/business/alternative-to-pap-test-is-approved-by-fda.

Pollock, Anne. 2008. "Pharmaceutical Meaning-Making Beyond Marketing: Racialized Subjects of Generic Thiazide." *The Journal of Law, Medicine, & Ethics* 36 (3): 530–36.

Pollock, Anne. 2012. *Medicating Race.* Durham, NC: Duke University Press.

Porter, Rachael M., Avnika B. Amin, Robert A. Bednarczyk, and Saad B. Omera. 2018. "Cancer-Salient Messaging for Human Papillomavirus Vaccine Uptake: A Randomized Controlled Trial." *Vaccine* 36 (18): 2494–2500.

Potts, Annie. 2000. "'The Essence of the Hard On': Hegemonic Masculinity and the

Cultural Construction of 'Erectile Dysfunction.'" *Men and Masculinities* 3 (1): 85–103.

Poynten, I. Mary, Andrew E. Grulich, Richard J. Hillman, Suzanne M. Garland, Christopher K. Fairley, Samuel Phillips, Sepehr Tabrizi, Annabelle Farnsworth, Andrew Carr, Dorothy A. Machalek, Monica Molano, Alyssa M. Cornall, Carmella Law, David J. Templeton, Jennifer M. Roberts, and Fengyi Jin. 2020. "The Natural History of Anal High-grade Squamous Intraepithelial Lesions in Gay and Bisexual Men." *Clinical Infectious Diseases* 72 (5): 853–61. https://doi.org/10.1093/cid/ciaa166.

Preda, Alex. 2005. *AIDS, Rhetoric, and Medical Knowledge.* New York: Cambridge University Press.

Prescott, Heather Munro. 2000. "The White Plague Goes to College: Tuberculosis Prevention Programs in Colleges and Universities, 1920–1960." *Bulletin of the History of Medicine* 74 (4): 735–72.

Prescott, Heather Munro. 2010. "Safeguarding Girls: Morality, Risk, and Activism." In *Three Shots at Prevention: The HPV Vaccine and the Politics of Medicine's Simple Solutions,* edited by Keith Wailoo, Julie Livingston, Steven Epstein, and Robert Aronowitz, 103–20. Baltimore, MD: Johns Hopkins University Press.

Proctor, Robert N. 1995. *Cancer Wars: How Politics Shaped What We Know and What We Don't Know about Cancer.* New York: Basic Books.

Rabin, Roni Caryn. 2011. "A Vaccine May Shield Boys Too." *New York Times,* July 18, Health. https://www.nytimes.com/2011/07/19/health/19garda.html.

Rabinow, Paul. 1996. *Making PCR: A Story of Biotechnology.* Chicago: University of Chicago Press.

Rabinow, Paul, and Talia Dan-Cohen. 2005. *A Machine to Make a Future: Biotech Chronicles.* Princeton, NJ: Princeton University Press.

Rahangdale, Lisa. 2012. "Pap Tests Every 3–5 Years: What Happens to the Annual Examination?" *Obstetrics & Gynecology* 120 (1): 9–11. https://doi.org/10.1097/AOG .0b013e31825bd729.

Rail, Geneviève, Luisa Molino, Caroline Fusco, Moss Edward Norman, LeAnne Petherick, Jessica Polzer, Fiona Moola, and Mary Bryson. 2018. "HPV Vaccination Discourses and the Construction of 'At-Risk' Girls." *Canadian Journal of Public Health* 109 (5–6): 622–32.

Reagan, Leslie. 1997. "Engendering the Dread Disease: Women, Men, and Cancer." *American Journal of Public Health* 87: 1779.

Reagan-Steiner, Sarah, David Yankey, Jenny Jeyarajah, Laurie D. Elam-Evans, James A. Singleton, C. Robinette Curtis, Jessica MacNeil, Lauri E. Markowitz, and Shannon Stokley. 2015. "National, Regional, State, and Selected Local Area Vaccination Coverage among Adolescents Aged 13–17 Years—United States, 2014." *MMWR Morbidity and Mortality Weekly Report* 64 (29): 784–92. https://doi.org/10.15585/ mmwr.mm6429a3.

Reich, Jennifer A. 2018. *Calling the Shots: Why Parents Reject Vaccines.* New York: New York University Press.

Reid, Richard. 1983. "Genital Warts and Cervical Cancer: II. Is Human Papillomavirus Infection the Trigger to Cervical Carcinogenesis?" *Gynecologic Oncology* 15 (2): 239–52. https://doi.org/10.1016/0090-8258(83)90080-X.

Reisner, Sari L., Madeline B. Deutsch, Sarah M. Peitzmeier, Jaclyn M. White Hughto, Timothy P. Cavanaugh, Dana J. Pardee, Sarah A. McLean, Lori A. Panther, Marcy

Gelman, Matthew J. Mimiaga, and Jennifer E. Potter. 2018. "Test Performance and Acceptability of Self- versus Provider-Collected Swabs for High-Risk HPV DNA Testing in Female-to-Male Trans Masculine Patients." *PLOS ONE* 13 (3): e0190172. https://doi.org/10.1371/journal.pone.0190172.

Reverby, Susan M. 2009. *Examining Tuskegee: The Infamous Syphilis Study and Its Legacy.* Chapel Hill: University of North Carolina Press.

Reverby, Susan M. 2010. "Book Review: Will This Be an Eternal Challenge?" *HEALTH AFFAIRS* 29 (4).

Reverby, Susan M. 2020. *Co-conspirator for Justice: The Revolutionary Life of Dr. Alan Berkman.* Chapel Hill: University of North Carolina Press.

Ries, L. A. G., D. Melbert, M. Krapcho, D. G. Stinchcomb, N. Howlader, M. J. Horner, and A. Mariotto, et al., eds. 2008. *SEER Cancer Statistics Review, 1975–2005.* Bethesda, MD: National Cancer Institute.

Riska, E. 2006. *Masculinity and Men's Health: Coronary Heart Disease in Medical and Public Discourse.* New York: Rowman & Littlefield.

Riska, Elianne. 2002. "From Type A Man to the Hardy Man: Masculinity and Health." *Sociology of Health & Illness* 24 (3): 347–58. https://doi.org/10.1111/1467–9566 .00298.

Riska, Elianne. 2010. "Coronary Heart Disease: Gendered Public Health Discourses." In *The Palgrave Handbook of Gender and Healthcare*, edited by Ellen Kuhlmann and Ellen Annandale, 158–71. London: Palgrave Macmillan UK.

Robbins, Hilary A., Ruth M. Pfeiffer, Meredith S. Shiels, Jianmin Li, H. Irene Hall, and Eric A. Engels. 2015. "Excess Cancers among HIV-Infected People in the United States." *JNCI: Journal of the National Cancer Institute* 107 (4). https://doi.org/10 .1093/jnci/dju503.

Roberts, Dorothy. 1997. *Killing the Black Body: Race, Reproduction, and the Meaning of Liberty.* 2nd edition. New York: Vintage Books.

Roche. 2011. "FDA Approves Roche's HPV Test for Identifying Women at Highest Risk for Cervical Cancer." Media release, April 20. https://www.roche.com/media/ releases/med-cor-2011-04-20/.

Roche. 2020. "Roche Receives FDA Approval for CINtec PLUS Cytology Test to Aid Clinicians in Improving Cervical Cancer Prevention." Media release, March 10. https://assets.roche.com/imported/01_Roche_MediaRelease_11032020_EN.pdf.

Roche. 2021. "CINtec * PLUS Cytology." Accessed February 3, 2021. https://diagnostics .roche.com/global/en/products/tests/cintec-plus.html#productInfo.

Rodriguez, Matthew. 2015. "Using What's in Your Underwear Drawer to Talk About Anal Cancer." TheBody: The HIV/AIDS Resource Center for Gay Men, January 12. https://www.thebody.com/article/using-whats-in-your-underwear-drawer-to-talk -about.

Rogers, Naomi. 1992. *Dirt and Disease: Polio Before FDR.* New Brunswick, NJ: Rutgers University Press.

Rose, Nikolas. 2001. "The Politics of Life Itself." *Theory, Culture & Society* 18 (6): 1–30.

Rose, Nikolas. 2007. "Molecular Biopolitics, Somatic Ethics and the Spirit of Biocapital." *Social Theory & Health* 5 (1): 3–29.

Rose, Nikolas, and Carlos Novas. 2003. "Biological Citizenship." In *Blackwell Companion to Global Anthropology*, edited by Aihwa Ong and Stephen Collier. Oxford: Blackwell.

Rosenberg, Charles. 2009. "Managed Fear." *The Lancet* 373 (9666): 802–3. https://doi
.org/10.1016/S0140-6736(09)60467-0.

Rosenberg, Charles E. 1962. *The Cholera Years: The United States in 1832, 1849, and 1866*.
Chicago: University of Chicago Press.

Rosenfeld, Arthur. 1962. "Clues to a Deadly Riddle: Scientists Find New Evidence That
Cancer Might Be Infectious." *Life*, June 22, 76–85.

Rosenfeld, Dana, and Christopher Faircloth. 2009. *Medicalized Masculinities*: Philadelphia, PA: Temple University Press.

Rosengarten, Marsha. 2009. *HIV Interventions: Biomedicine and the Traffic between
Information and Flesh*. Seattle and London: University of Washington Press.

Rosengarten, Marsha, and Mike Michael. 2009. "The Performative Function of Expectations in Translating Treatment to Prevention: The Case of HIV Pre-Exposure
Prophylaxis, or PrEP." *Social Science & Medicine* 69 (7): 1049–55. https://doi.org/
10.1016/j.socscimed.2009.07.039.

Rosenthal, Elisabeth. 2008. "Drug Makers' Push Leads to Cancer Vaccines' Rise." *New
York Times*, August 19. https://www.nytimes.com/2008/08/20/health/policy/
20vaccine.html.

Rotkin, I. D. 1973. "A Comparison Review of Key Epidemiological Studies in Cervical
Cancer Related to Current Searches for Transmissible Agents." *Cancer Research* 33
(6): 1353–67.

Rubin, Gayle. 2006 [1978]. "Thinking Sex: Notes for a Radical Theory of the Politics of
Sexuality." In *Culture, Society, and Sexuality*, edited by Peter Aggleton and Richard
Parker, 143–78. New Bunswick, NJ: Routledge.

Sagonowsky, Eric. 2016. "GSK Exits U.S. Market with Its HPV Vaccine Cervarix."
FiercePharma, October 21. https://www.fiercepharma.com/pharma/gsk-exits-u-s
-market-its-hpv-vaccine-cervarix.

Saguy, Abigail C. 2020. *Come Out, Come Out, Whoever You Are*. Oxford and New York:
Oxford University Press.

Samerski, Silja. 2018. "Individuals on Alert: Digital Epidemiology and the Individual-
ization of Surveillance." *Life Sciences, Society & Policy* 14 (1): 13. https://doi.org/10
.1186/s40504-018-0076-z.

Sankaranarayanan, Rengaswamy, Bhagwan M. Nene, Ketayun A. Dinshaw, Cedric
Mahe, Kasturi Jayant, Surendra S. Shastri, Sylla G. Malvi, Roshini Chinoy, Rohini
Kelkar, Atul M. Budukh, Vijay Keskar, Raghevendra Rajeshwarker, Richard Muwonge, Shubhada Kane, and Donald Maxwell Parkin. 2005. "A Cluster Randomized Controlled Trial of Visual, Cytology and Human Papillomavirus Screening for
Cancer of the Cervix in Rural India." *International Journal of Cancer* 116 (4): 617–23.
https://doi.org/10.1002/ijc.21050.

Sankaranarayanan, Rengaswamy, Bhagwan Nene, Surendra Shastri, Pullikotil Esmy,
Rajamanickam Rajkumar, Richard Muwonge, Rajaraman Swaminathan, Sylla
Malvi, Shubada Kane, Sangeeta Desai, Rohini Kelkar, Sanjay Hingmire, and Kasturi
Jayant. 2016. "Response to Article Titled 'US-Funded Measurements of Cervical
Cancer Death Rates in India: Scientific and Ethical Concerns' by Eric J. Suba."
Indian Journal of Medical Ethics 11 (3): 175–78.

Saraiya, M., E. R. Unger, T. D. Thompson, C. F. Lynch, B. Y. Hernandez, C. W. Lyu,
M. Steinau, M. Watson, E. J. Wilkinson, C. Hopenhayn, G. Copeland, W. Cozen,
E. S. Peters, Y. Huang, M. S. Saber, S. Altekruse, M. T. Goodman, and HPV Typing

of Cancers Workgroup. 2015. "US Assessment of HPV Types in Cancers: Implications for Current and 9-Valent HPV Vaccines." *Journal of the National Cancer Institute* 107 (6): djvo86. https://doi.org/10.1093/jnci/djv086.

Saslow, Debbie, Kimberly S. Andrews, Deana Manassaram-Baptiste, Robert A. Smith, Elizabeth T. H. Fontham, and the American Cancer Society Guideline Development Group. 2020. "Human Papillomavirus Vaccination 2020 Guideline Update: American Cancer Society Guideline Adaptation." *CA: A Cancer Journal for Clinicians* 70 (4): 274–80. https://doi.org/10.3322/caac.21616.

Saslow, Debbie, Philip E. Castle, J. Thomas Cox, Diane D. Davey, Mark H. Einstein, Daron G. Ferris, Sue J. Goldie, Diane M. Harper, Walter Kinney, Anna-Barbara Moscicki, Kenneth L. Noller, Cosette M. Wheeler, Terri Ades, Kimberly S. Andrews, Mary K. Doroshenk, Kelly Green Kahn, Christy Schmidt, Omar Shafey, Robert A. Smith, Edward E. Partridge, and Francisco Garcia. 2007. "American Cancer Society Guideline for Human Papillomavirus (HPV) Vaccine Use to Prevent Cervical Cancer and Its Precursors." *CA: A Cancer Journal for Clinicians* 57 (1): 7–28.

Scarce, Michael. 1999. *Smearing the Queer: Medical Bias in the Health Care of Gay Men.* New York: Hayworth Press, Inc.

Scheffler, Robin Wolfe. 2019. *A Contagious Cause: The American Hunt for Cancer Viruses & the Rise of Molecular Medicine.* Chicago: University of Chicago Press.

Schiffman, M., and D. Solomon. 2003. "Findings to Date from the ASCUS-LSIL Triage Study (ALTS)." *Archives of Pathology and Laboratory Medicine* 127 (8): 946–49. https://doi.org/10.5858/2003-127-946-ftdfta.

Schiffman, Mark, and M. Elena Adrianza. 2000. "ASCUS-LSIL Triage Study: Design, Methods and Characteristics of Trial Participants." *Acta Cytologica* 44 (5): 726–42. https://doi.org/10.1159/000328554.

Schiffman, Mark, Rolando Herrero, Allan Hildesheim, Mark E. Sherman, Maria Bratti, Sholom Wacholder, Mario Alfaro, Martha Hutchinson, Jorge Morales, Mitchell D. Greenberg, and Attila T. Lorincz. 2000. "HPV DNA Testing in Cervical Cancer Screening: Results from Women in a High-Risk Province of Costa Rica." *JAMA* 283 (1): 87–93. https://doi.org/10.1001/jama.283.1.87.

Schiffman, Mark, and Diane Solomon. 2009. "Screening and Prevention Methods for Cervical Cancer." *JAMA* 302 (16): 1809–10. https://doi.org/10.1001/jama.2009 .1573.

Schiffman, Mark, Nicolas Wentzensen, Michelle J. Khan, Philip E. Castle, David Chelmow, Warner K. Huh, Anna Barbara Moscicki, Colleen K. Stockdale, Teresa M. Darragh, Michelle Silver, and Richard S. Guido. 2017. "Preparing for the Next Round of ASCCP-Sponsored Cervical Screening and Management Guidelines." *Journal of Lower Genital Tract Disease* 21 (2): 87–90. https://doi.org/10 .1097/LGT.0000000000000300.

Schulman, Sarah. 2021. *Let the Record Show: A Political History of ACT UP New York, 1987–1993.* New York: Farrar, Straus and Giroux.

Schwartz, Stephen M., Janet R. Daling, Margaret M. Madeleine, David R. Doody, E. Dawn Fitzgibbons, Gregory C. Wipf, Joseh J. Carter, Er-Jia Mao, Shixuan Huang, Anna Marie Beckmann, James K. McDougall, and Denise A. Galloway. 1998. "Oral Cancer Risk in Relation to Sexual History and Evidence of Human Papillomavirus Infection." *JNCI: Journal of the National Cancer Institute* 90 (21): 1626–36. https:// doi.org/10.1093/jnci/90.21.1626.

SEER. 2021. "Cancer Stat Facts: Cervical Cancer." Surveillance Research Program, National Cancer Institute. Accessed November 16, 2021. https://seer.cancer.gov/statfacts/html/cervix.html.

SelfCollect. 2020. "HPV Home Test Kit." Accessed August 31, 2020. https://www.selfcollect.com/store/products/hpv-high-risk-virus.

Shah, Nayan. 2001. *Contagious Divides: Epidemics and Race in San Francisco's Chinatown.* Berkeley: University of California Press.

Sharma, Alankaar. 2010. "Diseased Race, Racialized Disease: The Story of the Negro Project of American Social Hygiene Association against the Backdrop of the Tuskegee Syphilis Experiment." *Journal of African American Studies* 14 (2): 247–62. https://doi,org/10.1007/s12111–009–9099–0.

Sharpe, Christina. 2016. *In the Wake: On Blackness and Being.* Durham, NC: Duke University Press.

Shibata, Darryl K., Norman Arnheim, and W. John Martin. 1988. "Detection of Human Papilloma Virus in Paraffin-Embedded Tissue Using the Polymerase Chain Reaction." *Journal of Experimental Medicine* 167 (1): 225–30. https://doi.org/10.1084/jem.167.1.225.

Shiels, Meredith S., Ruth M. Pfeiffer, Mitchell H. Gail, H. Irene Hall, Jianmin Li, Anil K. Chaturvedi, Kishor Bhatia, Thomas S. Uldrick, Robert Yarchoan, James J. Goedert, and Eric A. Engels. 2011. "Cancer Burden in the HIV-Infected Population in the United States." *JNCI: Journal of the National Cancer Institute* 103 (9): 753–62. https://doi.org/10.1093/jnci/djr076.

Shim, Janet K. 2005. "Constructing 'Race' across the Science-Lay Divide: Racial Formation in the Epidemiology and Experience of Cardiovascular Disease." *Social Studies of Science* 35 (3): 405–36.

Shim, Janet K. 2010. "Cultural Health Capital: A Theoretical Approach to Understanding Health Care Interactions and the Dynamics of Unequal Treatment." *Journal of Health and Social Behavior* 51 (1): 1–15.

Shoard, Catherine. 2013. "Michael Douglas: Oral Sex Caused My Cancer." *The Guardian,* June 3, 2013. https://www.theguardian.com/film/2013/jun/02/michael-douglas-oral-sex-cancer.

Shotwell, Alexis. 2014. "'Women Don't Get AIDS, They Just Die From It': Memory, Classification, and the Campaign to Change the Definition of AIDS." *Hypatia* 29 (2): 509–25.

"Should HPV Vaccines Be Mandatory for All Adolescents?" 2006. Editorial, *The Lancet* 368 (9543): 1212. https://www.thelancet.com/journals/lancet/article/PIIS0140673606694944/fulltext.

Shulman, L. P. 2006. "New Recommendations for the Periodic Well-Woman Visit: Impact on Counseling." *Contraception* 73 (4): 319–24. https://doi.org/10.1016/j.contraception.2005.10.008/.

Siers-Poisson, Judith. 2007. "Research, Develop, and Sell, Sell, Sell: Part Two in a Series on the Politics and PR of Cervical Cancer." *New Doctor* 87 (September): 6–9.

Silver, Michelle I., and Sarah Kobrin. 2020. "Exacerbating Disparities?: Cervical Cancer Screening and HPV Vaccination." *Preventive Medicine* 130: 105902. https://doi.org/10.1016/j.ypmed.2019.105902.

Silverberg, Michael J., Bryan Lau, Amy C. Justice, Eric Engels, M. John Gill, James J. Goedert, Gregory D. Kirk, Gypsyamber D'Souza, Ronald J. Bosch, John T. Brooks, Sonia Napravnik, Nancy A. Hessol, Lisa P. Jacobson, Mari M. Kitahata, Marina B.

Klein, Richard D. Moore, Benigno Rodriguez, Sean B. Rourke, Michael S. Saag, Timothy R. Sterling, Kelly A. Gebo, Natasha Press, Jeffrey N. Martin, Robert Dubrow, and the North American AIDS Cohort Collaboration on Research and Design of IeDEA. 2012. "Risk of Anal Cancer in HIV-Infected and HIV-Uninfected Individuals in North America." *Clinical Infectious Diseases* 54 (7): 1026–34. https://doi.org/10.1093/cid/cir1012.

Singer, Merrel, and Scott Clair. 2003. "Syndemics and Public Health: Reconceptualizing Disease in Bio-social Context." *Medical Anthropology Quarterly* 17 (4): 423–41.

Smith, Elaine M., Justine M. Ritchie, Kurt F. Summersgill, Jens P. Klussmann, John H. Lee, Donghong Wang, Thomas H. Haugen, and Lubomir P. Turek. 2004. "Age, Sexual Behavior and Human Papillomavirus Infection in Oral Cavity and Oropharyngeal Cancers." *International Journal of Cancer* 108 (5): 766–72. https://doi.org/10.1002/ijc.11633.

Snow, Anthony N., and Jennifer Laudadio. 2010. "Human Papillomavirus Detection in Head and Neck Squamous Cell Carcinomas." *Advances in Anatomic Pathology* 17 (6): 394–403. https://doi.org/10.1097/PAP.0b013e3181f895c1.

Somerville, Siobhan B. 2000. *Queering the Color Line: Race and the Invention of Homosexuality in American Culture.* Durham, NC: Duke University Press.

Songane, Mario, and Volker Grossmann. 2021. "The Patent Buyout Price for Human Papilloma Virus (HPV) Vaccine and the Ratio of R&D Costs to the Patent Value." *PLOS ONE* 16 (1): e0244722. https://doi.org/10.1371/journal.pone.0244722.

Sontag, Susan. 1989. *AIDS and Its Metaphors.* New York: Farrar, Straus and Giroux.

Stagg-Taylor, Joanne. 2012. "Writing Contagion as Cancer: Law, Gender and HPV Vaccination in Australia." *No Foundations* 13: 96.

Starr, Paul. 1982. *The Social Transformation of American Medicine.* New York: Basic Books.

Staton, Tracy. 2008. "Is Gardasil Worth the Cost?" *FiercePharma*, August 21, 2008.

Staton, Tracy. 2009. "Merck Readies Back-to-School Gardasil Push." *FiercePharma*, August 13, 2009.

Stein, Rob. 2005. "Cervical Cancer Vaccine Gets Injected with a Social Issue: Some Fear a Shot for Teens Could Encourage Sex." *Washington Post*, October 31. http://www.washingtonpost.com/wp-dyn/content/article/2005/10/30/AR2005103000747.html?noredirect=on.

Stein, Rob. 2007. "Virus Spread by Oral Sex Is Linked to Throat Cancer." *Washington Post*, May 10, 2007.

Stöckl, Andrea. 2010. "Public Discourses and Policymaking: The HPV Vaccination from the European Perspective." In *Three Shots at Prevention: The HPV Vaccine and the Politics of Medicine's Simple Solutions*, edited by Keith Wailoo, Julie Livingston, Steven Epstein, and Robert Aronowitz, 254–69. Baltimore, MD: Johns Hopkins University Press.

Stokley, Shannon, Jenny Jeyarajah, David Yankey, Maria Cano, Julianne Gee, Jill Roark, C. Robinette Curtis, and Lauri Markowitz. 2014. "Human Papillomavirus Vaccination Coverage among Adolescents, 2007–2013, and Postlicensure Vaccine Safety Monitoring, 2006–2014—United States." *MMWR. Morbidity and Mortality Weekly Report* 63 (29): 620.

Suba, Eric J. 2014. "US-Funded Measurements of Cervical Cancer Death Rates in India: Scientific and Ethical Concerns." *Indian Journal of Medical Ethics* 11 (3): 167–75. https://doi.org/10.20529/ijme.2014.046.

Suba, Eric J., R. E. Ortega, and D. G. Mutch. 2017. "Unethical Randomised Controlled Trial of Cervical Screening in India: US Freedom of Information Act Disclosures." *BMJ Global Health* 2 (2): e000177. https://doi.org/10.1136/bmjgh-2016–000177.

Suba, Eric J., R. E. Ortega, and D. G. Mutch. 2018. "Unethical US Government-Funded Cervical Screening Study in India: US Freedom of Information Act Disclosures." *Journal of Healthcare, Science, and the Humanities* 8: 57–78.

Suba, Eric J., R. E. Ortega, and D. G. Mutch. 2022. "The IARC Perspective on Cervical Cancer Screening." *New England Journal of Medicine* 386 (6): 607. https://doi.org/10.1056/NEJMc2119177.

Sulik, Gayle A. 2010. *Pink Ribbon Blues: How Breast Cancer Culture Undermines Women's Health*. Oxford: Oxford University Press.

Summers, Daniel. 2019. "Should Gay Men Be Getting Anal Pap Smears?" *Slate*, May 13. https://slate.com/human-interest/2019/05/gay-men-anal-pap-smear-cancer-hpv.html.

Sung, Hyuna, Jacques Ferlay, Rebecca L. Siegel, Mathieu Laversanne, Isabelle Soerjomataram, Ahmedin Jemal, and Freddie Bray. 2021. "Global Cancer Statistics 2020: GLOBOCAN Estimates of Incidence and Mortality Worldwide for 36 Cancers in 185 Countries." *CA: A Cancer Journal for Clinicians* 71 (3): 209–49. https://doi.org/10.3322/caac.21660.

Surveillance Research Program. 2019. "Cancer Stat Facts: Anal Cancer at a Glance." National Cancer Institute. Accessed April 30, 2019. https://seer.cancer.gov/statfacts/html/anus.html.

SurvivorNet. 2019. "Marcia Cross's Anal Cancer: Why We Need to Stop Using Words Like 'Taboo.'" SurvivorNet, June 19. https://www.survivornet.com/articles/marcia-cross-anal-cancer-why-we-need-to-stop-using-words-like-taboo/.

Swailes, A. L., C. E. Hossler, and J. P. Kesterson. 2019. "Pathway to the Papanicolaou Smear: The Development of Cervical Cytology in Twentieth-Century America and Implications in the Present Day." *Gynecologic Oncology* 154 (1): 3–7. https://doi.org/10.1016/j.ygyn0.2019.04.004.

Taylor, Rosemary C. R. 1982. "The Politics of Prevention." *Social Policy* 13 (1): 32–41.

Thomas, Karen Kruse. 2016. *Health and Humanity: A History of the Johns Hopkins Bloomberg School of Public Health, 1935–1985*. Baltimore, MD: Johns Hopkins University Press.

Thrasher, Steven W. 2022. *The Viral Underclass: The Human Toll When Inequality and Disease Collide*. New York: Celadon Books.

Thrift, Aaron P., and Elizabeth Y. Chiao. 2018. "Are Non-HIV Malignancies Increased in the HIV-Infected Population?" *Current Infectious Disease Reports* 20 (8): 22. https://doi.org/10.1007/s11908-018-0626-9.

Timmerman, Carsten. 2013. *A History of Lung Cancer: A Recalcitrant Disease*. Basingstoke and New York: Palgrave Macmillan.

Timmerman, Carsten. 2019. *Moonshots at Cancer: The Roche Story*. Basel: Roche.

Timmermans, Stefan, and Mara Buchbinder. 2010. "Patients-in-Waiting: Living between Sickness and Health in the Genomics Era." *Journal of Health and Social Behavior* 51 (4): 408–23.

Tolman, Deborah L., Meg I. Striepe, and Tricia Harmon. 2003. "Gender Matters: Constructing a Model of Adolescent Sexual Health." *Journal of Sex Research* 40 (1): 4–12.

Tom, Pamela. 2012. "Our Mission." HPVANDME. Accessed March 22, 2021. https://hpvandme.org/mission/.

Tranberg, Mette, Bodil Hammer Bech, Jan Blaakær, Jørgen Skov Jensen, Hans Svan-holm, and Berit Andersen. 2018. "Preventing Cervical Cancer Using HPV Self-Sampling: Direct Mailing of Test-Kits Increases Screening Participation More Than Timely Opt-in Procedures—A Randomized Controlled Trial." *BMC Cancer* 18 (1): 1–11.

Treichler, Paula A. 1999. *How to Have Theory in an Epidemic: Cultural Chronicles of AIDS*. Durham, NC: Duke University Press.

Tsu, Vivien, and Scott Wittet. 2009. "Appropriate Human Papillomavirus Vac-cination Strategies." *Lancet* 374 (9698): 1327–28. https://doi.org/10.1016/S0140-6736(09)61820-1.

Tuller, David. 2007. "New Vaccine for Cervical Cancer Could Prove Useful in Men, Too." *New York Times*, January 30, 2007. https://www.nytimes.com/2007/01/30/health/30virus.html.

UCSF Medical Center. 2008. "Anoscopy." Medical tests. Accessed November 30, 2022. https://www.ucsfhealth.org/medical-tests/anoscopy.

University of California San Francisco Department of Medicine. 2014. "How Is the Anus Examined?" Accessed November 11, 2014. http://id.medicine.ucsf.edu/analcancerinfo/diagnosis/examination.html.

US Citizenship and Immigration Services. 2021. "Policy Manual." Accessed January 20, 2020. https://www.uscis.gov/policy-manual.

US Food & Drug Administration. 2017. "Establishing the Performance Characteristics of In Vitro Diagnostic Devices for the Detection or Detection and Differentiation of Human Papillomaviruses: Guidance for Industry and Food and Drug Admin-istration Staff." Guidance document, September. Last modified August 24, 2018. https://www.fda.gov/regulatory-information/search-fda-guidance-documents/establishing-performance-characteristics-in-vitro-diagnostic-devices-detection-or-detection-and-0.

US Food & Drug Administration. 2020. "Letter to Merck Sharp & Dohme Corp., Supplement Accelerated Approval, STN 125508/868," June 12. https://fda.report/media/138949/June+12%2C+2020+Approval+Letter+-+Gardasil9.pdf.

"Vaccines and Immunizations." 2018. Centers for Disease Control and Prevention. Ac-cessed October 11, 2018. https://www.cdc.gov/vaccines/index.html.

Valier, Helen. 2016. "Conclusions: Medicine, Masculinity, and the Problems of the Prostate." In *A History of Prostate Cancer: Cancer, Men and Medicine*, 193–208. London: Palgrave Macmillan.

Vázquez-Otero, Coralia, Erika L. Thompson, Ellen M. Daley, Stacey B. Griner, Rachel Logan, and Cheryl A. Vamos. 2016. "Dispelling the Myth: Exploring Associations between the HPV Vaccine and Inconsistent Condom Use among College Students." *Preventive Medicine* 93: 147–50.

Ventola, C. L. 2011. "Direct-to-Consumer Pharmaceutical Advertising: Therapeutic or Toxic?" *P & T: A Peer-Reviewed Journal for Formulary Management* 36 (10): 669–84.

Virtanen, Mikko J. 2019. "What Kind of 'A Girls' Thing'? Frictions and Continuities in the Framing and Taming of the HPV Vaccine in Finland." *Sociology of Health & Ill-ness* 41 (4): 789–805. https://doi.org/10.1111/1467-9566.12853.

Wailoo, Keith. 2011. *How Cancer Crossed the Color Line*. Oxford: Oxford University Press.

Wailoo, Keith A. 2021a. "Epidemic Inequities: Pandemics, Policies, and the History of Structured Racial Inequalities." Powerpoint presentation at the NASEM Summit on

Diversity, Equity, Inclusion, and Anti-Racism in 21st-Century STEMM Organizations, June. https://www.nationalacademies.org.

Wailoo, Keith. 2021b. *Pushing Cool: Big Tobacco, Racial Marketing, and the Untold Story of the Menthol Cigarette*. Chicago: University of Chicago Press.

Wailoo, Keith, Julie Livingston, Steven Epstein, and Robert Aronowitz, eds. 2010. *Three Shots at Prevention: The HPV Vaccine and the Politics of Medicine's Simple Solutions*. Baltimore, MD: Johns Hopkins University Press.

Walboomers, J. M., M. V. Jacobs, M. M. Manos, F. X. Bosch, J. A. Kummer, and K. V. Shah. 1999. "Human Papillomavirus Is a Necessary Cause of Invasive Cervical Cancer Worldwide." *Journal of Pathology* 189 (1): 12–19.

Wald, Priscilla. 2008. *Contagious: Cultures, Carriers, and the Outbreak Narrative*. Durham, NC: Duke University Press.

Wang, Chia-ching J., Joseph Sparano, and Joel M. Palefsky. 2017. "Human Immunodeficiency Virus/AIDS, Human Papillomavirus, and Anal Cancer." *Surgical Oncology Clinics of North America* 26 (1): 17–31. https://doi.org/10.1016/j.soc.2016.07.010.

Washington, Harriet A. 2008. *Medical Apartheid: The Dark History of Medical Experimentation on Black Americans from Colonial Times to the Present*. New York: Random House.

Watkins-Hayes, Celeste. 2019. *Remaking a Life: How Women Living with HIV/AIDS Confront Inequality*. Oakland: University of California Press.

Waxman, Alan G., David Chelmow, Teresa M. Darragh, Herschel Lawson, and Anna-Barbara Moscicki. 2012. "Revised Terminology for Cervical Histopathology and Its Implications for Management of High-grade Squamous Intraepithelial Lesions of the Cervix." *Obstetrics and Gynecology* 120 (6): 1465–71. https://doi.org/10.1097/aog.0b013e31827001d5.

Weinbaum, Alys Eve. 2019. *The Afterlife of Reproductive Slavery: Biocapitalism and Black Feminism's Philosophy of History*. Durham, NC: Duke University Press.

Weir, Lorna, and Eric Mykhalovskiy. 2012. *Global Public Health Vigilance: Creating a World on Alert*. New York: Routledge.

Wemrell, Maria, Juan Merlo, Shai Mulinari, and Anne-Christine Hornborg. 2016. "Contemporary Epidemiology: A Review of Critical Discussions within the Discipline and a Call for Further Dialogue with Social Theory." *Sociology Compass* 10 (2): 153–71.

West, Paul. 2011. "Bachmann Keeps Up Attack on Perry over HPV Vaccine." *Tribune News Service*, September 13.

Whitemarsh, Ian. 2008. *Biomedical Ambiguity: Race, Asthma, and the Contested Meaning of Genetic Research in the Caribbean*. Ithaca, NY and London: Cornell University Press.

WHO. 2002. *Cervical Cancer Screening in Developing Countries: Report of a WHO Consultation*. Edited by Department of Reproductive Health and Research. Published collaboratively by Programme on Cancer Control, WHO. Geneva, Switzerland: WHO.

WHO. 2020. "Human Papillomavirus (HPV) and Cervical Cancer Fact Sheet." November 11. https://www.who.int/news-room/fact-sheets/detail/cervical-cancer/.

WHO. 2022. "Cancer Fact Sheet." February. Accessed May 2022. https://www.who.int/news-room/fact-sheets/detail/cancer.

Will, Catherine. 2009. "Identifying Effectiveness in 'The Old Old': Principles and Values in the Age of Clinical Trials." *Science, Technology & Human Values* 34 (5).

Will, Catherine, and Tiago Moreira. 2010. *Medical Proofs/Social Experiments: Clinical Trials in Shifting Contexts.* Farnham, UK: Ashgate Publishing.

Williams, Simon J., Paul Martin, and Jonathan Gabe. 2011. "The Pharmaceuticalization of Society? A Framework for Analysis." *Sociology of Health & Illness* 33 (5): 710–25.

Wingo, Phyllis A., Cheryll J. Cardinez, Sarah H. Landis, Robert T. Greenlee, Lynn A. G. Ries, Robert N. Anderson, and Michael J. Thun. 2003. "Long-term Trends in Cancer Mortality in the United States, 1930–1998." *Cancer* 97 (S12): 3133–3275. https://doi.org/10.1002/cncr.11380.

WNBA. 2005. "Top WNBA Athletes Urge Women to Ask for the HPV Test: WNBA Champions Cause to Eliminate Cervical Cancer." WNBA, April 20. Accessed August 30, 2021. https://www.wnba.com/archive/wnba/choose_to_know/announcement_042005.html.

Woo, Yin Ling, Liyann Ooi, and Marion Saville. 2021. "Program ROSE: A Revolutionary Strategy in Cervical Screening." *HPV World: The Newsletter on the Human Papillomavirus* 177. Accessed August 1, 2021. https://www.hpvworld.com/articles/program-rose-a-revolutionary-strategy-in-cervical-screening/.

Worden, Francis P., Bhavna Kumar, Julia S. Lee, Gregory T. Wolf, Kitrina G. Cordell, Jeremy M. G. Taylor, Susan G. Urba, Avraham Eisbruch, Theodoros N. Teknos, Douglas B. Chepeha, Mark E. Prince, Christina I. Tsien, Nisha J. D'Silva, Kun Yang, David M. Kurnit, Heidi L. Mason, Tamara H. Miller, Nancy E. Wallace, Carol R. Bradford, and Thomas E. Carey. 2008. "Chemoselection as a Strategy for Organ Preservation in Advanced Oropharynx Cancer: Response and Survival Positively Associated with HPV16 Copy Number." *Journal of Clinical Oncology* 26 (19): 3138–46. https://doi.org/10.1200/jc0.2007.12.7597.

World Health Organization. 2006. *Comprehensive Cervical Cancer Control: A Guide to Essential Practice.* Geneva, Switzerland: World Health Organization.

World Health Organization. 2020. Global Strategy to Accelerate the Elimination of Cervical Cancer as a Public Health Problem. Geneva, Switzerland: World Health Organization.

Wright T. C., L. Denny, L. Kuhn, A. Pollack, and A. Lorincz. 2000. "HPV DNA Testing of Self-Collected Vaginal Samples Compared with Cytologic Screening to Detect Cervical Cancer." *JAMA* 283 (1): 81–86.

Wright, Thomas C., Mark H. Stoler, Catherine M. Behrens, Abha Sharma, Guili Zhang, and Teresa L. Wright. 2015. "Primary Cervical Cancer Screening with Human Papillomavirus: End of Study Results from the ATHENA Study Using HPV as the First-Line Screening Test." *Gynecologic Oncology* 136 (2): 189–97. https://doi.org/10.1016/j.ygyn0.2014.11.076.

Yeh, Ping Teresa, Caitlin E. Kennedy, Hugo de Vuyst, and Manjulaa Narasimhan. 2019. "Self-Sampling for Human Papillomavirus (HPV) Testing: A Systematic Review and Meta-Analysis." *BMJ Global Health* 4 (3): e001351. https://doi.org/10.1136/bmjgh-2018-001351.

Yerushalmy, Jacob. 1947. "Statistical Problems in Assessing Methods of Medical Diagnosis, with Special Reference to X-ray Techniques." *Public Health Reports* 62 (40): 1432–49.

Yi, Doogab. 2011. "The Enemy Within? Oncogenes and the Demise of the Virus Cancer Program in the 1970s." Presentation at conference on Debating Causation: Risk, Biology, Self, and Environment in Cancer Epistemology, 1950–2000, Princeton University, October 21–22.

Zickl, Danielle. 2017. "Oral Sex with 5 or More Partners Could Up Your Risk of HPV." *Men's Health*, October 20, 2017.

Zimet, Gregory D., Rose M. Mays, and J. Dennis Fortenberry. 2000. "Vaccines against Sexually Transmitted Infections: Promise and Problems of the Magic Bullets for Prevention and Control." *Sexually Transmitted Diseases* 27 (1): 49–52.

Zola, Irving Kenneth. 1972. "Medicine as an Institution of Social Control." *Sociological Review* 20: 487–504.

zur Hausen, Harald. 1987. "Papillomaviruses in Human Cancer." *Applied Pathology* 5: 19–24.

zur Hausen, Harald. 2006. *Infections Causing Human Cancer*. Weinheim, Germany: WILEY-VCH & Co.

zur Hausen, Harald. 2009. "Papillomaviruses in the Causation of Human Cancers—A Brief Historical Account." *Virology* 384 (2): 260–65. https://doi.org/10.1016/j.virol .2008.11.046.

Index